MALACHY THE IRISHMAN *ON POISON*

Malachy the Irishman
On Poison

A Study and an Edition

R ALPH H ANNA

LIVERPOOL UNIVERSITY PRESS

First published in 2020 by
Liverpool University Press
4 Cambridge Street
Liverpool
L69 7ZU

British Library Cataloguing-in-Publication data
A British Library CIP record is available

ISBN 978-1-78962-219-5

Typeset by Carnegie Book Production, Lancaster
Printed and bound by CPI Group (UK) Ltd, Croydon CR0 4YY

Contents

Preface

Readers of Liverpool University Press's catalogue need offer no excuses for being quizzical on seeing this title listed for publication. Outside references buried in such standard bibliographical tools as Bloomfield *et al.*, Malachy the Irishman's *On poison* has had virtually no presence in the literary world for five centuries. The text has featured in only three article-length studies in the last century. Yet, paradoxically, *De ueneno* is very well known to (if not well read by) anyone who has nosed about in most major insular manuscript collections.

I first became acquainted with Malachy's work fifteen years ago in attempting to describe the glorious mess that is Oxford, Magdalen College, MS lat. 6. This binding includes six originally separate MSS of various dates, at least part of mid-fourteenth-century Irish origins. These discrete bits were perhaps gathered together by an early fifteenth-century fellow of Oriel College, one John Martell. Here the text keeps distinguished company; it sits, in the third of these separable productions, between copies of Richard Rolle's *Super nouem lectiones* and a single lection extracted from Robert Holcot's extensive *Super Sapientiam Salomonis*. (The copy of *De ueneno* is dated 1393 and provided with an equally distinguished ascription, to John of Wales.) Even had I been inclined to ignore Malachy here – I had more than two hundred other manuscripts to examine – the recurrence of his text in three other Magdalen manuscripts (MSS lat. 48, 200, and 202) reinforced a sense that this was an important text, worthy of considerable attention.

Exercises in this prefatory genre typically provide lengthy lists of friends and companions alleged to have been of incomparable aid in the production. Given the current (non-)state of Malachy studies, I can offer but two, the Richards. R. Newhauser long ago offered me his updated list of copies, and we discussed collaborating on an edition. Unfortunately, that connoisseur of late medieval materials for priests, far more knowledgeable about the field than I, is a busy man (a new edition of Peraldus and a *Chaucer Encyclopedia*, for example), and that plan was still-born. But R. N. has offered me ongoing encouragement, advice, and suggestions since I began this project in desultory fashion five or six years ago.

Equally encouraging and generous, and blessed with a meticulous knowledge of medieval Ireland, was the now unfortunately departed R. Sharpe. Early on, Richard gave me files he had assembled, including images of Malachy's one appearance in print and a transcript of Étienne's edition with notations of some of the sources. R. S. was constantly supportive in discussing details and answering queries of all sorts (evidence for word-spacing in Irish MSS? no, there is no Irish evidence for the episode Malachy attributes to St Columba), and he also subjected my introduction to his customarily incisive and meticulous scrutiny. I doubt that either of my helpful co-conspirators would approve, either in gross or in detail, with a variety of decisions I have made below, but I have benefited enormously from their comradeship and conversation, and, with the community of English manuscript scholars, deeply lament Richard S.'s passing.

I'm much indebted to the custodians of the books I have used in this study, most especially to Oliver Pickering at Leeds and to the good-humoured and welcoming Guy Mitchell and his staff at Gray's Inn. Subsequent to my submission of this book to the press, I have been delighted by the appearance of another scholar energetically committed to Malachy, Chris Tuckley of the York Archaeological Trust.

Finally, as always, I remain grateful to Liverpool University Press in all its various roles. The series editors, Gillespie (the *mafioso* of English medieval spiritual studies, known in the family as Big Vinnie) and his *capo*, Richard Dance, have, like R. S., read the text with great care. At the press, my editor Clare Litt and my production manager Patrick Brereton have offered their customarily excellent support. Words cannot express my admiration for and gratitude to my heroic typesetter, Rachel Clarke, who has, yet once again, turned a sow's ear, dodgy computer files, into the poison-free silk purse you are now holding.

Abbreviations

1518 or p	*F. Malachie Hibernici, ordinis minorum … Libellus septem peccatorum mortalium venena eorumque remedia describens, qui dicitur Venenum Malachiæ* (Paris: Henri Étienne, 26 April 1518)
BA	M. C. Seymour *et al.*, eds, *'On the Properties of Things': John Trevisa's Translation of Bartholomaeus Anglicus De Proprietatibus Rerum: A Critical Text*, 2 vols (Oxford, 1975), with *'On the Properties …', Volume 3* (Oxford, 1988). For my occasional references to the underlyng Latin, see *De proprietatibus rerum* (Nuremberg: Anton Koberger, 30 May 1483 [Bod-Inc-B-064])
Bod-Inc- …	Alan Coates *et al.*, *A Catalogue of Books Printed in the Fifteenth Century Now in the Bodleian Library, Oxford*, 6 vols (Oxford, 2005), online at incunables.bodleian.ox.ac.uk
BRUO	A. B. Emden, *A Biographical Register of the University of Oxford to A.D. 1500*, 3 vols (Oxford, 1957–59)
MMBL	Neil R. Ker (completed by A. J. Piper), *Medieval Manuscripts in British Libraries*, 4 vols (Oxford, 1969–92)
Neckam	*Alexandri Neckam De naturis rerum libro duo*, ed. Thomas Wright, Rolls Series 34 (London, 1863)
Patient	Ralph Hanna, *Patient Reading/Reading Patience: Oxford Essays on Medieval Literature* (Liverpool, 2017)
PL	*Patrologia Latina*
Tubach	Frederic C. Tubach, *Index Exemplorum: A Handbook of Medieval Religious Tales*, Folklore Fellows Communications 204 (Helsinki, 1969)
Walther *Sprich.*	Hans Walther, *Proverbia Sententiaeque Latinitatis Medii Aevi …*, 6 vols (Göttingen, 1963–69)

Introduction

The *De ueneno* attributed to a 'Malachias Hibernicus', generically a 'book of vices and (their contrasting) virtues', can scarcely be said to have left any impression on modern scholarship.[1] However, in the later Middle Ages it was a well-known and widely consulted text, one of the most successful of insular exports. *De ueneno* thus provides an outstanding example of a range of books typically invisible to modern scholars, but perceived as seminal by their contemporary audiences. Most directly addressed to preachers, *De ueneno* conveys views ubiquitously understood in the fourteenth and fifteenth centuries and shared potentially by 'lewed' as well as Latin-literate. It communicates, in readily available form, materials sophisticated and closely argued, but, in their original forms, restricted in their medieval circulation to learned textual communities. The text is thus representative of ubiquitous late-medieval 'popularising' modes by which a commonplace 'it-goes-without-saying', originally the property of closed communities, achieved global effect.[2] Moreover, as will appear below, any presentation of the text requires an engagement with some of the knottier issues of textual transmission and editorial theory.

The circulation of the text

The manuscript circulation testifies to the wide interest Malachy's text enjoyed. As Newhauser and Bejczy report, the fullest formal list

[1] For an introduction, sceptical as to whether such discussions constitute a genre, see Newhauser 1993.

[2] Insistence upon access to learned *originalia* has formed a commonplace misperception of the late medieval situation ever since Robertson's evocation of patristic exegesis as key to reading medieval texts. Popularising efforts, often rendering only snippets (sometimes in 'misquoted' citational forms) commonplace, have largely been ignored. The result, particularly in one exhibit offered here, *Piers Plowman*, has been a long sequence of studies erudite yet pretentious and misrepresenting the authors discussed.

of manuscripts, by Richard Sharpe, enumerates ninety-seven surviving copies of *De ueneno*; Sharpe extended earlier listings in Bloomfield *et al.* and in Thomson by finding fifteen copies unknown to either.[3] To this showing, Newhauser and Bejczy add an additional eight manuscripts (two of these in the Bodleian Library, and including Rome, Angelica 369, which Sharpe had rejected at 230). In addition, I am grateful to Newhauser for directing me to references to an additional six manuscripts, all these identified by Malachy's great scholarly devotee M. Esposito (one of them now destroyed):

Erlangen 739, fols 32^v–47 (s. xv) (the text here anonymous)

Maulbronn # (purchased from Arnsburg in 1439; the text attributed to Robert Holcot)

Münster, UB 541, fols 111^v–19 (s. xiv) (anonymous)

Regensburg, Alte Kapelle 1794, fols 171^v–80 (s. xv) (anonymous)

Vienna, ÖNB 14457, fols 140–49^v (s. xv) (anonymous)

Wrocław, BU Rehd Fol. 107 (s. xv) (attributed to Thomas Aquinas); while present when Esposito wrote, the Rehdigerani were all destroyed in World War II.[4]

Four further examples may be added to the list, bringing the total to 115 known copies (of these forty-six of insular manufacture):

Berlin, SBPK, Magdeb. 76, fols 156–61, s. xv med.

Göttweig, Stiftsbibliothek 369, fols 14 ff.

Innsbruck, Universitäts- und Landesbibliothek Tirol 311, fols 111^v–123^v, s. xv (attributed to Aquinas)

Jena, Thüringer Universitäts- und Landesbibliothek, MS Rec.adj o.2, fols 93^v–118, 1379.

In addition, Sharpe offers references to twenty-one copies now lost but appearing in medieval library catalogues. His references indicate the presence of multiple copies in several large and well-documented

[3] See Newhauser and Bejczy 289–90; Sharpe 218–45; Bloomfield *et al.* no. 5102; Thomson 268–70. For comparative data, see n.7.
[4] See Esposito 1933, at 247.

libraries, such as Durham Cathedral Priory and St Augustine's Abbey in Canterbury, an indication that the text was in persistent demand for reference purposes.[5]

Malachy's continental circulation appears to have begun in the later fourteenth century, and was especially marked in Bohemia.[6] In England, as Sharpe meticulously documents, *De ueneno* was frequently ascribed, whether explicitly or otherwise, to Robert Grosseteste, the great parochially engaged bishop of Lincoln; on the continent, readers were more apt to be informed that it was a work of an author no less respected than Aquinas. Such a broad dissemination and so distinguished a set of attributions would suggest that the work was widely perceived as conveying authoritatively useful materials of considerable sophistication.[7] The absence of *De ueneno* from virtually any sort of scholarly discussion since the text's single publication in 1518 suggests that at least something more than a modest reconsideration might be in order.

[5] Two additions: On 18 November 1491 a longtime fellow of Oriel College and later prebendary of Salisbury Cathedral, Richard Gardyner, deposited Bodleian Library, MS Bodley 442 in Oxford's Robury loan chest. The *cautio* note on the front pastedown indicates that Gardyner's security included two other manuscripts, one opening with a copy of *De ueneno*. For Gardyner, see *BRUO* 742–43. An early sixteenth-century inventory of the books of a Norfolk lawyer, Sir Robert Townshend, British Library, MS Additional 41139, fol. 23[v], lists a further copy at the head of a religious miscellany; see Moreton 346 (no. 44).

[6] Thus, Munich, BSB, CLM 16202 (from Passau OSA) is dated 1376, and Prague, Národní Knihovna V.G.21 (973), like the Jena copy noted above, 1379. Two dated Vienna copies are closely contemporary, ÖNB 4581 in 1387 and ÖNB 4686 in 1391. I have been unable to investigate the claim that Vorau, Stiftsbibliothek 362 might be of s. xiv[1/2]. Early Bohemian transmission might well qualify or extend Van Dussen's account of relations with England; Palmer describes another text of particular interest in assessing transmission of insular texts to Bohemia, a collection of *similitudines* constructed on principles different from Malachy's.

[7] Merely as a comparative, Goering and Mantello report that Grosseteste's own parochial classic, *Templum Dei*, survives in ninety-six copies; see their edition, 14–15. Their list can be marginally supplemented, e.g. with copies enumerated at Newhauser and Bejczy 338, and with Lambeth Palace 499, fols 70[v]–72 (excerpts); Arras, Bibliothèque municipale 753 (994), fols 41[v]ff.; Würzburg, Universitätsbibliothek, M. p. th. f. 55, fols 21–28. But the circulation still remains more than ten copies shy of the currently identified trove of books transmitting *De ueneno*.

The manuscripts used in this study

A text with so large a diffusion can obviously not be approached in its totality. I have begun my researches, originally as a way of confirming the usefulness of putting Étienne's edition into modern type, with the half-dozen oldest insular copies, all of those local manuscripts there is good reason to believe pre-date 1350.

A   London, British Library, MS Additional 46919

s. xiv in.; the book, Fr William Herebert's sermons, lyrics, and his collection of *praedicabilia*, must predate his death in 1333. Fols ii + 211. In the Malachy portion, where the leaves are somewhat smaller than elsewhere, overall 230 mm × 175 mm (writing area 175–80 mm × 120 mm). This portion in a not very narrowly datable textura. In 34 or 35 long lines per page.

Collation (this booklet only, fols 189–204): a single quire of 16. The concluding fols 203^v–4^v were originally blank; they now bear the start of a sequential index on fol. 203^v and theological notes 204^v (including, in Herebert's hand, Index of Middle English Verse 269.5).

A fascicular production, probably ten booklets, this the penultimate, preceding Herebert's autograph copy of his Middle English translations of Latin hymns. For Herebert, see *BRUO* 911–12 and Reimer extensively; he was in Paris in 1290, in Oxford by 1314 and a DTh by 1320, when he was lector of the Franciscan convent. After his death, the MS passed to his Hereford Franciscan brothers.

Described *British Library* 1:197–206; a good deal of further detail in 'Phillipps MS.'.

C   Durham University Library, MS Cosin V.ii.5

s. xiv in./med. (1325×40). Fols 198. Overall 240 mm × 165 mm (writing area in this portion 190 mm × 115–20 mm). In anglicana, by at least two different scribes. In 43 or 44 long lines to the page.

Collation (this booklet only, fols 41–58): 4^8 5^{10}.

The third of eight booklets; Piper and Doyle see close similarities with booklets 1, 2, and 7. The last transmits ps.-Ailred, Cassiodorus's 'De anima', and John of Wales's 'Breviloquium', on the whole the most interesting other contents (although booklet 4 includes a rare insular copy of Hugh of St Victor's *Didascalicon*).

From Durham Cathedral, with excised ex-libris probably of the house. Described in Piper and Doyle's draft catalogue.

D   Durham Cathedral Library, MS B.II.4

s. xiii/xiv or xiv in. (see further below). Fols 199. Overall 320 mm × 210 mm (writing area 265 mm × 155 mm). In textura rotunda, a script notoriously not narrowly datable, but implicitly so by other features: decorated top-line ascenders and extensive marginalia, in a single anglicana, s. xiv in. (? 1310×30). In double columns, 58 lines per page.

Collation: 1–16^{12} 17^{6+1} (+ 7) (Malachy at fols 128va–38va, in quires 10–11). The concluding text, selections from Gregory the Great's *Homeliae super Ezechielem*, beginning at the head of quire 15 (fol. 169), is apparently a quasi-independent extension. Following the end of Malachy's text, fol. 138va, a trial run at an alphabetical index, rather quickly breaking off at the column foot.

From Durham Cathedral.

Described Rud 99–101, an accurate listing of the largely patristic contents, mainly based on his own notes on fol. 199vb. I am grateful to Richard Gameson for sharing a draft description, to appear in his forthcoming catalogue of Cathedral MSS.

G   London, Gray's Inn, MS 23

s. xiv in./med. (1320×40). Fols 191. Overall 250 mm × 180 mm (in Malachy, writing area 220 mm × 140+ mm). In anglicana. In double columns, 50 lines per page. As Horwood notes, the bottom four or five lines of inner columns are often illegible from damp-damage.

Collation: 1–12^{12} [fol. 144, Nicholas of Gorran's *Distinctiones*] | 13–14^{12} 15^{12+1} (+13, fol. 181) [William of Lavicea's *Dieta salutis*, index, and sermon *themata*] | 16^{10}. Malachy begins at the head of fol. 181va, the concluding (originally blank?) side of quire 15; it ends at the top of fol. 190ra, where it is followed by a theological note and a text added later on leaves left blank.

One among at least eighteen Gray's Inn MSS (and twelve more at Shrewsbury School) associated with the Bostock family of Tattenhall (Ches.). All these with clear provenances came from religious houses in Chester (the total survival from the Chester Franciscans and Dominicans, a few books from the Benedictine St Werbergh's). This MS retains the original medieval binding of red skin (now rebacked, but apparently using the earlier six bands).[8]

Described summarily, *MMBL* 1:65–66 (and for the provenance, see 1:50–51, 4:288); Horwood, mounted on the library's website, mainly describes the contents.

L   Leeds University, Brotherton Library, MS 115

s. xiv in. (?; see further below). Fols 51. Overall 160 mm × 100 mm (writing area 110 mm × 60–65 mm). Like D, in relatively undatable textura, here

---

[8]   On the descent of this now divided collection, see Hanna forthcoming.

informal semiquadrata; but predating an added theme for a Latin sermon, with rhyming insertions in Yorkshire English, fols 49^v–50, in anglicana, s. xiv in./med. In double columns, 21 lines per page.

Putative collation (predicated on catchwords only): 1^8 2^{12} (one leaf lacking somewhere, a cancel with no text loss) 3^{12} 4–5^{10}. The MS is devoted to Malachy's text alone, followed by tables: an original one of further biblical examples of each sin (fols 48rb–49rb); the second a continental addition, a partial alphabetical guide to Malachy, mainly identifying *similitudines* (fols 50^v–51).

Although produced in England, later at Rooklooster/Rouge-Cloître, nr Auderghem, Brabant (Augustinian canons).

Only noted among the addenda at *MMBL* 5:14; cf. Pickering and Airaksinen 16–17.

S   Cambridge, Sidney Sussex College, MS 85
s. xiii/xiv or xiv in. (no later than the 1320s) and s. xiv$^{2/4}$ (fols 146–89 only). Fols iv + 222 + ii. Overall 230 mm × 155–60 mm (writing area in Malachy 180–90 mm × 125 mm). In three different anglicanas (fol. 98 a fourth hand that appears nowhere else). Since only frame-ruled, lines per page vary considerably (e.g. the primary scribe, responsible for fols 1–79, parts of 98^v–100^v, 100^v–44, and 190–222, within the same frame-rule writes 40 lines on fol. 214, but 30 on fol. 216). In Malachy, 39–42 long lines per page (this scribe, more current than the primary hand, copied fols 80–97^v and bits of 98^v–100^v).

Collation: 1^8 2^{14} 3–5^{12} 6–7^8 8^8 (lacks 6–8) [fol. 79, *Barlaam and Josaphat*] | 9^8 10 (the three single leaves, fols 88–90) 11^{18} 12^{10} 13^{12} 14^8 15^8 (lacks 7) [fol. 145, Malachy, followed by shorter texts, concluding with one of only four copies of John of St Edmunds] | 16–17^{14} 18–19^8 [fol. 189, Peter of Limoges's *Oculus*] | 20^{14} 21^{16} 22^6 (lacks 4–6) [Humbert of Romans's *De dono timoris*]. At the head, fols i–iv are the remains of an original eight-leaf quire (lacks 1, 5–6, 8), the first leaf probably an earlier pastedown; the two flyleaves at the end are probably singletons removed from this quire.

Fol. i has a contents table for the full volume, headed 'Liber domini Symonis de Gowshille canonici domus de Chikesond et quondam prioris eiusdem' (Chicksands, Beds., Gilbertine canons); as part of this indexing he foliated the volume (by the opening) to fols 209^v/210. A Simon is recorded as prior 1325×28 and 1334 (Smith and London 521). At the foot of the leaf, 'Constat Iohanni Stainborn monacho de Kyrkestall', s. xv (suburban Leeds, Cistercians).

Described James 1895, 68–71. The MS has been rebound since his inspection; at that time, quires 9 and 10 had apparently been reversed in the binding. This disruption had occurred in the Middle Ages, and fols 76–92 have notations of the proper ordering, the alphabetical sequence 'a–r' at the page foot.

In addition, I have consulted sporadically, for reasons that will shortly become clear, four further insular copies, all of the later fourteenth century:

B   Oxford, Bodleian Library, MS Bodley 122
One of four originally separate MSS, now bound together, this portion s. xiv/xv. Fols i (fol. 1) + 154. Overall 215 mm × 150 mm (writing area in Malachy 150–55 mm × 90 mm). Written in anglicana; the scribe signs the colophon to the single text (fol. 133^v), which includes extensive personal additions, 'quod R.P.'. In 35 long lines per page.

Collation: $1^{8?}$ (if so, lacks 1 to 5; now only fols 6–8) 2^{10} 3^{12} 4–5^{10} 6^4 [fol. 54, Peter of Limoges's *Oculus*, s. xiv med.] | 7–9^{12} [fol. 90, Rolle's 'Emendatio vitae' and Augustiniana] | 10–12^{12} 13^{10} (lacks 10, probably a cancelled blank leaf) [fol. 135, 'Malachy' only] | 14–15^{12} [Innocent III, *De contemptu mundi*, s. xv$^{2/4}$]; signatures indicate that the final three sections have been together since the Middle Ages, although not necessarily in this order.

In addition to the scribal signature there is a note added to the last line of the text, 'quod Thomas Moraunt sibi constans'. He is presumably the man who was principal of Hart Hall, Oxford in 1405 and 1406, subsequently vicar of Little/East Thurrock (Essex) until his death in 1413 (see *BRUO* 1300). His will, Commissary Court of London, Reg. 2, fol. 256, contains no reference to his books. The book came to the Bodleian from an unknown donor 1613×20.

Described Hunt *et al.*, no. 1985, 2, i, 146–47.

La   London, Lambeth Palace Library, MS 523
s. xiv/xv. Fols 139. Overall 190 mm × 115–20 mm (writing area in Malachy 130 mm × 70+ mm). In anglicana. In 35 long lines per page.

Collation: 1–10^8 | 11^8 (-8) [fol. 87, Peter of Limoges's *Oculus*; the final quire an index to his text, but mainly blank and filled with later notes] | 12^8 13–14^{12} 15^{12} (-12) [fol. 130; 'Malachy' runs from fol. 88, the head of this portion, to about the middle of quire 14] | 16^{10} (-8, mostly torn away); the MS tails off into raw notes.

One of only four copies with a correct ascription: 'Explicit. Malachias' is added in two different later hands, one word each, fol. 113. The ascription plausibly reflects accurate local knowledge, since *c.*1500 the book had some association with St Michan's church, Dublin, mentioned several times in the collection of notes at the end.

Described James and Jenkins 2:723–25.

R   London, British Library, MS Royal 7 C.i
s. xiv med. or xiv$^{3/4}$. Fols ii + 444. Overall 310 mm × 205 mm (writing area 230–40 mm × 140–45 mm). Produced by multiple hands, mainly anglicanas,

the portion with 'Malachy' a fere textura. In double columns, this portion around 50 lines per page.

For a detailed description and discussion of the production, at least partially from Oxford exemplars (and including Robert de Basevorn's exceedingly complicated *ars praedicandi*), see Hanna 2016. 'Malachy' appears, perhaps to fill out a quire, at the end of the first scribal stint (fols 1–90), following Peter of Limoges's *Oculus* and William of Lavicea's *Dieta salutis*, each in a separate fascicle. The book was produced for William de Kettering, monk of Ramsey (Hunts., OSB), and appears in the 1542 catalogue of the Royal Library.

V   London, British Library, MS Cotton Vitellius C.xiv

s. xiv med. or xiv³/⁴. Fols 210. A burned Cotton MS, badly shrunk at the top and without outer edges. Overall surviving 265 mm × 175 mm (in Malachy, surviving writing area 195 mm × 145 mm). In a variety of anglicanas. 'Malachy' in double columns, 64 lines per page.

Collation: The pages have been individually mounted and, given destruction and deterioration of the edges, there is no available production detail. The MS is clearly fascicular, in differing hands and formats, with blank leaves at the ends of the component units. The contents include works of Robert Grosseteste, Peter of Limoges's *Oculus*, the *ars praedicandi* customarily ascribed to John of Wales, William of St Amour, the exemplum book 'Convertimini' (often ascribed to Robert Holcot), and exemplary material drawn from Augustine's *De civitate Dei*.

At the end of the text an extensive ascription to Malachy, cited and discussed below.

Described Smith 89 and (the derivative) Planta 427.

The physical descriptions highlight one aspect of the transmission, the tendency, visible in all copies except D, for the text to occupy a more or less independent fascicle (mentioned Sharpe 238, 243). Here L, a pocket-sized volume dedicated to Malachy's text alone, is provocative; it suggests a book designed to be carried on the person for ready consultation. This feature points toward presumptive use by preachers (? perhaps Franciscan itinerants) seeking exemplary materials for that amplification of doctrinal points ceaselessly enjoined in manuals. It is certainly no accident, a feature particularly pronounced in the four ancillary MSS, that *De ueneno* regularly appears with widely transmitted texts customarily considered such 'handbooks for preachers', Peter of Limoges, William of Lavicea, and (once) Humbert of Romans.

Authorship

As I have already indicated, *De ueneno* routinely circulated with ascriptions to the great and good. As Esposito saw very clearly, and as Sharpe further elaborates, the only substantial evidence for the text's originator appears in the single printed edition of *De ueneno*, produced by Henri Étienne at Paris in 1518. While Esposito's account of this source and the inferences he draws from it remain authoritative, before considering his arguments at least one word of caution will be appropriate.[9]

As Sharpe implies (231, 236, and n230), Étienne's information is clearly derived from whatever manuscript he had used for copy. In this regard, the most proximate surviving copy of the text, one of only four sources Sharpe assembles with a correct authorial ascription, is that in V. In addition to the colophon naming an author, V is the only identified copy that shares with the print an otherwise unique explicit, in this burnt MS somewhat short of being legible.[10] I think it an inescapable conclusion that this unusual information, explicit and colophon, are linked, rather than independent, and that they came to Étienne together from a MS version resembling (but certainly not) V. The printer's information should thus be considered secondary, non-independent testimony; I doubt that Étienne can actually have known of his author any more than V's colophon offered him:

> Explicit tractatus qui dicitur Uenenum Malachie, editus a fratri Malachie de ordine minorum et prouincia Ybernie (cf. Sharpe 219).

Étienne's information, presented on his title-page, fragmentary though it is, is considerably in excess of this statement:

---

[9]   Esposito 1918. His account is so thorough that it has achieved an authority earlier historical bibliographers accorded to Étienne, and subsequent references to Malachy merely repeat his conclusions; see, for example, Fitzmaurice and Little 56–58; *BRUO* 1004; Cotter 91–92. In all my citations from the 1518 print I have normalised Étienne's varying presentations of medieval Latin 'e' (representing variously classical e, ae, and oe) as 'e'; and, as I do universally, except when citing printed authorities, I treat 'v' for 'u' and 'ij' for 'ii' as simply positional variants and reproduce the latter forms.

[10]   'Hec igitur dicta sufficiant secundum mei tenuitatem ingenii de predictis ad aliqualem instructionem simplicium qui habent populum informare, qui cum patre …' ('Therefore the things I have said here, so far as the slenderness of my wit allows, should be enough for some instruction of simple men who are appointed to teach the people); cf. Sharpe 236–37 n230.

F. Malachie Hibernici ordinis minorum, doctoris theologi, strenui
quondam diuini uerbi illustratoris, necnon vitiorum obiurgatoris
acerrimi libellus … qui dicitur Uenenum Malachie.

His colophon, in slightly different language, provides much the same
information, with one slight addition:

F. Malachie Hibernici, ordinis minorum, doctoris theologie ac
insignis diuini uerbi predicatoris, qui anno domini 1300 uigebat,
libelli qui uenenum peccatorum seu Malachie dicitur finis.[11]

If V's textual confirmations – an added sentence at the explicit plus
colophon – accurately represent what Étienne had received, much of this is
likely to represent only puffery. There is no evidence for Malachy at either
English university, or at Paris; the notion that he was a great preacher seems
only to reflect the obvious fact that he produced a handbook of *praedicabilia*, and thus must have known, from practice, what the task required.
A pointed tip-off appears in the printer's identification of Malachy as
'uitiorum obiurgatoris *acerrimi*'. This sounds suspiciously like an echo of
lines 46–47 in the text below; there, in a reading confined to the print and
those manuscripts I have surveyed most clearly related to Étienne's source
copy, S and B, Malachy urges *acrior* preaching against vice.[12]

Such qualifications being noted, Esposito saw very clearly that Malachy's
cognomen was accurate, and he printed all those passages in the text that
convey specifically Irish information. One can extend his evidence for an
Irish provenance; although Esposito found a good many manuscripts, he
relied solely on information provided by the 1518 print. He thus overlooked
the fact that in some copies (CDL, partially in V) one passage conveying
Irish material was considerably more extensive – and more locally pointed
– than the version printed in 1518, where only about ten rather more
summary lines occur (cf. the edition below, lines 871–79, with the textual
appendix, lines 362–91). Indeed, by the text's usual standards, this discussion
approaches digressiveness (one reason why, if Étienne knew it, he might have
substantially abbreviated it in his print). In addition, Esposito also pointed

[11] The colophon in V: 'Here ends the tract called "Malachy's poison", written by
Fr Malachy, a Franciscan from the Irish province'. Étienne's title and colophon:
'The little book called "Malachy's poison", by the Irish Franciscan Fr Malachy, a
Doctor of Theology, once a vigorous illuminator of God's word, as well as a very
harsh reprover of sins'; and 'Here ends the little book called "The poison of the
sins" or "Malachy's poison", by Fr Malachy, an Irish Franciscan, active around
1300, a Doctor of Theology, and an outstanding preacher of God's Word'.
[12] Not the majority *acucior*; V, which as will emerge, is at best a conflated
copy, here is illegible.

out that Franciscan origins are certainly at least hinted at in the text's single reference to the founder (lines 736–37), a conversational dictum of a sort that smacks of intra-ordinal biographical materials.[13]

Esposito also consulted with A. G. Little, the great historian of Irish Franciscans, and could offer one possible identification of the author of *De ueneno*. A Malachy, from the Franciscan convent at Limerick (founded 1267), was a candidate for election as bishop of Tuam, in neighbouring Connaught, in 1279/80; supported by a minority of the electors, although he pursued his claim in Rome, he withdrew his appeal in 1286.[14] The documents concerning the election include no references that would substantiate the details Étienne presents; strictly legal or jurisdictional in tenor, they never refer to a doctorate, to a preaching career, or to a battler against vice. Nor is there any surviving evidence of a scholar's career at either English university or at Paris. On the other hand, no other individual named Malachy, a name specifically Irish,[15] appears in any surviving Irish Franciscan documents down to 1450. Further, Esposito demonstrated that, so far as now appears, the remaining biographical accounts, including those of John Bale and Luke Wadding, can be seen, as I have argued of Étienne's details, as offering particularising probabilities predicated solely on Étienne's identification and lacking any external confirmation.

Thus, Bale, in his *Index*, must have certainly have recognised *De ueneno* from his manuscript researches, and knew the text on that basis as pseudo-Grossetestian ('Sunt qui hoc opus tribuunt Roberto Lincolniensi' [There are those who attribute this work to Robert, bishop of Lincoln]). But he appears to have known the author Malachy only through a copy of the 1518 print. This he found 'Ex officina Roberti Toye': i.e., in the shop of a London printer active 1542–55. He there ascribes Malachy a book of sermons, but that is simply an inference from Étienne's 'insignis prædicato[r]'.

In his later *Scriptores* Bale was prepared to be a little more fanciful, 'ut in quorundam Chronographorum scriptis habetur' (as is said in the writings of some historians). Here he tweaked the date of Malachy's floruit slightly, to 1310, and bestowed on him both an Oxford residence and a distinguished audience for his sermons, 'coram mundi principibus ac primatibus' (before worldly princes and prelates). In the absence of the 'Chronographi' Bale cites (although, given his Irish adventure, he might have known some texts

---

[13] One might also notice the injunction at lines 1065–66 (and my source note) and possibly the excessive modesty *topos* in the conclusion reported by both Étienne and V, cited in n.10 (although I suspect this a transmissional intrusion, rather than an authorial statement).

[14] For the documents, see Fitzmaurice and Little 46, 54–56.

[15] Cf. the 'double dactyl' claimed by 'Stately plump Buck Mulligan' at the opening of Joyce's *Ulysses*.

that are now lost), I find this only further puffery predicated on Étienne's materials, which Bale again cites here. He has managed to extrapolate from them what seems to him a nebulously appropriate career. Moreover, while Étienne's dating is plausible enough, a round number that might point to decades before and around 1300, Bale's dating is not, unless he refers to the preaching activities of a very old man. As I will show below, some evidence implies that *De ueneno* had been circulating, in an advanced textual state, by the 1290s.[16]

Esposito offers a rather minimalist identification, arguably generic (a late thirteenth-century Irish Franciscan), rather than personal. But, between them, both the dates of the earliest surviving manuscripts and at least some of Malachy's source materials suggest that Esposito's projected floruit, toward 1280, is just about right. The earliest copies of *De ueneno* date from just around and after 1300, and at least some materials I will discuss below would imply access to Franciscan texts composed or used in either Oxford or Paris in the period roughly 1260–80.

Malachy's work and its sources

Malachy is explicit about the method and purpose of his work, as well as its intended audience:

> Since I intend to speak about spiritual poison, I draw together metaphors from poisonous beasts, so that, the more pointed they are to preach and the more terrifying to hear, the more effectually they may penetrate the hearts of sinners. (lines 45–49)

This is not simply a work of vice and virtue, but a work designed to be used by preachers in their oral exhortation to good conduct. Here Malachy insists upon the key function of memorability – penetrating (and implicitly lodging in) sinners' hearts. He counts on the force of his metaphorical vehicle, its tactile frisson, the horror of dealing with venomous vermin, to underwrite that memorial function. Equally, his formulation makes clear that this is 'metaphor', analogy or similarity: sin and virtue are spiritual, his natural examples physical metaphors that offer a solid form to that detestation of sin that he seeks to inculcate.

Such metaphorical (or, to invoke the more usual medieval term, similitudinous) instruction is a well-established sermon technique, one Malachy

---

[16] For the texts, see Bale 1990, 286; and 1557–59, 2:242–43 (centuria decima quarta, cap. 91). But one might notice Sharpe's reference (232–33 n225) to Jean Garet of Louvain, who in 1561 dated *De ueneno* to 1308, although he may only be repeating information from a dated copy.

compactly, yet inexplicitly, invokes at the very opening of *De ueneno*. It is one standard ploy for the rhetorical amplification specifically enjoined on preachers by *artes praedicandi*. The Dominican Thomas Waleys, writing in the 1340s, offers particularly explicit instruction in the technique:

> Sometimes a preacher wants to extend a particular passage of scripture. One way of doing this is to draw upon the properties of those things to which the scriptural passage refers. For example, think about applying Isaiah 11:1, 'There shall come forth a rod out of the root of Jesse, and a flower shall rise up out of his root', to the Blessed Virgin and her Son. Then one might align with them the properties and nature of a rod, and the properties of a root, and those of a flower, and one might do this of either flowers generally or of some specific flower [presumably thinking of the common association of the Virgin with the lily].[17]

The salience of Waleys's persistent emphasis upon 'proprietas' will appear shortly. But, in the immediate context, one might well be reminded of Malachy's foundational explanation of his choice of similitudinous topic at the very opening of the text:

> Poison began in a rational creature, because, when pride was conceived in the angel's mind, it changed his most noble nature into that of a snake. For this reason, Apc 12:9 calls him 'the old serpent'. Also pride alone gave rise to every other poison. (lines 3–6)

Just as Waleys enjoins, Malachy presents his argument as arising from a metaphorical reading of a scriptural authority, here Apc 12:9. Satan/the devil is source of all evil, hence the antiquity ascribed him by the Revelator; and he is a snake, not simply on the warrant of the inevitably soon to be cited narrative of Gn 3, but because snakes have the 'property' of poisonousness, an indication of sin.

Following such an opening, Malachy's remaining exemplification, his persistent analogies between specific sins, spiritual poisons, and specific poisonous beasts, physical poisons (and, one should insist, their poison-derived remedies, their theriacs/*tiriaca* 'antidotes'), follows – dare one say? – quite naturally.[18] Customarily, however, Malachy's discussion is presented

---

[17] For the original Latin see Charland 396. Almost immediately after this passage, Waleys offers a careful explanation of the forceful utility of *similitudines*; see the citation and discussion at *Patient* 260–61, 326–30.

[18] Cf. Newhauser 1993, 159–60, where in a discussion of organisational metaphors in treatises on the virtues and vices he cites *De ueneno* as exemplary

in a differing, yet reasonably fixed order: it is pegged to vices or virtues; the natural-historical detail follows as exemplification of a specific spiritual state; and the local discussion is capped with an *auctoritas*, a specific illustrative citation to which the already presented analogy might be joined. Most of these *auctoritates* are, as Waleys suggests they should be, biblical citations, but many are not, and many are linked not with poisonous 'properties' per se but with the metaphorical tenors, the spiritual states, to which the specific poisons have been assigned.

These developed examples may then appear as delightful *memorabilia* in the amplification of sermon points. There traditionally the ordered presentation of *exempla ex scriptura*, *ex natura*, and *ex historia* have an outstanding place.[19] Malachy's conception, which begins with the most widely adaptable, most visually available, and least apparently dogmatic of the triad, is strikingly original, and the number of surviving copies shows the work was widely appreciated, largely for its diverting (and horrifying) scientific material.[20]

However, in addition to analysis of vice and virtue and the provision of amplificatory exemplary material, Malachy is, usually quite tacitly, engaged in a task he has promised in his opening. I have left my initial citation with an ellipsis; the contents there elided are rather telling, 'today, when usual forms of authorship have grown cold'. Implicitly, Malachy claims that there is a general need for the renovation of preaching and, in addition to its offering moralisable poisonous 'properties', the book is a very informal

of metaphors derived from medicine, in which the 'sins [appear] as wounds or illnesses, and the virtues as their corresponding remedies'. Newhauser suggests that the ultimate source is the good Samaritan of Luke 10 (cf. Wenzel 2008, 280–81, good background for Langland's treatment in *Piers Plowman* B 17). Newhauser also briefly refers to Malachy among his listing of examples of his genre at 35. On medical metaphors more generally, see McCann. Malachy's concern with antidotes, typically serpent-derived theriacs, draws upon a widespread approach to moralising nature, that the same being or object may have moral implications both *in malo* and *in bono*.

[19]   On the ordered presentation of exemplary material in sermon development, see the magisterial Wenzel 2015, 111–12 (the triad 'exempla ex natura, ex arte, et ex historia'). Wenzel 2008 offers a number of examples, e.g. 25–26, 141–42 (John Felton), 198 (Richard Fitzralph).

[20]   Cf. Newhauser: 'The frequent use of *exempla* as illustrative material in the representatives of the genre allied to the preparation of sermons and in late medieval exemplars of the genre which may have been suitable for private consumption hint at something approaching an aesthetic function ...' (1993, 65); and his comment (131) on the late medieval 'movement' of vice and virtue books 'towards greater homiletic usefulness'.

ars praedicandi with a range of helpful suggestions for pulpit performance. Although modestly billed as just some *similitudines* exemplifying variations on the metaphorical 'poison of sin', *De ueneno* offers a considerably broader and more informative preacher's toolkit.

Any reading of *De ueneno* should notice some rather malleable features of presentation. Far from everything here – particularly not Malachy's large-scale structural divisions of his argument – accords with the argumentative description I have just offered. Here I would draw attention to two particular gestures, neither signalled with any overtness but left as 'enhancing suggestions'. The first is fitful but fairly obvious, although perhaps not so to Malachy's 'chilled' practitioners; this involves structuring argument by, or offering citations from, Gregory the Great's seminal discussion of the sins and their 'parts' in *Moralia* 31.[21] These, I think, stand as signals to readers; following usual compilatory injunctions, one is not to be content with cited snippets, but seek *originalia* in their completeness.[22] Those places where Gregory is not explicitly invoked provide, every bit as much as do Malachy's overt Gregorian citations, materials useful for pulpit invention. Malachy's 'renovated preacher' might well seek out Gregory to fill the silences in the argument of *De ueneno*, and might use Malachy's developed Gregorian arguments as models for an original presentation of sins the author had not treated in this way.

The second feature, perhaps more persistent through the work, is most obviously present in Malachy's references to local, Irish conditions. Malachy offers a good deal of his argument not about sin *per se*, the sort of discussion his citations from Gregory underscore, but about specific social sites in which sin occurs. These are fairly predictable ones, lords associated with pride, merchants with avarice, for example. But they represent dips into materials that typify a specific pulpit genre, the *sermo ad status*, the sermon focussed upon a specific audience situation and the imagined temptations (and their execution) that might be appropriate to a specific social group. One should note that the majority of such surviving sermons are not addressed to society at large, but are rather *sermones ad cleros*. This fact not only accounts for Malachy's numerous applications of his poisons to sacerdotal misbehaviour but also, by implication, constructs a figure for the conscientious 'renovated' preacher whose absence Malachy is intent on filling, as well as offering that person pulpit strategies.

In addition to these features, Malachy offers other 'enhancing suggestions', again typifying a general *ars*, rather than specifically a 'book

---

[21] Insisting upon the importance of Gregory's discussion to the entire tradition is one of Bloomfield's major contributions.

[22] Cf. the discussion and citation from Thomas of Ireland's *Manipulus florum* at *Patient* 255–56.

of vices and virtues' or a collection of *similitudines* structured round the *proprietates* of natural beings. While I do find the tract consistently centred around such natural historical materials (and will revert to this point later), a good deal more is on offer here. Much of this natural history depends upon the observations of two classical figures, Aristotle and Pliny, and they here draw in their train a substantial amount of classical material. As one expects, the majority of Malachy's citations link his metaphors with biblical citations. But he also provides a quite substantial chunk of classical *auctoritas* on which to substantiate his moralisations, perhaps particularly citations from Seneca (and a certain amount of Cicero).[23] Nor is this all; at various points ancient history, moralising mythography, and Æsopian fable are drawn into the mix. While the book's centre may remain scientific, it is persistently suggesting materials potentially subject to similar moralising analogy, and at a variety of points offers implicit logics (or defences?) for such alien materials, or provides references to such justificatory accounts:

> If indeed a pagan [Socrates] avoided death in the name of a single god, what wonder is there if looking on the son of God on the cross should not free that person from death, once and for all? (lines 75–77, abbreviated)[24]

Esposito discussed Malachy's reading, based upon the author's overt citations of authority. His account was not absolutely accurate, but near enough to give some idea of the author's apparent range of reference. Sharpe comments that Malachy's 'moral and medical reading was wide though hardly recondite' (235). Unfortunately, neither Esposito nor Sharpe stopped to consider that *De ueneno* is a specifically tailored compilation,

---

[23]   This includes a healthy dose of materials 'Senecan' only, but regularly ascribed to the Stoic in the Middle Ages, particularly materials from proverb collections (echoing the author's terseness). It is possible that, like many medieval people, Malachy considered Seneca to be a Christian author, a perception based upon an apocryphal correspondence with St Paul.

[24]   Cf. a similarly 'classicised' group of sermon materials I will discuss further below, John of Wales's *Communiloquium*, here 1.3.3 (sig. b 4[va]), 'Et si tales fuerunt gentiles, quales debent esse principes fideles?' (And if pagan princes behaved [in this virtuous way], how ought Christian ones to behave?). Another 'enhancing suggestion' would be the inclusion of an encouraging reference to Augustine's discussion, *De doctrina Christiana* 2.16, the foundational justification of appropriations, for Christian edification, from scientific and pagan materials. I cite this important text in full below, in the notes on Malachy's sources, 1312–13.

designed to generate *similitudines* focussed, in the main, by a single topic: poison and the relevant remedies against infection.[25]

But this is a compilation. Malachy quotes and then moralises before moving on to a new topic; roughly half the work, the scientific information, is provided by the works he cites, and only his moralisations represent anything original (although they are often strikingly so). As the good Franciscan preacher he appears to have been, Malachy would have been intensely aware of other compilations from which he might derive relevant materials. As I will demonstrate shortly, compilation, as I have said elsewhere, is 'a gift that goes on giving'. While I do not wish to detract from the frequent homiletic effectiveness of the text, I must report that Malachy, however inventive his morals, is likely to have known no science at all, and that he certainly derived all those materials from careful consultation of a single source.

This is the great earlier thirteenth-century Franciscan compilation Bartholomew the Englishman's *De proprietatibus rerum*. I have checked all Malachy's scientific citations against BA, and, excepting a handful of isolated examples, every bit of this material in the text simply represents a quotation from information assembled by the earlier Franciscan. This dependence extends beyond what one might expect – for example, BA's identification of the authorities who provided his information carried over wholesale – to the actual language of the citations. BA frequently paraphrased his *auctores*, and Malachy's text reflects his language, not that of the sources.[26] Those citations original to Malachy are limited to his biblical references (although a small portion of these occur already in BA), his citations from the Fathers, and perhaps most of the classical material (particularly quotations from Seneca).[27]

---

[25] Peter of Limoges's *De oculo morali* provides an analogous example of such a focussed presentation, probably contemporary (1274×89) and considerably more widely transmitted. See Newhauser, trs.

[26] See, for example, the discussion below and textual note on 'lacteam saniem' (line 264). Particularly salient is the discussion of the Gregorian five parts of envy (lines 379–467), where the assignment to various species of asp follows both the order and information of BA 1134/37–1135/21 (with the material on the lynx at lines 443–50 intercalated from elsewhere in BA). A detailed account of the full range of materials derived from BA appears below, in the sequence of notes devoted to Malachy's sources.

[27] Malachy's reliance upon BA may suggest that, even if initially addressing an Irish audience, he had been continentally trained. As Seymour points out (1974, 156), only two thirteenth-century insular copies of the text survive, both late, one dated 1296. However, Richard Sharpe points out to me references to two lost copies certainly or possibly contemporary with Malachy: a book at

Choosing BA was, I should think, a 'no-brainer'. For not only is this a Franciscan text but it was deliberately compiled for just those purposes that led Malachy to seek it out. BA's prologue, in considerably more expansive language, outlines that use of *proprietates* I have already cited from Thomas Waleys:

> Est presens opusculum compilatum, vtile mihi, et forsitan alijs, qui naturas rerum et proprietates per sanctorum libros, necnon et philosophorum, dispersas non cognouerunt, ad intelligenda enigmata scripturarum que sub symbolis et figuris proprietatum rerum naturalium et artificialium a Spiritu Sancto sunt tradite et velate. (= BA 41/6–12)

or just a little later:

> Theologia prouide sacris et poeticis informationibus vsa est, vt et rerum visibilium similitudinibus allegorice locutiones et mystici intellectus transumptiones formentur, et sic carnalibus et visibilibus spiritualia et inuisibilia coaptentur. (= BA 41/22–27)

Malachy was astute and followed the programme, using BA in the way the author hoped it would be.[28]

Glastonbury 1274×91 and another limned and bound for Norwich Cathedral in 1300/1. For these, see Sharpe *et al.* 217, 299 (respectively, B40.13 and B57.24).

[28] Cf. the brief comments on BA, *Patient* 52–53, 301 and n27. I offer references to BA not from a Latin copy but from Seymour *et al.*'s edition of John Trevisa's Middle English translation (1398). This is, quite simply, an act of convenience; the Middle English is widely available, whereas reproductions of manuscripts or incunabula are not. Further, Trevisa was intensely conscientious and translated quite literally; as a result, his readings are an adequate guide to what Malachy should have found in a good Latin manuscript. (Moreover, Seymour *et al.*'s editorial practice renders the edition more like Latin manuscripts than many of the Middle English forms of the text do, largely through scribalisms.) Using this edition has the further advantage of absolving me of providing additional references to the primary sources that Malachy, however authoritative he may appear, knew only at second hand. Seymour *et al.* 1992 is largely given over to a line-by-line account of those primary sources BA combined in his tome, and there is no point reproducing its information here, when interested readers may seek it out themselves. The one addition to this useful index I would make concerns citations from Aristotle's *De animalibus*; references in this volume to Aristotelian *originalia* may be supplemented by the access to Michael Scot's translation, used by BA, afforded by its citation within Albertus Magnus's commentary (cf. the double citations in 1992, 60–76 passim).

For reasons that will be clear shortly, I would insist on Malachy's adherence to a Bartholomaean programme. Unlike many other books of this type, such as Peraldus's (Guillaume Peyraut's) particularly compendious *Summa*, Malachy is not producing an always expansible collection of useful citations, but is engaged in a narrowly focussed project, a book that steadfastly lays material poisons, their antidotes, and the animals responsible for them against their spiritual equivalents. He knew that, if one wanted simply the quotable – as opposed to his steadfast eye on Gregory's authoritative outline of the sins in *Moralia* 31 – there were plenty of places to find citations. The thirteenth century, following from Peter Chanter's *Abel*, had produced a great many alphabetical *distinctiones* collections, where one can uncover authoritative ammunition for constructing such discussions in plenty.

BA certainly represents Malachy's most abiding source. However, two other authors offered substantial contributions, both to the content and the mien of his text. The first, whom Malachy twice cites explicitly (lines 1039–41, 1628–38), was Alexander Neckam, in his *De naturis rerum*. One might see this work of *c.*1200 as a transitional text; it shares with the pre-scientific bestiary *Physiologus* an interest in moralising allegedly natural detail, yet Neckam also knows and draws upon reputable classical authority, principally Pliny. That recourse to the classics may well have inspired BA, who sought to update his predecessor through systematic recourse to standard thirteenth-century university curricular texts, principally Galenic medicine and Aristotelian natural history.

Neckam offers a variety of information comparable to Malachy's, but the later author's language nearly always follows what he found in BA. Neckam's influence is perhaps more general, yet in certain respects more specific. First of all, at 2.105–21 (pp. 187–99) he presents a sequence of discussions of various serpents, extensively paralleled in scientific material Malachy draws more directly from BA. Within this sequence, however, his 2.109 stands out. First of all, it provides a reference to a rather unusual text, the pseudo-Virgilian 'Culex', presented in a similar context in *De ueneno* (lines 100–4). But, more than that, Neckam's chapter includes a discussion of Christ as serpent that, at the very least, Malachy imitates closely:

Why is the Lord Jesus Christ compared to a snake? One may assign many causes for this. Just as the children of Israel in the desert, when they looked on the brazen serpent raised on a stake, were freed of the fiery bites of snakes, likewise people looking, with the eyes of faith and devotion, on Christ raised on the tree of the cross for us, will be freed from the attacks of the ancient enemy. For Christ is the theriac and antidote that expels the malice of the poison injected by the ancient enemy. Also Christ was our unharmed head, because his divinity was immune to suffering. Christ was also a snake in his prudence, since, in his humility, he evaded the subtlety of the prince of this world. (p. 192; cf. lines 50–68)[29]

Indeed, although I can, in this second instance, offer only rather fragmentary evidence, I should imagine that Malachy may actually have known independently only about as much about his 'authorities' as he did about his science. The signal that such might be the case is provided by two citations of John of Salisbury (lines 410–13, 1028–33). These potentially imply that Malachy is drawing not upon first-hand knowledge but upon a text thoroughly imbued with John's *Polycraticus*, John of Wales's *Communi-loquium*.[30] Such a source would explain a feature of *De ueneno* I have already mentioned, Malachy's use of the classics, not simply Seneca, but Cicero and, once (lines 1463–67), Valerius Maximus, a John of Wales favourite – and, rather surprisingly, perhaps, Fulgentian mythography. Were Malachy indeed a university figure, he might well have known John of Wales, as the author was a Franciscan attached to both Oxford and, from around 1270, Paris.[31]

I have surveyed carefully only the first part of John's *Communi-loquium*, but this portion alone throws up evidence provocative, even if not definitive. One has to say that in a handbook of these dimensions it is predictably not difficult to find citations common to both authors. Such isolated echoes, of which there are a fair number, prove very little, as both writers may simply respond to Franciscan preaching commonplaces.[32]

[29] 'Quid quod Dominus ipse Jesus Christus serpenti comparatur? Plures autem causas super hoc queunt assignari. Sicut enim in deserto, respicientes filii Israel in serpentem aeneum erectum in palo, liberati sunt ab ignitis morsibus serpentum, ita respicientes oculis fidei et devotionis in Christum in ligno crucis pro nobis erectum ab insidiis antiqui hostis liberabuntur. Christus etiam tiriaca est et antidotum ad expellendam malitiam veneni infusi ab antiquo hoste. Christi item caput illaesum erat, quia deitas impassibilis erat. Christus etiam erat serpens per prudentiam, cum in humilitate astutiam principis hujus mundi elusit'.

[30] For the only full-length study, see Swanson, perhaps less pointed than Pantin's essay. On the dating of John's texts, in the later 1260s, probably, but not definitively, in Oxford, see Swanson 4–10. Note particularly her comments on Bacon's discovery of Senecan texts in Oxford by 1258. My citation text represents the 'short' – and less inclusive – version of John's work.

[31] John might also underlie another of Malachy's 'enhancing suggestions' to his preacher readers, his allusion to Augustine's defence of fables in 'Contra mendacium' (lines 1238–42). See further my 2017.

[32] A few examples, with comments on the variable appearance of relationship: Malachy's lines 587–98 = John 1.4.4 (sig. d 1va, but in John paraphrased, whereas

However, either clumps or concatenations of citations common to both texts would imply very strongly that Malachy had recourse to John's collection. These certainly occur. In the discussion of flatterers, Malachy's lines 1017–21, 1026–33, and 1039–45 appear proximately in John's 1.8.2 (sig. d 6[rab]) – although Malachy supplies a different quotation from Juvenal and, as I have indicated, probably knew Neckam's text independently. More convincingly, Malachy's lines 1092–1105 offer the same citations as John's 1.3.8 (sig. c 1[rab]), and in the same order. Indeed, John's rendition confirms both that Malachy's text included the biblical citation absent in some manuscripts and that his assignment of one citation to Cicero's *De divinatione* (where it cannot be found) is incorrect. (It is, as John indicates, *De officiis* 2.55 – which he cites reasonably exactly, whereas Malachy paraphrases.) I think the question of 'Malachy's learning' probably should be left open, although I would argue that the author of *De ueneno* is considerably less erudite than it might appear at first glance.

Some users of *De ueneno*

Wide manuscript dispersal is one thing, a text's actual use another. I defer some of the most pregnant (and vexing) examples of the second to a discussion of the textual tradition. I here return to Malachy's statement of intent, and to the implicit general instructions for preachers included in the text passim. Without casting too wide a net, there are ample indications of the inspirational quality of *De ueneno*. One might note the number of manuscripts cited above that include at least incipient efforts at indexing (**ADL**), a gesture explicable only as an effort at preparing the text for ready consultation.

Signs of overt pulpit use begin very early in the tradition, with the MS I designate as **A**, William Herebert's collection of *praedicabilia*. Of course, **A** was produced by Franciscans (and certainly, after Herebert's personal use, institutionally owned), indeed by someone who inhabited locales associated with Malachy ascriptions (Paris and Oxford, see above). In addition to the text of Malachy, **A** also includes a sequence of Herebert's sermons, both in delivered and in outline form. These clearly demonstrate the purposiveness of his manuscript collection, as Herebert recycles materials he had collected for such use (and which appear elsewhere in the MS) in his pulpit performance.

Malachy has Seneca's language); 659–62 = 1.3.11 (sig. c 2[rb]); 1457–61 = 1.3.12 (sig. c 3[rb]); 1524–27 = 2.2.1 (sig. f 3[ra], where John supplies much of Jerome's discussion and I have, surprisingly, found no parallel in BA). At 664–70 = 3.7.2 (sig. i 1[vb]), John and Malachy offer differing degrees of exact citation and paraphrase for the same Senecan passage.

For example, Herebert's sermo 4 discusses the seven deadly sins. Over a protracted segment of the text (Reimer 82–86/315–461 passim) he chooses to develop his arguments with materials he has lifted from appropriate places in *De ueneno*.[33] One particularly telling moment in this appropriation is worth noting, 85/418–22; at the comparable point in *De ueneno* (lines 781–82) all the manuscripts, including A, ascribe the citation to Seneca, as is reasonably commonplace in the Middle Ages. Herebert demurs, because he recognises this statement as what it is, Gregory's *Moralia* paraphrased. He can stand as one example of a topic to which I will return, a reader who knows more than the supposed 'authority' on whom he draws.[34]

Given the paucity of published sermons, I can only gesture at further fragmentary evidence for the influence of *De ueneno*. Matters are not helped by the anonymity of Malachy's tract, so that one cannot search for indexed citations of the author. Nonetheless, there is one impressive published example, a sermon on the sins and their antidotes from the extensive Norfolk collection Cambridge, Jesus College, MS Q.A.13 (James's MS 13).[35]

I have unearthed a few further examples, all these, like that in Jesus College Q.A.13, in Middle English, certainly enough to imply the existence of a further extensive cache (especially in much less investigated Latin materials). Dublin, Trinity College, MS 241, fols 113–14 shows extensive knowledge of *De ueneno* similar to that on offer in the Jesus College MS. This sermon includes a protracted discussion derived from Malachy's opening, as well as examples of the *situla* and the basilisk. Again, the Shrewsbury preacher John Mirk, at British Library, MS Cotton Claudius A.ii, fol. 41, has the exemplum from lines 1106–13. While this is a commonplace kind of story, that Mirk specifically places his account in Ireland would indicate that he has derived it from Malachy. The same exemplum subsequently appears in a collection derived from Mirk's at British Library, MS Harley 2247, fols 36–38ᵛ.[36]

---

[33] Or again, at Reimer 86/457–61, he reproduces Malachy's lines 1457–61. Herebert similarly drew on his copy of Walter Map's 'Dissuasio Valerii' (now excised from the book); see Reimer 43–44/394–402, 65/234–36, 86–87/461–67. The second of these citations is instructive: the preacher's note to himself to extract relevant exemplary material from his copy of the original for insertion and development here.

[34] See further the textual note to line 825, where Herebert's knowledge exceeded not only Malachy's but that of Fulgentius's Teubner editor.

[35] Edited, with an important general discussion, in Newhauser 2008; on the MS, see further Wenzel 2005, 140–45, 505–25.

[36] For these examples, see O'Mara and Paul 269, 953, and 1113, respectively.

Other examples are somewhat more attenuated. The very sophisticated preacher of *Jacob's Well*, Salisbury Cathedral, MS 103, is perfectly capable of accessing Malachy's originals without prompting. His collection includes the similitude of lines 1308ff. (the serpent's skin-shedding as a figure for penance) at fols 128ᵛ–29; the material on harp-strings made of wolf-gut (lines 933–36) at fol. 30ᵛ, although probably, following his ascription, he has it directly from BA. More apt to be an incidental agreement in the commonplace is his association of anger, demonic possession, and the mad dog at fol. 34 (cf. Malachy's lines 621–25).[37] Finally, Worcester Cathedral, MS F.10, fol. 54, presents an image not directly borrowed from, but certainly inspired by, *De ueneno*. The preacher describes the lizard *stellio* that stares at its own beauty and thereby allows itself to be attacked by a scorpion, certainly consonant with Malachy's association of the scorpion and the flatterer. But this is perhaps a rather garbled memory of BA 1244/18–24.[38]

Provocative evidence of Malachy's diffusion and influence emerges from that connoisseur of the fourteenth-century commonplace, William Langland. After all, one of the poem's most well-known passages begins with the off-the-cuff reference to Malachy's founding metaphor:

For truþe telleþ þat loue is triacle of heuene:
May no synne be on hym sene þat vseþ þat spice. (B 1.149–50)

The allusion is consonantly used to introduce the theme of incarnation, which, as I have indicated above, is central to Malachy's generalised opening, inherited from Alexander Neckam.[39]

However, this allusion scarcely exhausts Malachy's potential influence on *Piers Plowman*. One discussion in *De ueneno* that seems particularly to have intrigued and energised Langland is Malachy's extensive material on Irish courtly flatterers, 'mimi et histriones'. While attacks on minstrelsy as the dark Other of properly moral sermonising are utter stocks, the sequence of materials in *Piers Plowman* is both intense and compelling.[40] Particularly in his C Version, where the poet-figure's moral status becomes a prominent issue, Langland offers an extensive effort at defining a purified poetry within the milieu of the courtly great house, with its contemporary swarm of 'fooles sages, flatereris and lieres' (B 13.421–56, reprised at C 7.81–118a).

---

[37] See O'Mara and Paul 2389, 2300, and 2302, respectively.

[38] See O'Mara and Paul 2626; and, on the MS, Wenzel 2005, 151–58, 607–25.

[39] For further commonplace antecedents to this passage see my 2019.

[40] For attacks on minstrels and their productions see, for example, Owst 10–16, 311–12, 327; or my 2005, 149–53 and nn.

Other probable borrowings come from Malachy's scornful discussion of the alleged pride-swelling panegyrics of popular lordly entertainment. These include a reprise of Malachy's lines 909ff., where the mis-limbed fox is offered as a figure for the *adulator*/flatterer:

> Kyndeliche, by Crist, ben such ycald lollares,
> As by þe Engelisch of oure eldres of olde mennes techynge.
> He þat lolleth is lame or his leg out of ioynte
> Or maymed in som membre, for to meschief hit souneth.
> Rihte so, sothly, such manere ermytes
> Lollen aȝen þe byleue and lawe of holy churche. (C 9.214–19)

Langland's 'Kyndeliche', of course, answers exactly the rhetorical end-product Malachy imagined for his entire discussion, the preachers' *exemplum ex natura*. The allusion – although, again, it is commonplace[41] – interfaces with the earlier discussion of flatterers, as Langland invokes Malachy's fox to describe wheedling, begging false hermits, parading an ingratiating fake-piety. Further, Malachy's flatterer materials recur in the poem in a passage unmarked as pertaining to the topic but overtly from Malachy – and within the same (protracted) discussion (lines 1162–65):

> 'Thoruȝ experience', quod heo, 'I hope þei shul be saued;
> For venym fordooþ venym, and þat preue I by reson.
> For of alle venymes foulest is þe scorpion;
> May no medicyne amende þe place þer he styngeþ
> Til he be deed and do þerto; þe yuel he destruyeþ,
> The first venymouste, þoruȝ venym of hymselue …' (B 18.150–55)

One should again note the introduction, 'Thoruȝ experience', yet another parallel to *exemplum ex natura*. Of course, this brings this brief discussion of *Piers Plowman* full circle, as Mercy is here discussing the Incarnation as the antidote, the 'theriac', to man's fall. It is, further, not amiss to recall Langland's most prominent constructive minstrel-figure, Patience, virtually defined by his penchant for encouraging natural figures. Certainly, *Piers* was a text where the 'literary' and Malachy's more humble offering interfaced.

However, Langland is scarcely Malachy's most sophisticated reader (and difficult author). The Oxonian Robert Holcot OP silently invokes Malachy's materials at the head of his commentary on the prophet Joel (MS Bodley 722, fol. 37ᵛ). He there begins by quoting extensively from Jerome's association of the four beasts in Joel 1:4 with four successive

---

[41]   It appears, for example, in the bestiary *Physiologus*.

conquests of Judea (*PL* 25:951–52). But he further develops Jerome by analysing the biblical *eruca* with language borrowed from Malachy's lines 695–702. Again, when his discussion moves on to the *dentes leonis* of Joel 1:6, he offers a version of details Malachy associates with the 'formicoleon' (lines 851–64). This is largely based upon Malachy's moralisation that, as lesser predators, they represent bailiffs. Simply on the basis of the scrappy examples I have assembled, Malachy's reach would appear to have been long indeed.

The text: some general textual observations

Malachy's *De ueneno* is not simply an excellent example of compilation and an amusing work popular in the Middle Ages and now ignored. On inspection, attempting to identify the work's parameters engages the researcher in a thorny (and theoretically revelatory) editorial project. For a variety of reasons, one cannot recover a securely authorial text of *De ueneno*.

An initial difficulty is signalled by a range of persistently routine variations among the copies. An already packed *corpus lectionum* might be further expanded by inclusion of a wide, if not, in the main, meaning-effecting, range of variation. In many instances, the scribes would appear to have accommodated the text to stylistic formats with which they were comfortable, irrespective of whatever had been communicated to them. Tracking, much less recording, such variation is fruitless, but, by the same token, one is left in doubt as to what Malachy's own practice might have been.[42]

One can specify a sequence of repeated variations among copies that should be ignored in any analysis. First of all, authorial word-order is probably unrecoverable. Generally, copyists manage to include the complete substantive text, but not necessarily with attention to the order of its elements. One might note that Herebert's copy **A** is particularly errant in this regard.

Editors may justifiably disagree about whether prose word-order represents substantive variation. However, in a wide variety of other instances, certainly substantive, the manuscripts persistently communicate variants on the whole indifferent, and thus irresolvable. Again, authorial practice is in all these instances indeterminate. Examples liberally evidenced across the manuscripts include the following, all here ignored:

How are sentences and clauses to be connected? Is it igitur? ergo? uero? Or etiam? enim? autem? Or qui? quia? quod?

---

[42] With the following discussion, cf. Lutz's editorial exclusions from her variant corpus, *Remigii* 59, analogous to the procedures adopted here.

What preposition is intended? These are subject to persistent variation across the copies, as well as (secondary) variation in the cases governed. Equally persistently, there is variation between prepositional phrases and unmarked ablatives/locatives.

Are punctuational features such as 'scilicet' and 'id est' necessary? These are sometimes present, sometimes not.

Which synonym is intended? The text is littered with simple substitutions, usually not affecting sense, e.g. a persistent waveryness over 'bestia' and 'bestiola' or variations involving one or another *nomen divinum*.

What is the verb? The manuscripts hesitate over the supply or absence of *esse* in contexts where it is obvious. There is persistent minor variation over verbal prefixes and alternation between verb moods and tenses. Thus, the MSS rather indifferently use the subjunctive or indicative in cases such as *cum*-clauses, where classical Latin has the former. They also routinely alternate between imperfect, perfect, and future perfect. Frequently, particularly with compound subjects, the singular appears, where a grammarian would insist upon the plural.

Particularly vexing in a text given over to quotation is widespread variation in the presentation of citations. How are invocations of authority to be introduced? 'Sicut dicit'? 'Est notandum quod X dicit'? 'Vnde dicit'? Or simply the name of the authority, with implicit following colon? Does one need to mark the end of an extended example with 'Hec ille'?

Reference forms universally vary. Is it 'Isidorus, libro 12' or 'Isidorus, *Ethimologiarum* 12'? Are books to be numbered in roman or arabic? As expected, book and chapter references are frequently and hopelessly inaccurate. Moreover, there are reasonably persistent confusions of normal forms of reference for authorities, e.g. Pliny ('secundum Plin") and Aristotle ('secundum phm"), or 'Augustinus' ('Au') and 'Anselmus' ('An').[43]

A further difficulty, predictably enough for an initially Franciscan audience adept with Scripture, concerns biblical citations. How abbreviated should these be? Can one count on readers recognising a reference through citation of biblical book and three or four words of a text? Should the whole verse be cited, often in a severely abbreviated form?[44]

I choose to present none of these variations, frequent as they may be. Any text in these (and analogous) instances must present 'copy-text' only.

---

[43]   Not typically a problem in Latin texts, but here exacerbated by a number of citations from the latter author's *Hexameron*.

[44]   The 1518 print's neat chapter divisions are considerably more careful, and their rubrics usually more extensive than the early MS versions. V, for example, offers no divisions between the sins and their contrary virtues. While A, particularly early, erratically marks some inner divisions of chapters, it agrees with GS in providing no rubrics at clear chapter divisions.

Whatever textual basis is chosen, its forms are to be taken as 'representative' (not 'definitive') of what Malachy wrote. In a broad number of instances, one cannot find an authorial text.

Having noted these exclusions, the remaining corpus of variants does allow some definitive conclusions. An initial collation of copies reveals the broad outlines of transmission.[45] The six manuscript versions here examined in detail profusely and consistently, as an inspection of the collations to any single paragraph in the edition below will indicate, fall into three groups:

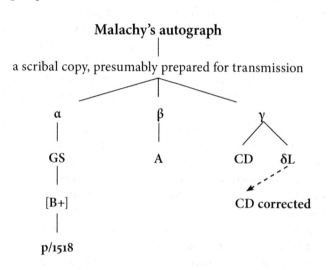

Malachy's autograph

a scribal copy, presumably prepared for transmission

α   β   γ

GS   A   CD   δL

[B+]   CD corrected

p/1518

One must hypothesise a transmissional copy, a version of the text not Malachy's autograph but the source of the surviving MSS. Whatever their form of descent, a wide scatter of universally transmitted readings is manifestly erroneous. For example, at line 1415 all six copies read 'tunc ducit unum ex eis ad locum proprium'. On this showing, 'locum proprium' was certainly the reading of αβγ. But the source here, BA 1248/25, reads the considerably more pointed 'a drye place', i.e. 'ad locum siccum', and presumably represents Malachy's reading. However, the only connection I can draw between the received reading and what should have been in Malachy's autograph is an unattested 'locum suum' in a copy preceding αβγ. In such an account, the received reading has emerged

---

[45]   On those occasions when all six copies are presenting comparable materials, they are clearly responding with reasonable accuracy to the same original text. On only five isolated occasions, at lines 649–54, 1236–41, 1425–30, 1609–17, and 1629–38, do the MSS differ from thorough-going paraphrase of ostensibly similar materials (usually as the result of inadvertent omissions and some further effort at repairing the sense).

from a homeographic representation of the source (confusion over an abbreviated form, perhaps *s^cum*?). This reading has been subjected to a 'second-generation' homonymous substitution in the copy underlying αβγ. On the basis of such local analyses, it is further evident, as none is the source of any of the others, that the copies that survive for scrutiny are at best fourth-generation representatives of whatever Malachy wrote. During the two or three decades between its composition (late 1270s or 1280s?) and the extant copies, the text had an exuberant, and only fitfully visible, transmission, a topic that will occupy us further in a moment.

The stemma above also displays some important details about the surviving copies and their interrelationships. Both C and D were copied from the same (surely, given their provenances, Durham) source. In addition, both have been corrected, C extensively and meticulously, D a bit sporadically. These corrections again reflect a common source, not the original exemplar underlying both, but a copy I designate δ, which resembled L.[46]

Most of the readings communicated in p are ancient in the tradition and most consistently reflected in S. However, B here stands in for a later fourteenth-century manuscript that was Étienne's immediate source or its ancestor. Such a conclusion is mandated by the extensive variation of the S intrusion following line 541, where B shares an intrusion of the same dimensions as that of S, but lacking that manuscript's eccentricities, as also does p. (Of course, the variations in S, which include at least one clear example of homeoarchy, indicate that that scribe, no later than the 1320s, was already copying from a manuscript scribal and yet interpolated.)

The textual proximity and persistent collective deviance of CDL creates one problem. The persistence of these three MSS in shared unique readings unhelpfully weights the sample and renders any statistical showing of other relations among the copies difficult. Here the principal problem concerns where to place Herebert's A. Agreements of the type AGS are

---

[46] C has been corrected by at least three different hands, one the original scribe, another with tiny marginalia of s. xv. C thus is a problem; I have obviously provided all its relevant variants, but finally (because they are systematic, and thus profuse, and will simply clutter the collation with a variety of readings that failed to convince the correcting hands of the MS) have usually reported only its 'final text'. Thus, with C I follow a widely honoured rule of textual criticism, that 'the readings of MS X' represent the text as presented by the last medieval hand operating on the book. However, C is, in the nature of things (three correcting hands) in fact hyper-corrected, and the quality of these revisions suffers from the fact that none of the correctors had available anything but an already-related copy (δ, itself a derivative of the original scribe's γ exemplar), and thus no access to potentially better readings confined to αβ.

unhelpful, as they potentially are only setting off readings that were in the archetype at the head of transmission, passed without change indifferently to all hyparchtypes, and only showing variation because of innovations introduced in γ. They will not prove **A** a descendant of α. Moreover, across the whole text – and leaving aside the issue of correctness of readings – **AGS** agreements are distinctly recessive. Agreements of **A** with the majority of **CDL**, whether or not erroneous, occur more than twice as frequently as do those of **AGS**.

However, one should note that this is probably a false, if a sobering, dilemma. Joining **A** with either α or γ in fact undermines the very logic for presenting a stemma. It constructs a descent through two branches, each dependant upon a single hyparchetype. As has long been recognised, such a presentation of textual transmission, persistently mandated, offers no guidance to an editor. Any decisions about what underlies α and γ, the nature of the text preceding the extant copies, can be forthcoming only as the product of what any stemma seeks to exclude from editorial consideration, 'ratio', 'iudicium', or 'ingenium'. For, in all disputed passages, the bifid stemma is a statement that there are only two readings to choose between, and it is up to the editor – not to the transmissional evidence – to so choose. The editor must be guided either by 'usus scribendi' (the author's normal practice, which I will invoke with a heavy hand below) or, as is evident from my discussion of 1415 'proprium' above, by identification of the 'lectio difficilior', conjoined with a demonstration of the (hypothetical) generation from it of all other readings. Depressingly, the arguments underlying such decisions, whatever their intelligence, usually turn out to be reversible: e.g., is an apparent example of homeo-archy/-teleuthon indeed an accidental omission, or rather a clarifying insertion?[47]

But, ultimately, from a stemmatic point of view, placement of **A** with either α or γ will achieve exactly the same end results as identifying this copy with an independent line of transmission. The apparent resolution of the bifid dilemma, that three lines of descent will allow an automatic editorial decision on the basis of 'majority rule', is a fake. That is, in a bifid stemma, in a reading where **A** agrees with α, the stemma will mandate that reading as correct, even if it displays **A** to be a descendant of γ (and vice versa, were **A** to agree with γ, even if the stemma shows it as descending from α). In this stemmatic logic a single member of one family agreeing with the reading of the other family is construed to indicate that, whatever the majority reading

[47] I am simply restating here Joseph Bédier's 'loi suprenante', which led him to suggest that one simply provide as edition 'the best MS' (on what basis would one know?). See Timpanaro 79 on the antiquity of this perception (it predates Lachmann), as well as his frequently exemplary discussion at 157–87, and particularly his response to Michael Reeve at 207–15.

of the first family, the single manuscript must be transmitting a reading originally common to both branches (and that the majority of the first family innovates).[48] But these are exactly the same results as the stemma would direct were **A** to represent an independent line of descent. Presenting the descent as trifid obviates the difficulties traditionally associated with a two-branch stemma and shows agreement between **A** and either family as determining a correct reading. In this account, the only doubtful readings should occur when all three hyparchetypes offer different readings (a result that would be replicated in a two-branch stemma, wherever one decided to place **A**).[49] I will return to the helpfulness of these findings in a moment.

Provenance detail historicises the situation the stemma represents and may offer confirmation of Irish origin. Only one of the MSS is fully associable with the south (and with centres of learning), Fr Herebert's **A**.[50] The remaining copies, so far as traceable, are all Northern, **CD** from Durham Cathedral Priory. **G** is one of a group of nearly thirty books divided between Gray's Inn and Shrewsbury School in the early seventeenth century; all of them show signs of having passed through a single religious house, inferentially Chester Cathedral (St Werbergh's, Benedictines). As noted above, **L**, although its marked institutional ownership is continental, has added sermon notes, partly in English – and this of a distinctly Yorkshire stripe.[51] And **S**, although it had been produced in the south earlier (Chicksands [Beds., Gilbertines]), was subsequently in the Cistercian house of Kirkstall, suburban Leeds. The later copies, excepting **V**, have clear (and dispersed) provenances: **B** owned by an Oxford figure; **La** in a Dublin church *c.*1500; **R** produced at Ramsey (OSB, Hunts.), in part from Oxford exemplars.

The northern **CDL** offer one textual feature germane to Malachy's geographical transmission. At line 872 (Appendix 362–77) they share an addition, ostensibly designed to distinguish two sets of 'Scoti', the (Ulster) Irish and the Scots. The passage invokes a Scots myth of foundation that seems to have its roots in the history ascribed to the mythical 'Nennius'. This is suitably obscure material – except that this foundation-story was invoked by Scottish polemicists in the 1290s in order to counter Edward I's claim to the overlordship of Scotland. This feature certainly indicates that

---

[48] Cf. Timpanaro's discussion, 106–7, 109–12.

[49] Since, were **A** to descend from α, one could resolve its disagreement with **GS** only through 'ratio' (and only then determine which of α or γ were correct by that same means). And, by the same token, were **A** to descend from γ one could again determine the text only by two analogous exercises of 'ratio'.

[50] The trilingual **A** is more extensively Anglo-Norman than Latin. One might note particularly Nicole de Bozon's rhymed sermons; he will have been among Herebert's Oxford Franciscan colleagues.

[51] See Pickering and Airaksinen 16–17.

within two decades of composition Malachy's text was subject to intrusions. Yet, equally, this implies that either γ or a predecessor had passed through a locale at least Scot-sympathetic; the reference to *Ultonia* 'Ulster' might imply transmission through what formed a transoceanic community, particularly embracing the Lordship of the Isles and the Glens of Antrim. The only likely Franciscan connection would be through the house in Dumfries, on the edge of the lordship of Galloway (site of the Bruce's murder of John Comyn, 1306).[52] However, as the Durham Benedictine provenance of C and D would imply, this version of the text early escaped any specifically ordinal transmission.

G points to a differing route of direct exportation. Chester was a normal port of embarkation for adventurers in Ireland, and there is plenty of information pointing to cross-channel exchanges between northern England and Hibernia. Much of this comes from vernacular texts that moved from Northern locales to Ireland (e.g. the English verses embedded in the Bridlington monk Pierre Langtoft's chronicle in Cambridge University Library, MS Gg.1.1).[53] But obviously the trade might well have gone either way, and brought codices produced in Ireland to Great Britain.

There is a certain amount of passing evidence that the original exemplar of all copies was indeed Irish and that it has left sporadic marks on the surviving MSS. Perhaps unusually in the copying of British Latin, D regularly follows an old-fashioned system of word-division in which frequently prepositions are not separate from their objects, but prefixes are from their roots. I am grateful to Richard Sharpe for his suggestion that I examine Bodleian Library, MSS Laud misc. 460 (s. xii/xiii, from Armagh) and Rawlinson B.485 (s. xv, Irish). Neither has word-division between prepositions and their following objects; in the former, neither the Tironian nota 'et' nor 'non' is separated from what follows either. This seems to be an Irish convention – classical Irish does not separate prepositions from their objects – sometimes reproduced, yet occasionally capable of tripping up English scribes.[54]

However, having a model for textual descent does not get a student of Malachy's text out of the woods: far from it. One rather quickly discovers that the procedures normally mandated by a stemma are of limited value. Even in the presence of three lines of descent, the possibility that a substantial number of variants might be resoluble proves the proverbial 'forlorn hope'. A relatively brief yet heavily contested sample passage (lines 252–76) will demonstrate the difficulties:

---

[52] See Hanna 2005, 89–95 and nn.; and, for connections between Irish Franciscans and Scots independence, Gallagher.

[53] For further discussion and references, see *Patient* 175 and esp. 175–76 n. 32.

[54] See further the textual note to line 22.

Superbie uirus intumescit ex professionis (1) **sublimitate**, et hoc est pessimum uenenum, superbire scilicet de statu sublimi, quando (2) **uota et uita** + repugnant. Hoc uenenum est falsorum religiosorum qui comparantur salamandre, que est secundum Isidorum, libro 12, bestiola uenenosa uiuens in solo igne; ignis tamen incendia non tantum non (3) **adurit**, immo extinguit. Sic mali (4) **religiosi** in medio sunt ignis gratie, sicut de principe eorum dicitur Ezechielis 28, 'In medio lapidum ignitorum ambulasti'. Regnat tamen in eis uenenum malitie que extinguit omnem effectum gratie, non tantum in se per malam uitam, sed in aliis per malam doctrinam. Sicut dicit Plinius de ista bestiola, libro 4, quod nunquam apparet extra furnum, nisi cum pluit. Cuius tactus est frigidus ut glacies ita ut ignem extinguat, et de ore eius (5) **lacteam** saniem euomit, ex cuius contactu calorem corporis inficit. Hec ibi. Sic falsus religiosus apparet ad pluuiam carnalitatis et extinguit in aliis (6) **per prauum exemplum** donum gratie. Pretendit lacteam, et uenenosam saniem doctrine que postmodum auditores exemplo praue uite magis inficit quam conuertit. Sed quam nociuum est istud uenenum patet per Isidorum, ubi supra; qui dicit quod uenenum aliorum serpentum singulos inficit, salamandra multos simul interimit (7) **que si ita** irrepserit arbori, poma eius inficit et comedentes omnes interimit. Si in puteum cadat, omnes potantes inficit. Sic predicator (8) **prauus** secundum Anselmum, *Libro de similitudinibus*, quod more medici bene (9) **instruit**, sed ipse herbam uenenatam assumit et se et alios postmodum (10) **inficit**.

In these twenty-odd lines of text ten significant variations occur. I here present the variation through an abbreviated table. The full variation is available in the *corpus lectionum* accompanying the text below, and the logic by which I have determined rectitude of readings is discussed in the textual notes, for this passage more detailed than usual.

	Correct	In error
1	γ	αβ
2	α/β	γ [uota α, uoto β]
3	L	GβCD/S
4	αβ	γ
5	α	βγ
6	αβ	γ
7	αβ	γ
8	αβ	γ
9	αD	CL/β [D a correction, originally as CL?]
10	αβCL	D

In addition to these readings, the passage contains further variations, all limited in attestation and all pretty certainly wrong; these appear in A 3×, D 3×, G 5×, and S 5×. These are noteworthy because they offer evidence as to how much trust one might repose in individual copyists. As these are individual efforts, they indicate the degree to which individuals might feel free not to represent what they had before them in exemplars – and thus, the degree of trust to be extended to their isolated efforts. One might note that among the 'significant variations' I cite, D and A/β again offer individual efforts, D in 9 (where it does not preserve γ), and 10; A in 2 and 9.

In a general way, the stemma appears 'useful'. That is, in these major readings, genetic lines of descent are typically respected (and they equally indicate the erroneous quality of the sixteen further isolated readings mentioned above).[55] However, the value of this trifid descent for producing an authorial version (what Malachy wrote) might be described as 'compromised'. In only six of the ten major readings (all examples of αβ agreement, or alternatively isolated error in γ) does the stemma actually mandate the authorial text. On four occasions (1, 3, 5, and 9) Malachy's text is attested by a reading the use of the stemma would mandate as secondary. Moreover, correct readings appear in places that would appear inherently unlikely: L errs in eight of the major readings, but uniquely preserves something approximating Malachy in 4; D also errs in eight examples – and has additional unique errors – but emends its original reading to a correct one in 9. One cherished goal of stemmatic editing, the 'eliminatio lectionum singulorum', is here utterly impossible. As a consequence, there is no way to edit the text, except to address every variant on its own merits.

Thus, one is persistently faced with what I have come to consider 'mixed blessings'. As the following brief example (lines 1330–35) will indicate, one routinely discovers that the MSS, in short compass, are equally prone to offer readings compelling – and disastrous. At this point, my edited text reads:

Generale enim remedium contra uenenum in cibis sumptum est uomitus; sic uenenum spirituale, detestatum per contricionem, uomitur per confessionem. Gregorius, de ulceribus Lazari, 'Quid est', inquit, 'peccatorum confessio, nisi quedam uulnerum ruptio? Quia peccati uirus salubriter aperitur in confessione quod pestifere latebat in mente'.

[55] The only exception is that, through the second half of the text, there is persistently sporadic evidence, variations joining CDGL, that G was consulting simultaneously both his usual exemplar and a copy derived from γ.

Malachy here cites Gregory, *Homiliae in evangelia* 2.40 (*PL* 76:1302, on Luke 16:20–21):

> Quid est ergo peccatorum confessio, nisi quaedam vulnerum ruptio? Quia peccati virus salubriter aperitur in confessione, quod pestifere latebat in mente.

The associated variant corpus includes:

> 1–2 Generale … confessionem] *om.* A, an eye-skip, following the use of *confessionem* at the end of the preceding sentence 1 uenenum] *adds* gule S 2 detestatum per contriccionem] *om.* GSp (detestatum *corr. from* -tant C, *from* -tatur D) 3 ulceribus] uulneribus G 4 peccatorum] *om.* ACD, peccatoris p uulnerum] ulcerum p 5 uirus] uulnus L

In the second line I have, unusually, taken the γ reading, not as this family's frequent fastidious clarification, but an authorial statement predicated upon the chiastic phrasing of the preceding sentence, 'peccati uomitus et detestacio, scilicet per contricionem et confessionem'. This interpretation both answers (and, in its turn, mandates as 'fact') a view that α + p have omitted the phrase through a skip between two examples of phrases ending *-ionem*. (The absence of the phrase in A is completely independent, a product of that scribe's having already skipped a larger portion of the text – but with an analogous stimulus.) In line 4, *uulnerum* is confirmed by the Gregorian source; here p has been attracted to the earlier use of *ulcer-*. Yet, in the next member, Gregory confirms p (and most others) in reading *uirus*, and L, which appears the most accurate copy throughout this selection, here errs, attracted to the earlier use of *uulnus* – accidentally echoing G, also attracted to *uulnus*, but, in this case, for earlier *ulcer·*. In addition, Gregory also confirms αL's plural *peccatorum*. The word is absent in δ (=CD), which had earlier correctly provided the phrase skipped in α + p. This word does not appear in A/β either, which, at least at this moment, might appear the least trustworthy of all the copies (although, over the full text, its readings are generally more reliable than those provided by α).

   Given that so much of Malachy's text is citation, there is a check on this impasse, as the preceding paragraph suggests. Quite simply, the guarantor of many conflicted readings is provided by Malachy's sources. The logic underlying citation in a work like this is what it has always been (and remains for us): that citations are rendered authoritative and readily repeatable by virtue of their *ipsissima verba*; one should expect Malachy to have provided the most accurate renditions he could. Thus, wherever possible, I have judged the variants against the readings of the originals, always bearing in mind the possibility that Malachy might have been looking at a copy scribally disfigured.[56] But the reader should understand that this is an edition predicated largely upon 'ingenium', a hypothesis, rather than an authoritative demonstration.

Split transmission or interpolation?

Editorial reliance upon 'ingenium' is particularly necessary because, as some statements above will have implied, determining local readings is scarcely the sole problem in constructing a text of *De ueneno*. The difficulty turns out to be quite other, a variousness that brings into question whether there is a single text here. It is no exaggeration to say that *every witness of De ueneno* has different textual dimensions. The readiest quick demonstration is to point out that the text extends to around 1,390 typescript lines in my initial transcription from the 1518 print, but to only around 1,170 in a comparable transcription from A. Somewhere along the line, the text has either been substantially augmented or substantially reduced, by about 20 per cent.

This is not just a case of what I have elsewhere described as 'the insouciance of Latin scribal traditions', but should be seen as reflecting the compilational nature of *De ueneno*. Malachy's book has actively engaged its users; after all, most of the copies I have used here represent collections of *praedicabilia*. Malachy's intended audience of preachers has sought to increase the usefulness of their copies either by inserting, as they have variously deemed appropriate, material germane to the discussion of virtues and vices, or by deleting materials in which they had minimal interest.[57]

With the exception of β/A, all versions of the text, representatives of α and γ, appear to be copies supplemented to some degree. Intrusions into the latter, excepting the Scottish example I have already mentioned, are rather restrained in size, but utterly persistent across the text – the supply of qualifying connectives (frequently introduced by 'scilicet') absent from α, and frequently vacuous or repetitive. A few of these are reasonably

---

[56]   I cite my patristic texts from *PL*, rather than meticulously edited editions such as *Corpus Scriptorum Ecclesiasticorum Latinorum* or *Corpus Christianorum*. Migne's texts are derived, sometimes at a remove, from incunables; these were, for compositorial ease, set from contemporary, i.e. late medieval, copies (the *recentiores* rejected by modern editors). Thus, Migne more closely reflects what Malachy will have had to hand than do modern scholarly texts. (An example: Migne's Jerome mainly reprints Domenico Vallarsi's mid-eighteenth-century edition. But Vallarsi was himself only offering a reprint – from some descendant of the first book printed in Rome [1469], itself reproducing a surviving Florentine manuscript of s. xv in.)

[57]   Cf. Lutz's comments on the '"living" text', *Remigii* 50.

extensive, a sentence or so (for example, a reference to John the Revelator at line 75 or to Becket at 215), but scarcely so, in comparison to what one finds in the α manuscripts.

Before turning to some specific examples of α's expansiveness, I would offer a further observation. Generally, textual editing proceeds on the assumption that authors are beings distinctly better endowed than those who transmit their works. This is the principle underlying the ancient rule 'Lectio durior potior est', implicitly a statement that scribal transmission is predicated on misunderstanding and simplification. But, in the case of Malachy's *De ueneno*, such a distinction (and division of labour) cannot be sustained. As the early manuscripts show, the scribes who transmitted this work – in many cases they will have been owners/users like Herebert, intending to mine the text for the practical homiletic aims for which Malachy had constructed it – were trained similarly to Malachy. His early audience, inferentially his Franciscan brethren, shared a common ordinal education, one that encouraged their access to the same texts Malachy had used. Moreover, they appear to have viewed his work pragmatically, as a portable *vade mecum* for ready consultation on any topic related to vices and virtues (Malachy's spiritual analogues to poisons and their antidotes). Consequently, they took steps to render their slim quires of *De ueneno* texts that would be more useful in their professions. Indeed, I would suspect that a number of them may have been more adept seminarians than was Malachy himself.

One can easily demonstrate the point from one example early in the text, in the books I have surveyed, a presentation unique to B. This MS is a *recentior*, from a point advanced in the transmission, and, particularly given its text generally, the reading represents an individual intrusion. At the conclusion of the opening chapter (line 49), B adds:

> Because my tract gathers examples of poisonous snakes according to the differences between them, one should know that Isidore says, in *Etymologies* 12.4, that there are as many poisons as there are kinds of snake, as many destructive behaviours as there are species, as many injuries as there are colours – and I will align these with the poisons associated with the various sins.[58]

On the one hand, this passage shows a tendency that appears across a variety of manuscripts in similar situations. Malachy's *On poison* is legitimately

---

[58] 'Et quia tractatus noster sumit exempla de serpentibus uenenosis secundum eorum differentias, sciendum est secundum Ysidorum, *Ethimologiarum* 12 libro, capitulo 4, quod tot sunt uenena quot genera, tot pernicies quot species, tot dolores quot colores, quibus adaptabimus uenena peccatorum diuersorum'.

'compilational', a gathering of quotations from others, with interstitial materials largely provided by Malachy's suggested moralisations of scientific material (before he returns to yet another moralisable nugget from Pliny or Aristotle). The text is rather formless and, on many occasions, users with a stronger sense of the literary than Malachy have sought to build in conclusive statements at chapter ends. (The signal example is the final sentence, attested only in V and the 1518 print.) This addition, in other words, displays a sense of literary sophistication stronger than that of the original 'author'.

But, more soberingly, this B passage sounds very much like something Malachy should have written. It relies on the same ultimate source he (along with all medieval literates) knows is the first port of call for anyone seeking 'the nature of things', Isidore of Seville's *Etymologies*. Moreover, the language here is, at least possibly, not Isidore's at all, but that of the source I have already indicated that Malachy used again and again, BA (cf. BA 1125/7–10). Here only belatedness and transmissional isolation would indicate that this passage indeed represents 'insertion', not text. However, the passage indicates an ongoing quandary: separating Malachy himself from his mirroring users, some, like Herebert, a great deal more learned than he, is a chancy procedure.

From a very early point, the α transmission is marked by isolated blocks of extra materials like this one, some very extensive indeed. They are regularly present in S and often (sometimes only incipiently) in G. My selective examination of four late fourteenth-century copies suggests that at least some materials included in the 1518 print were alive (and developing further offshoots) from this relatively early date, and thence features integral to the later transmission.

A revelatory example of such behaviour appears following line 302 (Appendix lines 5–20). This passage will indicate the layering, the successive provision of unique materials, that typifies the α tradition (and many later manuscripts). At this point, the end of a discussion attacking false judges and their diabolical worldly knowledge, five of the ten MSS I have surveyed (α+LaRV), as well as the 1518 print, include (as copies frequently do elsewhere) a conclusive summarising sentence:

> Non infletur ergo iudex falsus siue aduocatus malus, si sit ut serpens callidus, quia nullam ueram sapientiam habet.

The statement is not only conclusive but echoes the opening of the paragraph and thus rounds off the argument. Although Malachy's discussion explicitly addresses only false judges, the head of the discussion (line 292) is introduced by a reference to 'falsi iudices *et garruli aduocati*'. The concluding statement reinforces what is not clearly present in the discussion: that what one might say about bad judges would be equally true of lawyers.

However, the summary sentence at line 302 was not quite enough for some scribe within the early α tradition. Three of the witnesses, S, R, and the 1518 print, offer further materials here (see the Appendix). Apparently the doubled reference to lawyers suggested that they should receive treatment analogous to that extended to judges. S *et al.* 'remedy the deficiency' by offering *after* the concluding sentence discussed above a developed paragraph on voluble lawyers.[59]

Yet this addition still was not enough for someone in the tradition underlying S, although not that underlying R and the print. The 'garruli aduocati' material common to all three MSS offers a *similitudo* or *figura*, a moralisable titbit suitable for a provocative point in a sermon. Lawyers' tongues are like a balance beam (a pun, also a *lingua*), capable of swinging one way or the other, depending on the money placed in the balance's pan. One good figure may easily generate another, and thus S provides a further example, not altogether consonant with what has preceded, to demonstrate the wastefulness of litigiousness. This final extension was either unique to an isolated branch of the α tradition or, if not, suppressed in the production of R and the print. For the moment, I will simply observe that none of this material, however potentially edifying and diverting it may be, has anything much to do with Malachy's poison or his snakes.

In this context, the state of affairs in B is telling. This MS is especially prone to provide extra materials, for, not only does this textual rendition include a variety of extensive materials reproduced in the 1518 print, it has been swollen by a number of *figurae/similitudines* the scribe-owner found germane instances to have at hand in a vices and virtues context. Moreover, there is evidence, perhaps a bit tenuous, that these additive behaviours were being carried on in the act of copying the instant MS. In the main, these intrusions offer similitudinous readings, moralised biblical narratives (e.g. Haman, following 119 'uenenum', or Ahab following 132 'permittit'). But far from all are so predicated (and a few extend for so long as a full folio); for example, following 156 *Pastorali*, the MS expatiates at length on one 'natural inequality':

> Consequently, a man should remain in his proper station, and a woman in hers, nor should either of them, through pride, take up the station appropriate to the other. But this happened once with queen Semiramis; after the death of her husband, Bil', the king of Babylon, in order to rule longer, she married her own son Ninus and had a son by him. But since she and her husband-son

---

[59] S's readings are scribally deviant from the other copies, even including a unique bit of Anglo-Norman, and had been received in his exemplar, not innovated in his copying.

looked very alike, she forced him to remain in a private room, as if he were the queen, and she herself rode about with the Babylonian magnates, as if she were the king. Down to that time, people had not worn trousers, but she made herself a pair, so that, when she mounted her horse, she would not be judged to have a woman's figure. She also thought to herself, 'If my men should now pay attention and see me wearing trousers around my loins, which they do not wear, they will suspect me'. And having considered the plan, she commanded that everyone in the kingdom should wear trousers. And thus, as one reads in *The ecclesiastical history*, she invented wearing trousers. But, because it says in Deuteronomy (cf. 22:5), 'It is an abomination before God that a man should wear a woman's clothing, and vice versa', God roused an evil spirit against her, for her son-husband, who had remained closeted up in the palace as if he were the queen, rebelled against his mother and killed her. See what a vengeance follows upon prideful self-glorification![60]

These intrusions are limited to B, but isolated unique examples occur in La as well. One such, following line 196 'species reguli', begins:

For this reason, Virgil says, 'Every *cerastes* covers its body to deceive birds; it only bares its body to seize a wretched fowl'. This snake also indicates lechery, for women solicit youths through the

[60] '... vt homo, scilicet staret in gradu suo et mulier in suo, ne scilicet neuter eorum ambiret per superbiam statum alterius. Sicut fuit de quadam regina nomine Semirande que post mortem mariti sui, scilicet Bil' regis Babilonis, ut posset diucius regnare, nupsit proprio filio suo \Nino et ex eo habuit filium/. Set quia similum (?) erant mater et maritus, fecit filium in camera remanere tanquam reginam, et ipsamet (?) equitauit cum proceribus terre \tanquam/ rex esset. \Set/ quia tunc temporis adhuc non erat usus bra<ct>arum, ipsa uero fecit sibi bractas, ne ascendendo equum perpenderetur figura mulieris. Item cogitauit inter se, dicens, "Si homines de regno modo aduertant et uideant me habere bractas circa lumbos, quibus ipsi non utuntur, habebunt me suspectam"; et ex cogitato concilio, indixit toti regno quod uterentur bractis, et sic inuentus fuit usus bractarum, ut legitur in *Historia ecclesiastica*. Sed quia scribitur in Deuteronomii, "Abhominabile est apud Deum ut uir utatur ueste feminea, et e conuerso", suscitauit Deus spiritum malum aduersus eam. Nam filius eius qui et maritus, qui domi sic remansit incameratus tanquam regina, surrexit contra matrem suam et interfecit eam. Ecce qualis uindicta ex superba elacione'! I do not find B's reference; Orosius, *Historiae* 1.4 (*PL* 31:699–700), offers a scathing account of Semiramis's reign (as Ninus's *widow*) as a time of licence, but does not mention her alleged sartorial inventiveness.

horns on their heads and other hair-dos. (about 40 per cent of the
full insertion)[61]

Here one might notice that telling 'eciam'/'also'. The subject here is pride,
and particularly hypocrisy, but the 'horns' of the snake *cerastes* remind
this scribe of a completely alien (yet widely rebuked) kind of 'horns', those
in women's hair-dos. As his 'eciam' indicates, even while providing the
material La is aware that this discussion more properly belongs somewhere
else in Malachy's text (for example, at lines 1416–19).

I am inclined to take all such material, generally of isolated attestation
and resembling the examples in B and La, to be practitioner-added supple-
mentation of Malachy's original text. The clearly personalised presentation
in B is telling in this regard, for this copy often offers signs of overt
interpolation. For example, the scribe frequently acknowledges (perhaps
representing inadvertent homeoarchy?) that he is inserting material; he
often repeats Malachy's readings from the point where he began inserting
his unique extra materials at their conclusion, as in examples following
132 'permittit' or 176 'prolem'. Again, following 219 'dentes illos', amid a
paragraph in which he contrasts Josephus's report of endemic Roman
bribery with the injunctions of Ps 1, he inscribes a signal that he is aware
that the discussion has gone off-track, 'Set redeamus ad propositum de
serpente ceraste ...' (But let us return to the point, which was about the
snake *cerastes*).

Similarly, a variety of shorter material, variously attested, is marked as
having been incorporated from marginal notations. For example, at line 104
(Appendix 1–4) La precedes a widely attested concluding trio of sentences
(both α copies, all four *recentiores*, and the print) with: 'Insere hic contra
nolentes audire uerbum <Dei?> et odientes predicatores' (Here insert this
statement against those who don't wish to hear the word of God and who
hate preachers).[62] Similarly, at line 73, a reading that appears in the text
in γ occurs marginally in B (and appears in the text in some later copies I
have scanned). Or, at line 215, L includes a reference to Becket in the text;

---

[61] 'Unde Uirgilius, "Decepturus aues corpus tegit omnis cerastes; corpus
denudat miserum uolatile raptat". Per hunc serpentem significatur eciam luxuria,
que crinibus et cornubus in capitibus mulierum adolescentes solicitat ...'. The
leonine hexameters are, of course, certainly not Virgil, but see James 1913, at
293, lines 61–62. James knew the poem, which draws its snake-lore from Lucan's
famous description, *De bello civili* 9.700–838 (cf. BA 1129/24–25, 1135/22–23),
from five MSS; Walther adds five further copies at nos 8095 and 18131.

[62] The form of this note implies that a scribe in the tradition underlying La
was comparing two different versions of the text, one without this material, and
marking his copy so as not to overlook it.

comparable material appears as a marginal note in the heavily corrected C, but is absent altogether in D.

I have surveyed my selected *recentiores*, and I am afraid that they offer no guidance on how to proceed here. They serve only to identify passages intruded in early stages of the transmission and subsequently in the text available to Étienne for his print. In their varying provision of materials originally limited to α or to γ, they also indicate that the tradition had become hopelessly conflated. That is, every MS I have examined includes at least one bit from both traditions. Apparently scribes recognised that the text was of variable dimensions, consulted multiple copies for a sense of its contents, and took from these materials that seemed useful to them. It should go without saying that, on the basis of this showing, these books' local readings should probably be ignored as secondary.[63]

Here one can speak only of tendencies. In light of the previous discussion it will occasion no surprise to find that B is the most indifferently acquisitive of all the copies I have examined. This MS includes in some form virtually all the extensive α materials, as well as having (marginally – R is nearly equally so profuse) more distinctive γ material than other copies. The other MSS surveyed are much more restrained; they typically convey, on no very predictable basis, perhaps 50–60 per cent of the distinctive α material and relatively few of those readings early limited to γ. One should draw attention here to V, which has a relatively small γ component, but is unique, among all copies I have surveyed, in including one large γ insertion (at line 876, Appendix 379–91). Instructively, this describes Hiberno-English settlers as 'poisonous' (and thus addresses a Malachian topic). But, equally instructively, V's text is scribally advanced from that in early γ MSS, and the scribe has either overlooked or chosen not to integrate in his copy the equally extensive γ intrusion that immediately precedes (at line 872, Appendix 362–78).

Although one can identify a number of these extra bits as entering the English α tradition from a very early date, these do not form the bulk of the massive additions that have swollen the 1518 print out of any recognisable shape. On occasion, this activity is explicit; for example, a large intrusion follows line 541 (Appendix 21–112) in S, B, and the print. Roughly corresponding to a point at which the interpolation ends in the MSS, the print includes what must have originally been an editorial note to the compositor, 'Sequitur aliqua addicio' ('a further addition follows', Appendix 91). Or again, the discussion following line 556 (Appendix 113–29) has certainly been interpolated, as it interrupts a numbered argument,

[63] A single example, from a book I have examined only cursorily, Cambridge, Queens' College, MS 10 (of the 1360s, perhaps Oxford Franciscans): for variant 5 in the passage analysed above, it offers 'lactaneum sanguinem'.

Malachy organising his discussion through the five Gregorian parts of wrath. The passage is comprised entirely of biblical citation with connective tissue.

Here I think we have another case of compilation as the gift that goes on giving. In preparing the 1518 print, Étienne inserted his own handbook material from searches in pre-existing compilations. I would read his presentation as a final echo of earlier textual intrusions. The print continues ongoing behaviours evident in *De ueneno* from its initial composition: Malachy constructing his original text from compilations, a number of his earlier readers/transmitters providing further, perhaps marginally germane, materials from similar sources.

Here the question of the germane is telegraphed by Étienne's reliance on biblical citation. An easy demonstration of the foreignness of these add-ons appears in the print's extra paragraph at the end of chapter about patience, the tonic for wrath, after line 680 (Appendix 244–56). This differs rhetorically from Malachy's usual mien, his 'usus scribendi'. Rather than piling up strings of allegedly authoritative citations, the author typically offers carefully chosen proof-texts that 'clinch' a preceding argument predicated on moralised natural history. Implicitly, *De ueneno* was to appeal by organising underutilised poison/theriac material and by bringing this into contact with authoritative biblical texts, far from all of them obvious analogues. Like all such efforts, its appeal was to be its novelty, the new information it might show as relevant to the discouragement of vice and the exercise of virtue. In contrast, Étienne's offerings here are utterly pedestrian. The citations are scarcely recondite or surprising; they are, rather, the utterly ubiquitous commonplaces that a competent Franciscan preacher could probably pull up from memory – and that a less adept one could have found in any preacher's notebook under 'paciencia'.[64]

So far as my researches allow conclusions, Étienne's primary source for this intruded material appears to have been the master-work in the field, no less than Peraldus's *Summa*. A few examples I have identified include:

As I have indicated, the material following line 556 in 1518 is clearly interpolated, as it interrupts a numbered argument, Malachy running through the five Gregorian parts of wrath. The passage is comprised entirely of biblical citation with connective tissue. The same citations, although in a different order and with different connectives, appear at *Summa de vitiis* 8.1 (sig. R vj$^{ra–va}$).

The last portion of the addition following line 630 (from Appendix 148) cites seven biblical passages or authorities (the Hugh of St-Victor here) paralleled at *Summa de vitiis* 8.2 (sig. R vj^{va}–vij^{rb}).

---

[64] For an introduction to the commonplaces see *Patient* 271, 297–300, with further references.

The full paragraph introducing a substantial intrusion in the print in the addition following line 713 (Appendix 258–65) reproduces, in condensed form, the discussion at *Summa de vitiis* 5.2 (sig. H viij^rab).

Material unique to 1518 may easily be rejected as offering evidence only for Étienne's desire to bloat his text, perhaps with an eye to what would make up a volume of saleable dimensions. As I have indicated, the material stands out as intrusive, and frequently commonplace. None of it resembles what appears Malachy's 'usus scribendi' as attested elsewhere (and not even in B's individualistic narrativised materials that frequently appear mixed with materials also included in the 1518 print).

However, particularly given my demonstration above, materials in early MSS represent a provocative and troubling case. As I have shown, stemmatic isolation is valueless in determining whether a reading is authorial. Thus, particularly in the case of extensive materials attested only in α, sometimes in S alone, one is persistently faced with the issue of the extent of the text. Have these been intruded by α, or one or another scribe in that tradition? Or is their absence from γ (and usually β) a mark of editorial abbreviation – usually the passages offer no signal that they have been omitted through skips of like to like? Similarly, although here the extra material is limited to phrasal insertions, has γ (and often β) introduced clarifications, or has α suppressed some often fussy material that was nonetheless Malachy's own?

Given that attestation (and even minority attestation) is valueless in this context, one must clearly consider each example on a case-by-case basis. As I have already argued, this can proceed on only two grounds – 'ratio' or a sense of authorial 'usus scribendi'. An example of the first would be my logic for excluding the γ reading 'quoad corpus', variant 4 in the passage analysed above: I quite simply can find nothing sensible in a statement that priests 'stand *bodily* in the fire of grace' (although Richard Rolle might disagree). At the same time, given Malachy's insistence upon his offering material/physical referents for spiritual states, I can understand why one might wish to insist on the point, given the clerical moral corruption described here. However, as the text, in all its copies, says, ordination should have conferred grace;[65] and, indeed, as the passage develops, it is the material, bodily behaviour of bad priests that shows their indifference to this spiritual presence. A number of my textual notes will argue out analyses of this sort.

But, more generally, with respect to the more extensive readings, particularly those of α, I invoke 'usus scribendi' (perhaps like a meat-cleaver). My reading of the text finds Malachy's argumentative mode generally

---

[65] The 'uota/o' that the priests have forgotten – and that in variant 2, γ has converted into the bathetic and over-emphatic 'tota' (rejecting this variant on these grounds is another example of the exercise of 'ratio').

consistent. He relies, reasonably exclusively, upon moralised *naturalia*, illustrative of poison or its antidotes. This exemplary material is customarily accompanied by either a proof-text and/or an authoritative citation offering an explanation for the appended moral. Other modes of presentation are simply alien to this repeated core, and I identify them as non-authorial and consign them to a textual appendix. Even though some α additions include a certain amount of moralised *naturalia* (e.g. the mole at Appendix line 53 or the hedgehog at lines 150–58), I find such echoes of Malachy's procedures echoic only. This is a text about poisons and their antidotes, not just animals arbitrarily.[66]

The presentation here

The following edition presents, with the exclusion of the variants noted above, a full report of the textual transmission, as revealed in seven central copies, the early MSS and the 1518 print (p), together with a facing-page translation. As I have argued, substantial portions of the text communicated by these witnesses represent interpolation; material that I judge to represent such user-behaviour I have removed from the text. Shorter examples, up to two or three sentences, appear in the collations beneath the text, there typically headed in bold-face and the rejected reading set off as an insert paragraph. Longer interpolations, with their facing-page translations, appear in an Appendix following the primary edited text; their presence is signalled in the text itself by paraphs (₡). The Appendix also records the presence of materials early interpolated in the four secondary copies I have examined. I thus include all analogues from BLaRV, but not, for example, any further taste of B's individual insertions.

The edition has the form of a copy-text version of what, in my view, Malachy originally wrote, a hypothetical reconstruction. Were one to choose a copy-text from among the MSS, the most logical choice would be to present A. It is free from most of the materials I identify as interpolated, and in some sense is the most 'neutral' copy. It is also the one firmly datable copy, written before 1333 and produced by or for a Franciscan conversant with locales associated with Malachy ascriptions (Paris and Oxford), and within the kind of book for which Malachy imagined his text.

In spite of these benefits, I have chosen instead to present a corrected version of the *textus receptus*, Étienne's print. There are two reasons for this. First, leaving aside excision of non-authorial material, p does not require much more emendation than presenting A would have done. Second, given

---

[66] Although one can adduce marginal cases, e.g. the serpent *prester* in Appendix lines 137–40.

the hypothetical nature of my text, this decision allows me to present in a single format the entirety of p, so that readers can see (and probably disagree with) what I have excised from my hypothetical authorial text. The reader should recall the transcription rules from n.9 above. In my collations, I use the bar '|' to indicate a reading at or split at the line-end (a notorious spot for variation).

While in my edition below I follow my copy-text, with its frequently erroneous references, all biblical passages are identified in the facing-page translation, the books indicated by the abbreviations used in the Stuttgart Vulgate. (With the exception of biblical passages, where I follow the Douai-Rheims version, all translations are my own.) The edition and translation are supplemented by three further forms of annotation. First comes a conventional series of notes on textual matters, explanations of my editorial choices. As the length of the collation shows, an editor is persistently faced with decisions, and this account is extremely selective. The textual notes are followed by a consecutive account of the 'fontes', an outline of the sources of Malachy's extensive references, mainly, of course, ones to BA. Finally, I provide three comprehensive indexes, including the materials I present in the Appendix, as well as my hypothetical authorial text: first, of biblical passages cited, in the order of the Vulgate; second, ignoring BA, laid under contribution persistently, of other authors cited, alphabetically ordered; finally, an alphabetical list of Malachy's *similitudines*.

Bibliography

(With the exception of BA, editions of Malachy's sources are identified in that index.)

Albertus Magnus, *De animalibus libri xxvi ...*, ed. Hermann Stadler, Beiträge zur Geschichte der Philosophie des Mittelalters 15–16, 2 vols (Münster i. W., 1916–20).

Bale, John, *Index Britanniae Scriptorum: John Bale's Index of British and Other Writers*, ed. Reginald L. Poole and Mary Bateson, with introduction by Caroline Brett and James Carley (Woodbridge, 1990).

—, *Scriptorum Illustrium Maioris Brytanniae ... Catalogus*, 2 vols (Basel, 1557–59).

Bédier, Joseph, *La Tradition manuscrite du Lai de l'ombre: réflexions sur l'art d'éditer les anciens textes* (Paris, 1929; repr. 1970).

Bloomfield, Morton W., *The Seven Deadly Sins: An Introduction to the History of a Religious Concept ...* ([East Lansing, MI], 1952).

—, et al., *Incipits of Latin Works on the Virtues and Vices, 1100–1500 A.D ...* (Cambridge, MA, 1979).

The British Library Catalogue of Additions to the Manuscripts 1946–1950, 3 vols (London, 1979).

Charland, Th.-M., *Artes praedicandi: Contribution à l'histoire de la rhétorique au moyen âge* (Paris and Montreal, 1936).

Cotter, Francis J., ed. Roberta A. McKelvie, *The Friars Minor in Ireland from their Arrival to 1400* (St Bonaventure, NY, 1994).

Esposito, M., 'Friar Malachy of Ireland', *English Historical Review* 33 (1918), 359–66.

—, 'Notes on Latin Learning and Literature in Medieval Ireland – III', *Hermathena* [Trinity College, Dublin] 48 (1933), 221–49.

Fitzmaurice, E. B., and A. G. Little, eds, *Materials for the History of the Franciscan Province of Ireland, A.D. 1230–1450* (Manchester, 1920).

Gallagher, Niav, 'The Franciscans and the Scottish Wars of Independence: An Irish Perspective', *Journal of Medieval History* 32 (2006), 3–17.

Grosseteste, Robert, *Templum Dei*, ed. Joseph A. Goering and F. A. C. Mantello, Toronto Medieval Latin Texts 14 (Toronto, 1984).

Hanna, Ralph, '"Classicizing Friars", Miscellaneous Transmission, and MS
    Royal 7 C.i', *Journal of the Early Book Society* 19 (2016), 97–123.
—, 'The Descent of Some Chester Libraries', forthcoming in *The Library*.
—, *London Literature, 1300–1380* (Cambridge, 2005).
—, '"Put the Load Right on Me": Langland on the Incarnation (with
    apologies to The Band)', *Notes and Queries* ns 66 (2019), 197–201.
—, 'The Wisdom of Poetry: John of Wales's Defense', *Journal of Medieval
    Latin* 27 (2017), 303–26.
Horwood, Alfred, *A Catalogue of the Ancient Manuscripts Belonging to the
    Honourable Society of Gray's Inn* (London, 1869), online at https://www.
    graysinn.org.uk/library/medieval-manuscripts.
Hunt, R. W., *et al.*, *A Summary Catalogue of Western Manuscripts in the
    Bodleian Library at Oxford*, 7 vols in 8 (Oxford, 1895–1953).
James, Montague R., *A Descriptive Catalogue of the Manuscripts in the
    Library of Sidney Sussex College, Cambridge* (Cambridge, 1895).
—, 'Ovidius De Mirabilibus Mundi', in *Essays and Studies Presented to
    William Ridgeway* ... (Cambridge, 1913), 286–98.
—, and Claude Jenkins, *A Descriptive Catalogue of the Manuscripts in
    the Library of Lambeth Palace*, 2 vols (originally 5 fascicles; London,
    1930–32).
John of Wales/Waleys, *Communiloquium siue summa collationum*
    (Strasbourg, 25 May 1489; rep. The Phoenix Series 1, East Ardsley, 1964).
Langland, William, *Piers Plowman: The B Version*, ed. George Kane and
    E. Talbot Donaldson (London, 1975).
—, *Piers Plowman: The C Version*, ed. George Kane and George Russell
    (London and Berkeley, 1997).
McCann, Daniel, *Soul-Health: Therapeutic Reading in Later Medieval
    England* (Cardiff, 2018).
Moreton, C. E., 'The "Library" of a Late-Fifteenth-Century Lawyer', *The
    Library* 6 ser. 13 (1991), 338–46.
Newhauser, Richard, *The Treatise on Vices and Virtues in Latin and the
    Vernacular*, Typologie des sources du Moyen Age occidental 68
    (Turnhout, 1993).
—, 'Preaching the "Contrary Virtues"', *Mediaeval Studies* 70 (2008), 135–62.
—, and István P. Bejczy, *A Supplement to Morton W. Bloomfield et al.
    Incipits* ... (Turnhout, 2008).
O'Mara, V., and S. Paul, *A Reportorium of Middle English Prose Sermons*,
    Sermo 1, 4 vols (Turnhout, 2007).
Owst, G. R., *Literature and Pulpit in Medieval England* ... (Cambridge, 1933).
Palmer, Nigel F., 'Das Exempelwerk des englischen Bettelmönchen: ein
    Gegenstück zu den *Gesta Romanorum*?', in *Exempel und Exempel-
    sammlungen*, ed. Walter Haug and Burghart Wachinger (Tübingen,
    1991), 137–72.

Pantin, W. A., 'John of Wales and Medieval Humanism', in *Medieval Studies Presented to Aubrey Gwynn*, ed. J. A. Watt *et al.* (Dublin, 1961), 297–319.

Peraldus, William (Guillaume Peyraut), *Summa aurea de virtutibus et vitiis* (Venice: Paganinus de Paganinis, 20 December 1497 [Bod-Inc-G-334]).

Peter of Limoges, tr. Richard Newhauser, *The Moral Treatise on the Eye*, Medieval Sources in Translation 51 (Toronto, 2012).

'Phillipps MS. 8336 …', Robinson's of Pall Mall catalogue 79 (London, 1950).

Pickering, Oliver, and Katja Airaksinen, 'The Medieval Manuscripts in Leeds University Library', *Bulletin of International Medieval Research* 14 (2008), 3–23.

Piper, A. J., and A. I. Doyle, draft catalogue of Durham University Library Cosin MSS, online at https://www.dur.ac.uk/library/asc/theme/medmss/apvii5/.

Planta, Joseph, *A Catalogue of the Manuscripts in the Cottonian Library, deposited in the British Museum* ([London], 1802).

Reimer, Stephen R., ed., *The Works of William Herebert, OFM*, Studies and Texts 81 (Toronto, 1987).

Remigii Autissiodorensis Commentum in Martianum Capellam Libri I–II, ed. Cora E. Lutz (Leiden, 1962).

Robertson, D. W. Jr., *A Preface to Chaucer: Studies in Medieval Perspectives* (Princeton, NJ, 1963).

Rud, Thomas (d. 1732), ed. James Raine, *Codicum Manuscriptorum Ecclesiae Cathedralis Dunelmensis Catalogus Classicus* (Durham, 1825).

Seymour, M. C., 'Some Medieval English Owners of *De Proprietatibus Rerum*', *Bodleian Library Record* 9, iii (1974), 156–65.

—, et al., *Bartholomaeus Anglicus and his Encyclopedia* (Aldershot, 1992).

Sharpe, Richard, *Titulus. Identifying Medieval Latin Texts. An Evidence-Based Approach* (Turnhout, 2003).

—, et al., *English Benedictine Libraries: The Shorter Catalogues*, Corpus of British Medieval Library Catalogues 4 (London, 1996).

Smith, David M., and Vera C. M. London, *The Heads of Religious Houses: England and Wales II, 1216–1377* (Cambridge, 2001).

Smith, Thomas, introd. Colin G. C. Tite, *Catalogue of the Manuscripts in the Cottonian Library 1696 …* (Cambridge, 1984).

Swanson, Jenny, *John of Wales: A Study of the Works and Ideas of a Thirteenth-Century Friar* (Cambridge, 1989).

Thomson, S. Harrison, *The Writings of Robert Grosseteste, Bishop of Lincoln 1235–1253* (Cambridge, 1940).

Timpanaro, Sebastiano, ed. tr. Glenn W. Most, *The Genesis of Lachmann's Method* (Chicago, IL, and London, 2005).

Van Dussen, Michael, *From England to Bohemia: Heresy and Communication in the Later Middle Ages* (Cambridge, 2012).

Walther, Hans, *Initia Carminum ac Versuum Medii Aevi Posterioris Latinorum* ... (Göttingen, 1959).

Wenzel, Siegfried, *Latin Sermon Collections from Later Medieval England* ... (Cambridge, 2005).

—, *Medieval* Artes Praedicandi: *A Synthesis of Scholastic Sermon Structure* (Toronto, 2015).

—, *Preaching in the Age of Chaucer: Selected Sermons in Translation* (Washington, 2008).

Malachy the Irishman,
On poison:
text and translation

Quod triplici racione omne peccatum ueneno comparatur.
Capitulum I.

Racio ueneni potissim[e] conuenit peccato prioritate +
originis, generalitate infectionis, difficultate cure et medicationis.
+ Uenenum incepit a [cre]atura rationali, quia quando concepta
est [superbia] in mente angeli, naturam eius nobilissimam mutauit
5   in serpentinam. Unde dicitur 'serpens antiquus', Apocalypsis 12.
Illa etiam superbia originauit omne [ali]ud uenenum. Augustinus,
De ciuitate, libro 14, capitulo 3: 'Omnium', inquit 'malorum, tam
spiritualium quam + carnalium, est superbia origo prima'. Nam
antequam diabolus effunderet suum uirus per serpentem, dicitur
10   quod nullum animal fuit uenenosum, uel si fuit, homini non
noceret. Unde in testimonium status innocentie, serpens adhuc
formidat hominem nudum et insilit in uestitum, secundum
Isidorum, libro 12, capitulo de animalibus. Saliua etiam hominis
ieiuni est uenen[um] serpenti, secundum Plynium et philosophum,
15   *7 de animalibus*. Congrue tamen permissus est diabolus uenenum
refundere per serpentem, + quod natura[lis astutia] serpentis
conueniret transfuse malitie. Unde Genesis 3, 'Serpens erat
callidior cunctis animantibus', et quod exterior serpentis forma
corresponderet cogitate nequitie. Dicitur enim serpens, eo quod
20   occultis serpat accessibus, secundum Isidorum, libro 12. Sic et
tentatio a sensualitate serpit ad rationem, et etiam quod uenenum
materiale esset in [testimonium] ueneni spiritualis.

---

heading] *om.* AG, Incipit tractatus de ueneno CLS, De ueneno in generali D
   1 potissime] *om.* A, potissima L, potissimum p   2 originis] originationis p
  • cure et medicationis] curacionis S, *adds* Primo enim p   3 incepit] cepit G
  • creatura] natura p • quia quando] quia que A, quando CDL, quod
quando S   4 superbia] *om.* Ap   6 aliud] illud p • uenenum] *om.* A, uenū C,
peccatum S   8 carnalium] corporalium S, corporalium siue carnalium p
11 serpens] *om.* A   14 uenenum] uenenosa p   16 refundere] infundere CDL,
effundere GS • serpentem] *add* ut pateret GSp • quod] Tamen ut ACDL,
nam ut G • naturalis astutia] natura p • serpentis] *adds* quecunque G
18 et quod] Tamen ut ACDL   19 cogitate] cogitatui CDL, cogitanti G
  • nequitie] malicie S   20 occultis] occulte A   21 tentacio] de peccato quod A
  • et etiam quod] tamen ut A, Tum eciam ut CDL   22 in testimonium]
intellectui S, intellectiuum p

Every sin is compared with poison for three reasons.
Chapter 1.

Reason most powerfully shows the accord between sin and poison: in the priority of its origin, in the universal nature of its infection, and in the difficulty of curing and healing it. For poison began with a rational creature, because when pride was conceived in the angel's mind, it changed his most noble nature into that of a snake. For this reason, Apc 12:9 calls him 'the old serpent'. Also pride alone gave rise to every other poison. Augustine, *On the city of God* 14.3, 'Pride is the first beginning of every evil, both spiritual and bodily ones'. For before the devil poured out his poison through the serpent, it is said that there was no poisonous animal – or, if there were, it was not harmful to man. For this reason, as a witness to the state of innocence, the serpent to this day fears a man when he is naked and assails him when he is clothed, according to Isidore, *Etymologies* 12, in the chapter on animals. Also according to Pliny and Aristotle, *On animals* 7, the saliva of a fasting man is poisonous to a snake. Nevertheless, it was appropriate that the devil be allowed to pour out his poison through a snake, because the snake's natural cunning would accord with its communicating malice. For this reason, Gn 3:1 says, 'The serpent was more subtle than any of the beasts of the earth', and because a snake's external shape should correspond with its considered malice. For it is called a serpent because it creeps in (*serpat*) by secret passageways, according to Isidore in book 12. Likewise a sensual temptation creeps into the reason, just as if a physical poison should testify to a spiritual poison.

Secundo, principaliter dicitur peccatum uenenum generalitate
infectionis. Uenenum enim secundum Isidorum, ubi supra, dicitur
25   quasi 'uenas uectens'. Currit enim subito per uenas ad cor. Omne
enim uenenum est frigidum et ideo humane nature contrarium,
et extinguit calorem cordis et expellit animam, que secundum
Isidorum et Papiam, ignee est nature, cuius uita est in calore. Sic
uenenum peccati transiens per uenas anime, id est affecciones,
30   extinguit calorem charitatis et priuat animam uita sua, que
est Deus.

Tertio, peccatum dicitur uenenum propter difficultatem +
medicationis. Uenenum namque corporale, recto incessu transiens
per uenas ad cor, extinguit calorem uite. Sed uenenum spirituale,
35   prius inficiens naturam angelicam, per serpentem infecit primum
hominem, tanquam unam personam, in qua tota erat humana
natura infecta, et per naturam infectam inficitur omnis humana
persona. Unde circulari incessu transit spirituale uenenum. Et quia
secundum philosophum, uulnera circularia tardius curantur quam
40   oblonga, uenenum spirituale + difficilius curatur quam corporale.

Patet igitur quid sit principaliter uenenum, quia peccatum.
Quis primo ueneficus, quia demon. Que res primo uenenata, quia
illa in qua coniectum est uenenum, scilicet serpens, per quem
transit uenenum ad hominem. In cuius signum, adhesit sibi
45   semper uenenum [corpor]ale. Dicturi igitur de ueneno [spirituali],
metaphoras sumimus a creaturis uenenatis, ut [e]o sint ac[uc]iores
ad predicandum et horribiliores ad audiendum, tempore isto
quo s[t]ilus tepescit communis, eo possint penetrare efficacius
corda peccatorum.

---

24 ubi supra] *om.* ACDL, *adds* et Papiam G(+B)   25 subito] semper L   28 ignee]
igne| L   •   est¹] eius L   29 uenas] *adds* ad cor L

32 dicitur] *adds* proprie G   33 medicacionis] curacionis S, cure et medicationis p
35 serpentem] illam S   35–36 primum hominem] unum hominem scilicet
Adam CDL   36 qua] qua quia A, quo CDGL   •   tota erat] scilicet homine
erat omnis CDL   37 et per … infectam] *om.* A   37–38 per … persona] *om.* G
38 persona] natura siue persona S   39 tardius] prius tardius A   •   curantur]
sanantur S   40 difficilius] tardius S, tardius et difficilius p

41 quia peccatum] *om.* GS   42 primo] uero S   •   demon] poor (*expunged*) demon A,
dyabolus CDL   43 est] *adds* primo A   43–45 scilicet … corporale] *om.* G
45 semper] sepe L   •   corporale] materiale Sp   •   igitur] *add* aliquid CDL
45 spirituali] *om.* p   46 sumimus] sumemus A, sumamus CDL   •   eo] *om.* G,
quo Sp   •   sint] *add* sermones CDL   •   acuciores] acriores Sp   48 stilus]
salus S, silus p   •   communis] *om.* S   48 eo … efficacius] quatinus (quamuis L)
ea pocius CDL   •   possint] eciam A

[23] The second main point is that sin is called poison from the universal nature of its infection. For venom, according to Isidore, is called that as if it were drawing along the veins (*uenas uectans*). Thus it runs immediately from the veins to the heart. For every poison is cold and therefore is opposed to human nature. For it extinguishes the heat of the heart and drives out the soul, whose life is in heat, for according to Isidore and Papias, the soul has a fiery nature. Likewise the poison of sin, passing through the veins of the soul, that is through the desires, extinguishes the heat of charity and takes away the soul's life, which is God.

[32] Third, sin is called a poison on account of the difficulty of healing it. For a physical poison, passing by a direct entryway through the veins to the heart, extinguishes the heat of life. Likewise spiritual poison, having first infected the angelic nature, through the serpent infected the first man as if he were a single person. But through him all human nature was infected, and through his infected nature, every human person in turn is infected. Thus spiritual poison passes by a circular entryway. And since, according to Aristotle, circular wounds are healed more slowly than are slits, spiritual poison is cured more slowly than is bodily poison.

[41] Thus it is evident what the greatest poison is: it is sin. And the first poison-bearer: the devil. And the first thing that was poisoned: the serpent, the thing in which poison was inserted and through whom it passes to man. As an indication of this, physical poison has always adhered to the serpent. Therefore since I intend to speak about spiritual poison, I draw together metaphors from poisonous beasts, so that, the more pointed they are to preach and the more terrifying to hear, the more effectually they may penetrate the hearts of sinners. This is needful today, when usual forms of authorship have grown cold.

Triplex remedium contra peccatum in generali ponitur.
Capitulum II.

50   Remedium contra uenenum peccati est triplex. Primum est
remedium curatiuum, scilicet erigere serpentem salutiferum
contra + antiqui [serpentis] uenenum. Numerorum 21, 'Fac
tibi serpentem eneum et pone eum pro signo, ut qui percussus
a serpente prospexerit eum uiuat'. Glossa: 'Serpens in ligno
55   suspenditur quando filius Dei cruci affigitur, qui uenena serpentis
antiqui exclusit et [percussum] sanitat[i] restituit'. Serpens enim
secundum philosophum, libro 10, de medulla hominis mortui
gignitur. Et congrue secundum Isidorum, libro 12, quia sicut
per serpentem mors homini propinata est, sic per hominem
60   mortuum, scilicet Christum, mors morituro serpenti propinari
debuit. Christus ergo dicitur serpens propter similitudinem
carnis peccati. Sed dicitur 'eneus', quia secundum glossam, ubi
supra, 'Es, quod durabilius est omnibus metallis, sign[ific]at
corpus Domini nostri Iesu Christi, quod per inhabitantem
65   diuinitatem uiuit in eternum'. Remedium ergo quod curat
uenenum peccati est aspectus filii Dei per fidem in cruce.
Ioannis 3, 'Sicut exaltauit Moyses serpentem in eremo +, sic
exaltari oportet filium hominis etc.'.
        Nec mirum quia, sicut narrat commentator super Boetium,
70   *De disciplina scholarium*, 'Cum Socrates esset accusatus quod
librum fecisset de Deo et non de diis, compulsus fuit haurire
uenenum in nomine Dei, quo hausto nihil sibi nocuit. Et postea
fuit co[mpuls]us haurire in nomine deorum et mortuus [est]. Unde
Seneca, 'Socratem calix uencnatus transtulit de carcere in celum'.

---

heading] *om.* AGS, Contra uenenum peccati triplex remedium CD, Triplex
    remedium contra uenenum L
50 remedium] *om.* CDGL   **52** antiqui serpentis] diaboli id est antiqui hostis
    (serpentis G) GSp   **54** Glossa] *om.* ACDL   **55** cruci affigitur] crucifigitur D
    56 antiqui] *adds* hostis et L   • percussum sanitati] percussum hominem
    sanitati CDL, sanitatem GSp   **59** homini] *om.* L   **62** Sed] *add* serpens iste CDL
    63 Es] *om.* AD   • significat] signat p   **65** diuinitatem] ciuitatem L
    66 filii] *om.* L   **67** eremo] deserto S, *adds* in ligno p
69 narrat] refert G   **71** librum] unum librum A   • fecisset] confecit G   **73** fuit
    compulsus] compulsus est A, compulsus CDGL, fuit coactus Sp   • est] *om.* A,
    fuit statim Sp   **75** de carcere] *om.* A   • celum] CDL+B (*the last marginally*)
    add: (*om.* pAGS+LaRV)
        Item nota de (de beato L) Iohanne euangelista qui bibit (bibebat B) uenenum
    in nomine Domini et nichil sibi nocuit (*from* uenenum] etc. L)

He offers here a threefold general remedy against sin.
Chapter 2.

[50] The remedy against the poison of sin is threefold. First there is a remedy that cures, namely to raise the salvation-bringing serpent against the poison of the old serpent. Nm 21:8 says, 'Make a brazen serpent and set it up for a sign; whosoever being struck by a snake shall look on it, shall live'. The gloss explains, 'The serpent is hung up on a tree when the Son of God is fixed to the cross, for he shuts out the poisons of the old serpent and restores the person bitten to health'. According to Aristotle, in book 10, a snake is bred from the marrow of a dead man. And this is appropriate, according to Isidore, book 12, because just as death was ordained for man through a snake, so through the dead man Christ, death should be prepared for the snake who is to die. Therefore, Christ is called a serpent because of his likeness to our sinful flesh. But that same gloss says he is called 'brazen', because 'Brass, which is harder than all other metals, indicates the body of our Lord Jesus Christ, because he lives eternally through his indwelling divinity'. Therefore the remedy that cures the poison of sin is looking upon the Son of God on the cross with faith. Io 3:14 says, 'As Moses lifted up the serpent in the desert, so must the Son of man be lifted up [that whosoever believeth in him may not perish, but may have life everlasting]'.

[69] And this is not at all wondrous, for it is just as the commentator on Boethius's *De disciplina scholarium* tells. 'When Socrates was accused of having made a book about God, and not the gods, he was forced to drink poison in God's name, and after he had drunk it, it did not hurt him at all. And afterwards, he was forced to drink in the name of the gods, and he died'. For this reason, Seneca says, 'A poisoned cup transported Socrates from a prison to heaven'.

75   Si ergo paganus euasit mortem in nomine unius Dei, quid mirum
si aspectus filii Dei in cruce pro salute hominis pendentis liberet
ipsum hominem [finaliter] ab omni morte?

Secundo + requiritur contra uenenum remedium
restauratiuum, quia de serpente inficiente fit tyriaca contra
80   serpentis uenenum. Isidorus, libro 12, capitulo tyriaca, 'Tyri[a]ca
est antidotum serpentium, quo uenena pelluntur ut pestis peste
sanetur'. Sic de serpente eneo, scilicet Christo crucifixo, fit tyriaca
peccati. Unde Augustinus, 'Caro medici facta est medicamentum
egroti', secundum illud Ioannis 6, 'Caro mea uere est cibus', scilicet
85   ad saluandum animam.

Tertio requiritur contra uenenum remedium conseruatiuum,
quod est gratia interioris illu[min]ationis et exterioris predicacionis.
Unde narrat Isidorus, libro 12, quod saura quedam bestiola
naturaliter est inimica serpentibus, et quando homines dormientes
90   in desertis et syluis habent ora aperta, serpentes, naturaliter
calorem diligentes, attentant intrare ora [dormientium]. Sed
saura ascendit faciem dormientis et scalpit eam quousque
excitet a somno, significans interiorem gratiam sti[mu]lantem
+ conscientiam et exteriorem predicatorem semper clamantem
95   [ad animam in peccati miseriis dormientem], secundum
illud Ephesiorum 1, 'Surge qui dormis et exurge a mortuis, et
illuminabit te Christus'.

Sed ingrati expellunt gratiam excitantem et admittunt
serpentem uenenosum, [gratuita occidentem et naturalia
100   uulnerantem]. Sicut narratur de Uirgilio quod dum dormiisset
et serpens sibi appropinquasset, musca eum in fronte pupugit, ut
ipse collisa manu ad frontem muscam interfecit. Expergefactus
uero et uidens serpentem, doluit de morte musce que ipsum fecit
euadere mortem, et ideo fecit librum de laude musce. ℭ

---

75 unius] huius AS   77 finaliter] fidelem GS, *om.* p
78 Secundo] *adds* sequitur siue p   79 restauratiuum] restauracionis L   80 serpentis
uenenum] serpentem uenenantem C (*corr. to* uenenantem C, uenenum *a corr.* D)
• Isidorus] *om.* A • Tyriaca²] Tyrica p   81 pelluntur] p̄stantur (? *for*
prestantur) A   84 egroti] egrotis CD   85 saluandum] sanandum A
87 illuminacionis] illustracionis AGSp   88 narrat] dicit A   88 (and 92) saura]
lamia A   89–90 dormientes, habent] dormiunt, habentes ACDL   90 desertis et]
om. S   91 intrare] *om.* S • dormientium] *om.* Ap, aperta G   92 faciem] super
corpus CD, *om.* (*with following acc.*) L   93–94 stimulantem conscientiam] *om.* L
93 stimulantem] stillantem in Sp   94 predicatorem] predicacionem CDS
95 ad animam … dormientem] secundum illud ASp, *om.* G
99–100 gratuita … uulnerantem] *om.* AGSp

Therefore, if a pagan avoided death in the name of a single God, what wonder is there if looking upon the Son of God, hanging on the cross for man's salvation, should not free that person from death, once and for all?

[78] Second, poison requires a restorative remedy, since theriac, the antidote against a snake's poison, is made from the infecting snake. Isidore, book 12, 'Theriac is an antidote for snakes that drives out their poisons, so that one plague may be healed by another'. In just the same way, the antidote for sin is made from the brazen serpent, Christ crucified. For this reason, Augustine says, 'The physician's flesh is made the drug for the sick man', in accord with Io 6:56, 'My flesh is meat indeed', that is for saving the soul.

[86] Third, poison requires a preserving remedy, and that is grace from inner enlightenment and external preaching. For this reason, Isidore tells in *Etymologies* 12 that the lizard is a certain kind of small animal, by its nature inimical to snakes. When people are asleep in deserts and wild places and leave their mouths open, snakes, who naturally love heat, try to get into their mouths. But the lizard climbs up on the sleeper's face and scratches it until it may rouse them from their slumber. This shows both the inner grace stimulating their conscience and the preacher always crying out to that soul, asleep in the wretchedness of sin, in accord with Eph 5:14, 'Rise thou that sleepest and arise from the dead, and Christ shall enlighten thee'.

[98] But ungrateful people drive out the grace that should be stimulating them, and they let in the poisonous snake, which destroys gracious things and wounds natural ones. Likewise, there is a story about Virgil that, while he was asleep and a snake approached him, a fly kept stinging his forehead. He slapped his forehead with his hand and killed the fly. But awakened and seeing the snake, he lamented the death of the fly that made him escape death, and therefore he made a poem in praise of the fly. ℭ

De primordiali ueneno peccati et principali, scilicet superbia.
Capitulum III.

105   Uenenum superbie est primum + a quo cetera oriuntur.
        Unde Augustinus, *De ciuitate Dei*, libro 12, capitulo 6, 'Hic
        primus defectus, hec prima inopia, et cui omnia famulantur'.
        Et Gregorius, libro *Moralium* 31, 'Regine superbie omnia uicia
        famulantur tanquam duces [sue]'. Ad huius ueneni euidentiam
110   notandum quod occasionem primam habuit ex collata bonitate,
        quia naturalis bonitas angelo indita fuit occasio eius ruine,
        secundum A[nselm]um, libro *De casu diaboli*. Et ideo uirus
        superbie irremediabilius, quo de bono collato extollitur et 'supra
        statum suum graditur'. Inde [enim dicitur superbia] secundum
115   Anselmum, libro *De similitudinibus*, quod 'Superbia super Deum
        extollitur secundum eundem ibi[dem] uolendo', scilicet quod
        Deus non uult eum uelle.
            Sic collata bonitas et data potestas dominis, regibus, et
        principibus terrenis conuertitur eis in superbie uenenum. Unde
120   dominus terrenus comparatur basilisco, qui idem est quod regulus
        Latine. Qui secundum Isidorum, libro 12, 'quoad uirus, rex est
        omnium serpentium; ita eum omnes timent propter [ex]cessum
        ueneni'. Unde dicitur super illud Esaie 11b, 'In cauerna reguli
        mittet manum suam qui oblactatus fuerit', dicit glosa quod
125   'Regulus flatu et uisu occidit omne uiuum et etiam + uolantes
        aues'. Dicit enim Plynius, libro 4, quod est serpens semipedalis

---

105 Uenenum superbie ACDL, *om.* GS • primum] *add* omnium ASp, *adds*
    omnium principium G • cetera] *add* uicia CDL **107** omnia] *add* mala CDL
    • famulantur] falerantur S **108** Et] *add* loquitur de superbia et CDL
109 famulantur] falerantur et famulantur S • duces sue] duces AGSp, ducisse
    sue CD • ueneni] *om.* AD, *add* scilicet superbie CL • euidentiam] *om.* D
111 naturalis] *om.* S (*at line-break*) • indita] indicia G **112** Anselmum]
    Anselm' ACDL (*over eras.* CD), Au'/An' G, Ans' S, Augustinum p **114** statum]
    gradum CDLS • enim … superbia] notandum Sp **115** Superbia] *om.* AG
116 ibidem] ibi p
119 principibus] *add* potestatibus ACDL • terrenis] *add* si ea abuntantur CDL
    • superbie] *adds rubric* De superbia dominorum comparata basilisco A
120 dominus] *om.* S • terrenus] *add* abutens suo dominio CDL **121** Latine]
    om. L, *adds* basilicus enim Grece idem est quod regulus Latine G • secundum]
    om. D **122** omnes] *add* serpentes CDL • excessum] in eo excessum CDL,
    recessum p **123** cauerna] camera CD **125** et uisu] *om.* S • occidit] interficit S
    • et etiam] *om.* A, eciam autem S **125–26** uolantes aues] superuolans A,
    aues desuper uolantes Gp, *skips to* **128** et aues … L, desuper uolantes aues S

On pride, the original and principal poison of sin.
Chapter 3.

[105] The poison of pride is the first, from which the other poisons all spring. For this reason, Augustine, *On the City of God* 12.6, says, 'This is the first failure, the first helplessness, and all others are related to it'. And Gregory, *Morals* 31, says, 'All vices consort with pride the queen as if they were her generals'. And one should notice what is evident about this poison, that it had its first occasion from goodness God had conferred, for the natural goodness passed on to the angel was equally the occasion for his fall, as Anselm says in his book *On the devil's fall*. Therefore the poison of pride is more resistant to being cured insofar as it is raised up as a result of the good conferred and 'advances above its proper station'. Thus, 'Anselm', in his *Book of likenesses*, says that 'pride is raised up above God in accord with what the proud person wishes there', that is what God doesn't want him to wish.

[118] Likewise, lords, kings, and worldly princes change the goodness conferred and the power granted them into the poison of pride. For this reason, an earthly lord is compared to the basilisk, which is the same as the snake called *regulus* 'little king' in Latin. According to Isidore, book 12, 'this snake, so far as its venom is concerned, is the king of all snakes, so that all fear it because of the excessive quality of its poison'. For this reason, in the gloss on Is 11:8, 'The weaned child shall thrust his hand into the den of the basilisk', it says, 'The snake *regulus* with its breath and sight kills every living thing, even flying birds'. Also Pliny says in book 4 that it is a snake half a foot long

in cuius cauerne circuitu nichil uirescit, omne uiuum quod primo
uidet interimit, et aues uolantes flatu suo uel uisu occidit.

130   + Hic est tyrannus et terrenus dominus circa cuius cauernam
siue curiam nihil pauperibus uirescit. Omne etiam animal uiuum
in predam sibi arripit, immo aues, id est religiosos uiuere non
permittit. Et tantum inualuit uenenum talium tyrannorum quod
religiosi illi qui totum mundum calcant, quibus promittitur 'super
aspidem et basiliscum ambulare etc.', nichil in eis proficiunt.

135   Unde glosa dicit ibidem quod 'Membra Christi, id est p[erfec]ti,
potestate[m] calcant + inimici, conuertendo', scilicet membra
diaboli ut fierent membra Christi. Sed modernos dominos nec
sanctitate uite nec ueritate doctrine conuertunt, ut impleatur illud
Hieremie 8, 'Mittam eis serpentes pessimos (alia littera, "regulos"),

140   quibus non est incantatio'. Glosa, 'Qui Dei precepta et diuina
eloquia contemnunt, contrariis potestatibus traduntur'. Unde
ratio est quare uerbum Dei in eis nihil efficit, quia ue[nen]um
superbie eos [tantum] inficit et cecitatem interiorem inducit ita
quod hereditatem temporalem et eternam amittere facit. Dicit

145   enim Hieronymus de Nabugodonosor super illud Esaie 14,
'Perdidisti terram tuam etc.', quod superbia unius hominis
gentem, prolem, imperium destruxit, et imperium Chaldeorum,
quod secundum Orosium, per 154 annos durauit, [ex]terminatum
fuit. Ecclesiastici 10, 'Sedes superborum destruxit Dominus'.

150   Uenenum superbie inficit ex generis nobilitate, et hoc
uenenum est contra naturam, quia [non] habet + gradum. Origo

---

127 quod] *adds* regulus A • uirescit] uiridescit CD, L *om.* **128** flatu suo]
om. L • flatu … occidit] *om.* CD (uisu suo interimit *int. corr.* C) • occidit]
interimit L

129 Hic] Moraliter hic p **130** uirescit] uiridescit CDL **131** immo] ī̄m|os C, (?)
neruos D • aues] *adds* uolantes L • religiosos] *add* et contemplatiuos CDL
133 calcant] calcauerunt ACDL **134** nichil … proficiunt] *om.* AL, et
con[culcabis] le[onem] et dra[conem] CD (et con] etc. D) (*extending the citation
of Ps 90:13*) • proficiunt] *add* sed per tales miseros dominos nimium sunt
oppressi CDL **135** perfecti] prelati Sp **136** potestatem] potestate GSp
• calcant] *add* uirtute (uirtutem Sp) GSp **139** littera] *add* habet CDL
• regulos] religiosos G **142** nihil] *om.* G • in eis, efficit] efficit in eis ASp,
eis proficit CL, in eis proficit D, eis deficit G • uenenum] uerbum Sp
143 eos … inficit] eos exteriore infecit A, quod in eis est tantum proficit et
ita eos CDL, eos ex toto infecit (inficit p) GSp **148** Orosium] Originem CDL
• 154] 1064 CDL • durauit] *om.* S • exterminatum] exterminauit, *corr. to*
exterminatum fuit C, interminatum p
151 non habet] habet nobilitatis GSp

and that nothing lives in the neighbourhood of its cave, that it kills
every living thing it sees first, and that it kills flying birds with its breath
or sight.

[129] The *regulus* is a tyrant or worldly lord around whose court
– it would be better called a cave – nothing lives for the poor. Also it
seizes every living beast as its prey, even birds; that is, it does not allow
religious people to live. The poison of such tyrants has been so very
powerful that those religious people who trample upon everything that
is worldly, those to whom Ps 90:13 promises, 'Thou shalt walk upon the
asp and the basilisk[,and thou shalt trample under foot the lion and
the dragon'], may not succeed in their works. For this reason, the gloss
on this verse says, 'The limbs of Christ, that is those who are perfect,
trample on their enemy's power'; that is to say that they convert their
enemies, the limbs of the devil, so that they become limbs of Christ.
But these days they do not convert lords, either by the sanctity of their
lives or by the truth of their teaching. Thus, Jeremiah's prophecy (8:17)
is fulfilled, 'I will send among them [the worst] serpents – in another
reading, basilisks – against which there is no charm'. The gloss here
says, 'Those who disdain God's precepts and divine eloquence are given
over to perverse powers'. This, then, is the reason why the word of God
achieves nothing in them: the poison of pride infects them completely
and produces inner blindness that causes them to lose both their worldly
and their eternal inheritance. Also Jerome says of Nebuchadnezzar
concerning Is 14:20, 'Thou hast destroyed thy land', that a single person's
pride has destroyed people, offspring, and empire. The empire of the
Chaldeans, which, according to Orosius, lasted 154 years, was ended.
Sir 10:17 says, 'God has overturned the thrones of the proud'.

[150] The poison of pride infects through nobility of lineage, and
this poison is unnatural, because nature is without class. For the origin

enim omnis humane nobilitatis, qua unus extollitur alteri, aut
ex tyrannide par[ent]um, sicut Nemphroth, Genesis 10: oppressit
multos et eis prefuit. Et de tali nobilitate gloriari superbire est de
155   malitia et contra naturam, que omnes genuit equales, secundum
Gregorium in *Pastorali*. Uel astuta sapientia [filiorum], et hec
gloria serpentina. Unde narrat Plinius, libro 8, quod ru[bet]a siue
bufo est quoddam genus rane uenenose quod habitat in paludibus.
Inueniens oua aspidis, fouet ea, et ex tali ouo generatur regulus,
160   qui et basiliscus, solo uisu interficiens omnia. Et quando generatur,
in suum fotorem primo exercet malitiam; quam cito enim
recipit a natura uisum, nutritorem suum primo inspicit et ipsum
interimit. Sic est origo nobilitatis mundane qua parens uel nutritor
uenenatu[s], informans prolem ad sapientiam animalem, terrenam,
165   et diabolicam, imbuit eam ueneno.

Et non solum, ut dicit Hieronymus, de parentibus uenenatis
nascuntur filii uenenati, sed etiam aut ex terrena substantia, quod
enim unus fuerit pulchrior et nobilior altero. Hoc est [a dieta],
quia, secundum Isaac, ex subtili cibo generatur subtilis sanguis, et
170   si talis cibus daretur filio pauperis, esset subtilis complexionibus.
Unde talis gloria oritur ex terreno stercore. Et de hiis omnibus
intelligitur illud Esaie 59, 'Quod confotum est', scilicet de ouis
aspidis, 'erumpet in regulum'; glossa, 'Ex ouis aspidis generatur
regulus, qui et basiliscus'. Sic et ex malignis parentibus uel

---

152 omnis] tocius S • omnis … nobilitatis] hominis seu humane nature aut
nobilitatis G • humane] *om.* S • extollitur] superextollitur AGS
153 parentum] personarum Sp   **155** malitia] natura G   **156** astuta] astu|cia D
• sapientia filiorum] sapiencia AGSp, superbia (superba D) filiorum DL (*corr. to*
sapiencia C)   **157** serpentina] *om.* CD, serpentis L • rubeta] *om.* A, rudeca p
160 uisu] *add* ut predicitur CDL • interficiens] interficit A, inficiens S
• omnia] hominem ACDGL • quando generatur] generatus CDL
161 fotorem] nutritorem A • primo] *add* deseuit et suam … primo CD, *add*
suam ALS • quam cito] quando S   **162** recipit] procedit et accipit A
• a natura] *om.* L • inspicit] respicit ACDGL   **163** interimit] interficit ACDL
• mundane] humane G • parens] pater L   **164** uenenatus] uenenatur Sp
• prolem] pueros (*and* 115 eos) ACD, *om.* L • sapientiam] *add* mundanam ACDL
166 Et non solum] *om.* G   **167** etiam] *add* suo ueneno parentes inficiunt et
occidunt CDL   **168** unus] adds uideatur G • nobilior] decenter \cor/pulencior
(*originally* opulencior) CD, et decencior corpulencior L • a dieta] *corr. from*
adita C, *corr. from* adiecta (?) D, ad|iecta G, ex adiecto Sp   **169** cibo] *add* quia
ex subtili cibo CDL   **172** confotum] fotum GS   **173** regulum] regulus C,
regulos DL • aspidus] aspidum confotis A   **174** qui et basiliscus] *adds*
uocatur A, *om.* CDL

of all human nobility, in which one person is raised up over another, comes first from the tyrannous behaviour of one's parents, like Nimrod (Gn 10:8–9): he oppressed many and put himself ahead of them. And to rejoice in such nobility is to be proud, and it comes from malice and is unnatural, for nature produced us all equal, according to Gregory in his *Pastoral rule*. Alternatively, it is the result of children's crafty wisdom, and this is a snake's glory. For Pliny tells in book 8 that the toad *rubeta* is a particular kind of poisonous frog that lives in swamps. When one finds an asp's eggs, it broods on them, and such an egg produces a *regulus*, the same as the basilisk – a basilisk kills everything with its sight alone. And when it is born, it first uses its malice on its own 'nurse', for just as soon as it receives its sight from nature, the first thing it does is to look at its nurse, the toad, and kill it. This is the source of worldly nobility by which a poisonous parent or nurse, moulding their offspring to worldly wisdom, both beastly and demonic, suffuses it with poison.

[166] And as Jerome says, it is not just that poisonous children are born from poisonous parents, but they are also poisoned by their earthly substance. For one of them will be more beautiful or more noble than another. This comes about from their diet, because as Isaac Israeli says, fine blood is made from fine food and if such food were given to a poor person's child, it would be fine in its 'complexions'. For this reason, such glory arises from worldly shit. Is 59:5, 'That which is brought out', that is from an asp's egg, 'shall be hatched into a basilisk' is understood to refer to all these cases; the gloss there says, 'From an asp's egg is born a *regulus*, just the same as a basilisk'. Thus, an even more malign inheritor

175   nutritoribus exit malignior successor; propter hoc, non est
gaudendum quod mal[us dominus] gignit prolem. Sicut
in *Apologiis Aesopi* narratur quod filius fuit natus cuidam
tyranno, et cum quidam exultassent, dixit sapiens, 'Audite',
inquit, 'gaudium uestrum. Sol genuit solem, et omnes creature
180   ge[m]uerunt, dicentes, "Unicus sol erat nobis hactenus, et uix
pre calore eius uiuere potuimus. Nunc autem sol multiplicatus
tollet uitam nostram". Sic', inquit, 'est gaudium uestrum. Unus
tyrannus nos omnes oppressit; quanto magis multiplicatus in
filiis uenenatis tollet uitam nostram? Si dicat filius quod gloriatur
185   de parentum bonitate, non nobilitate, dico quod sic inaniter
gloriatur, si non sit talis [quales] illi [sunt]. Sicut si gloriaretur
lutum uile de radio + solari qui transit super ipsum; sic bonitas
parentum transit super malum filium, sed non decorat ipsum'.
Unde demon posset sic gloriari de sola sua bonitate prima.
190   Hoc uenenum superbie etiam inficit ex collata dignitate,
tanto periculosius, quanto sub specie pietatis uenenum infundit.
Quia secundum Gregorium in *Pastorali*, 'Nemo in ecclesia Dei
magis nocet quam qui sub specie sanctitatis peccat'. Et de hoc
intelligitur illud Genesis penultimo, 'Fiat Dan sicut coluber in uia
195   et sicut cerastes in semita'; alia translacio, 'sicut regulus in locato'.
Cerastes enim est serpens [et species reguli] et habet, secundum
Isidorum, libro 12, corpus paruum et duo cornua ad modum
arietis; corpus autem totum in uia occultat sub arena, solis
cornibus derelictis sine operculo. Et tunc auicule, credentes
200   quod cornua sint uermes mansueti, dum eis refici nituntur,

---

175 exit] erit S • malignior successor] malignitas successorum CDL, peior s. S
176 malus dominus] m. terrenus d. G, malis terrenis deus p, *adds* malam A
178 quidam] *adds* de hoc multum A, *add* ex hoc CDL **180** gemuerunt]
genuerunt p • hactenus] nocens G, accensus S **181** Nunc] ‖ Unicus L
182 nostram] *adds* totam G **185–89** sic … gloriari] *om.* A **186** si … quales]
sic gloriatur sicud G, sic inaniter gloriatur p **186** quales illi sunt] quales illi
D, sicut illi Sp **187** radio] *adds* solis uel p **188** malum] *om.* CDL **189** de sola]
scilicet de A, *add and canc.* scilicet sobrietate CD

190 Hoc … etiam] Item est uenenum quod inficit ACDL • superbie] *om.* GS
(*at line end* S) • dignitate] *add* et hoc CGL, et hoc ‖ et hoc D **191** pietatis]
proprietatis L **193** magis] *om.* S • qui] que D • sanctitatis] proprietatis L,
pietatis S **195** translatio] *add* habet sic CDL **196** locato] *adds* \id est peccato/ G
• serpens] *om.* G • et species reguli] *om.* (*at line boundary*) Sp **199** derelictis
sine operculo] non coopertis CD, d. s. opertitulo S • auicule] *add* mansuete
CDL **200** refici] uesci S

will come from malign parents or nurses; for this reason, one should not rejoice that an evil lord produces an heir. Likewise, Æsop's fables tell that a son was born to a certain tyrant, and when some people had rejoiced, a wise man said, 'Listen to this about your joy. The sun gave birth to a sun, and all creatures lamented, saying, "Until now we had only a single sun, and we might scarcely live on account of his heat. But now this multiplied sun will take away our lives". That's what your joy is all about', he said. 'A single tyrant has oppressed us all; how much more will he bear away our life when he is multiplied in poisoned children? If a son should say that he rejoices in his parents' goodness, rather than their nobility, I say that he rejoices foolishly, if he is not such as they are. It is just as if a vile bit of mud would rejoice about the sun's ray that passes over it; likewise the parents' goodness passes over a bad child, but it does not confer honour on him'. Following this reasoning, the devil might rejoice, simply because of his original goodness.

[190] The poison of pride also infects from dignity that has been conferred, the more dangerously so, the more the poison is poured in under a guise of piety. For according to Gregory in his *Pastoral rule*, 'No one in God's church does more harm than the person who sins in the guise of holiness'. And Gn 49:17 is understood to refer to this point; it says, 'Let Dan be a snake in the way, a serpent in the path' – in another translation, 'a basilisk in the place'. *Cerastes* (the biblical 'snake' here) is also a snake, a kind of basilisk, and according to Isidore, book 12, it has a small body and two horns like a ram; but it hides its whole body under sand in the road, leaving only its horns uncovered. Then small birds, thinking that the horns are humble worms, while they try to eat them,

a doloso serpente + interimuntur. Dicit enim glossa, ubi supra,
quod 'tante perniciei est quod si eius uenenum ungulam equi
tetigerit, ipsum cum equite interimit'. Sic malus prelatus totam
malitiam cor[d]is sui cooperit sub falsa specie alicuius commodi
205   ecclesie, cornua sue auctoritatis sub specie pietatis pretendens,
in quibus pauperes, sanctitatem et pietatem inuenire credentes,
penitus decipiuntur. Ita quod quicunque uenenum malorum
dominorum fugit, uenenum malorum prelatorum incurrit,
secundum illud Esaie 19, 'Quod a malo recessit, prede [patuit', id
210   est qui uenenum regalium et laycorum euadit, prede] prelatorum
patuit. Immo in dominis terrenis est aliqua misericordia, sed in
malis prelatis nulla, nisi uiderint munera. Sicut refert Seneca,
epistola 18, 'Reges Parthos non poterat salutare quis sine munere'.
Sic nemo potest accedere ad curiam prelatorum, nisi deferat
215   munera, quoniam sentiet in cornibus uenena. Et hoc est contra
natura cornuum, quia dicit philosophus, libro 13 *De animalibus*,
quod animal habens cornua non habet dentes in superiori
mandibula, quia non debetur ei uiuere de rapina. Unde, ut dicitur,
propter hoc subtrahit ei natura dentes illos.
220   Superbia etiam inficit ex apparente pulchritudine corporis.
Et hoc est uenenum *scitalis*, qui est serpens, secundum Isidorum,
libro 12, prefulgens in tergo omnium colorum uarietate ita quod
ob gratiam sui omnium aspectum facit admirari. Et quia tarde
+ repit, quos gradiendo inuadere nequit, miraculo sui coloris
225   sistere facit et postea occidit, et quanto magis est discolor, tanto
nequior. Hoc est uenenum meretricis, que ex falso fulgore

201 doloso] solo L • interimuntur] perimuntur ACDL, subito interimuntur p
202 quod] *add* cerastes CDL   203 interimit] *add* et sic nimirum ascensor equi
retro cadit (*continuing the citation of Gn 49:17*) CDL   204 cordis] corporis
AGSp, cordis et corporis CDL • cooperit] *om.* A • falsa] aliqua falsa CDL
(falsa *over eras.* C, fal\s/a D)   205 auctoritatis] auctoritatem scilicet suam
(*a corr.*) CL, auctoritatem D   206 pauperes] *add* et mansueti CDL
207 decipiuntur] accipiuntur D   208 fugit] effugit A • malorum] *om.* AG
209 (and 210) prede] *corr. from* pede CD   209–10 prede … prede] prede GSp
210 regalium] regularium L   212 malis] *om.* A   213–14 poterat … potest]
poterat G   213 sine] nisi uiderunt S   214–15 nisi … munera] sine munere S
215 cornibus] corporibus L • **uenena**] *adds* L (*marg. note* C, *these generally
ignored*) (*om.* ADGSp+BLaRV):
Memorandum (Me L) de beato Thoma Cantuar'
216 libro] *om.* D   218 mandibula] *om.* S   219 illos] *om.* CDGL, *adds rubric*
Superbia ex pulcritudine A
220 corporis] *om.* CDL   221 uenenum scitalis qui] *om.* L • scitalis] situle CD
224 repit] recipit p • coloris] corporis ADL   225 occidit et] *om.* A

are killed by the treacherous snake. The gloss to the passage says, 'This snake is of such viciousness that if its poison has touched a horse's hoof, it kills it, along with its rider'. Likewise, a bad priest covers all the malice of his heart under the false appearance of some behaviour useful to the church, and sticking forth the horns of his authority under the guise of piety, poor men, believing they have found holiness and piety there, are completely deceived. Thus, whoever flees the poison of evil lords encounters the poison of evil priests, according to Is 59:15, 'He that departed from evil lay open to be a prey', that is the person who escapes the poison of noble laymen has laid himself open to be the prey of priests. Even in worldly lords there is a little mercy, but there is none in evil priests, unless they have seen bribes first. It is just as Seneca says in epistle 18, 'No one might greet the Parthian kings without a bribe'. Likewise, no one can approach an episcopal court, unless he hands out bribes, for he will perceive the poison in the horns. This runs quite contrary to the nature of horns, for Aristotle says, *On animals* 13, that an animal with horns does not have teeth in its upper jaw, because it is not appropriate for such to live by prey. For this reason, as he says, nature has taken these teeth from them.

[220] Also pride infects through the visible beauty of the body. This is the poison of the *scitalis*; according to Isidore, book 12, it is a snake brightly shining with the variousness of every colour on its back, and on account of its beauty, it makes everyone looking at it marvel. Because it crawls slowly, it is unable to assault them by swift motion, but through the wonder of its colours, it makes its victims pause and then kills them, and the greater its variety of colour, the more harmful it is. This is the poison of a whore, who infects onlookers with her false outer sheen,

[ex]teriori inficit [intuentes], quia 'propter speciem mulieris multi
perierunt', Ecclesiastici 9. Quere plus de hoc capitulo de luxuria.
    Superbia inficit ex apparenti sanctitate, ut in hypocritis,
230 qui comparantur cameleoni, que est bestiola transformans in
se omnem colorem sibi appositum. Secundum Augustinum,
libro 11 *De trinitate*, capitulo 1, ['Res cupide aspecta, ubi
non occurrit durior pinguiorque materies, tocius corporis
informantis est informatiua et in sui similitudinem, speciem,
235 et colorem est commutatiua. Sicut corpusculum camaleontis ad
colores, quos cupide intuetur, facillima conuersione uariatur'.]
Uel secundum Isidorum et Auicennam et Aristotelem, gyrat
oculos suos frequenter circumquaque, quia hypocrita arrogans
attribuit sibi omnem sanctitatem et [simulat] opera aliorum. Et
240 secundum Plynium, libro 12, alteratur ei color quando corium
eius sufflatur; sic hypocrita eleuatur + quando commendatur.
Dicit etiam Esicius super 4 capitulo Leuitici quod pre
infirmitate fingit se manusetum, cum sit crudelis bestia; ita
hypocrita pius est in uerbis sed crudelis in factis. Esaie 9,
245 'Hypocrita est nequam', secundum unam litteram. Dicit enim
Plynius, ubi supra, de hoc animali quod uis eius est maxima
contra accipitres, quia eos uolantes ad se trahit ut dilacerat.
Sic hypocrita uiros uirtuosos diffamat et eorum uirtutes sibi
arrogat. Unde fur uel predo uocatur, Iob 17, 'Que est spes
250 hypocrite si auare rapiat?' Unde Gregorius, 'Rapit de presumpta
sanctitate laudem aliene uite'.
    Superbie uirus intumescit ex professionis sublimitate, et hoc
est pessimum uenenum, superbire scilicet de statu sublimi,

227 exteriori] interiori p, *add* sui corporis CDL   227–29 inficit … inficit]
inficit A   228 intuentes] *om.* GSp
229 ut] *add* patet CDL   232 *De trinitate*] *om.* A   232–36 Res … uariatur] *om.* GSp
233 -que] *over eras.* C, *inserted beween words* D   234 informantis] -atis A
236 conuersione] uariacione L   238 frequenter] *add* usquequam et CDL
• quia hypocrita] *om.* D 239 attribuit] tribuit CDL   • simulat] fingit L,
transumit Sp   240 corium] corun A   241 eleuatur] *adds* per superbiam p
• quando] *add* laudatur et CDL   242 Esicius] Augustinus G   245 Hypocrita]
Omnis hypocrita CDGL   • unam] aliam ACDL   245 de hoc animali]
om. CDL   247 trahit] attrahit G   248 Sic … diffamat] uirtuousos … diffamat
marg. corr. C, Sic … dilacerat *marg. corr.* D   • uirtuosos] *add* dilacerat et ACDL
249 spes] species DL   250 si auare] nisi ut auare rem CD, nisi ut auaros L
• auare] auarus S   250–51 de … laudem] sub specie sanctitatis laudem sibi
ascribit G   251 uite] *adds rubric* \Superbia ex professione/ A
252 sublimitate] subtilitate AGS   253 uenenum] *om.* G   • sublimi] subtili G

because 'Many have perished by the beauty of a woman', Sir 9:9. See the further discussion of this point in the chapter on lechery.

[229] Pride also infects through visible sanctity, as in hypocrites. They are compared to the chameleon, a small animal that changes itself into any colour put next to it. According to Augustine, *De trinitate* 11.1, 'Anything observed with desire, unless a harder or denser material is interposed, has the power to form perception and to change the entire body into its own likeness, appearance, and colour. Likewise the chameleon's tiny body changes to those colours that it looks at avidly in an easy transformation'. Alternatively, according to Isidore, Avicenna, and Aristotle, the chameleon frequently revolves its eyes every which way, because the arrogant hypocrite attributes all sanctity to himself and imitates other people's works. And according to Pliny, book 12, its colour changes when it puffs out its skin; likewise the hypocrite is raised up with pride when he is complimented. Also Hesychius says in the gloss on Lv 11 that the chameleon pretends to be meek on account of his weakness, while it is really a savage beast; likewise a hypocrite is pious in his words but cruel in his works. Is 9:17 says, 'Every hypocrite is wicked', according to one reading. Pliny also says of this animal that it exerts its greatest strength against sparrowhawks, because it draws them in their flight so that it can tear them to pieces. Likewise, a hypocrite defames virtuous people and claims their virtues as his own. Thus, he is called a thief or a pillager; see Iob 27:8, 'For what is the hope of the hypocrite, if through covetousness he take by violence?' For this reason, Gregory says, 'He seizes from his presumed sanctity the praise befitting another person's behaviour'.

[252] The poison of pride swells up from the height of profession, and this is pride's worst poison, that is pride concerning an elevated place,

quando uota et uita repugnant. Hoc uenenum est falsorum
255   religiosorum, qui comparantur salamandre, que est secundum
Isidorum, libro 12, bestiola uenenosa uiuens in solo igne; ignis
tamen incendia non tantum non [adur]it, immo extinguit. Sic
mali religiosi in medio sunt ignis gratie, sicut de principe eorum
dicitur Ezechielis 28, 'In medio lapid[um] ignitorum ambulasti'.
260   Regnat tamen in eis uenenum malitie, que extinguit omnem
effectum gratie, non tantum in se per malam uitam, sed in aliis
per malam doctrinam. Sicut dicit Plinius de ista bestiola, libro 4,
quod nunquam apparet extra furnum, nisi cum pluit. Cuius tactus
est frigidus ut glacies ita ut ignem extinguat, et de ore eius lacteam
265   saniem euomit, ex cuius contactu calorem corporis inficit. Hec ibi.
Sic falsus religiosus apparet ad pluuiam carnalitatis et extinguit
in aliis per prauum exemplum donum gratie. Pretendit lacteam et
uenenosam saniem doctrine que postmodum auditores exemplo
praue uite magis inficit quam conuertit. Sed quam nociuum est
270   istud uenenum patet per Isidorum, ubi supra; qui dicit quod
uenenum aliorum serpentum singulos inficit, salamandra multos
simul interimit, que si ita irrepserit arbori, poma eius inficit et
comedentes omnes interimit. Si in puteum cadat, omnes potantes
inficit. Sic predicator prauus secundum Anselmum, *Libro de*
275   *similitudinibus*, quod more medici bene instruit, sed ipse herbam
uenenatam assumit et se et alios postmodum inficit.
        Superbie uirus surgit de scientie subtilitate et astutie
calliditate, quod est proprie proprium serpentis qui, secundum
Plynium, libro 1 *De animalibus*, est naturaliter astutus, sicut

254 uota] uoto A • uota … repugnant] tota uita repugnat CDL   256 bestiola]
animal S   257 adurit] L, admittit ACDG, sentit Sp   258 religiosi] *add* quoad
corpus CDL   259 lapidum] lapidis p   264 lacteam] *om.* ACDL   265 saniem]
fumum D • inficit] extinguit S   267 per prauum exemplum] *om.* CDL
268 saniem] sanguinem G • auditores] audi\res/ C, au|di^{tes} (= audientes?) D
269 Sed] O Sp   270 patet] *om.* S   272 interimit] interficit A • que si ita] quia
si CDL (si] *a corr.* D), que si illa S • irrepserit] resparserit G, repserit S
274 prauus] prauus est A, qui malus est in uita et facundus in lingua CDL,
prauus qui G   275 instruit] instructi A, instituit CL (inst\r|u/it D)   276 et alios]
ita A, ex alios D • inficit] *adds rubric* \Superbia de sciencia/ A; **D+B** *add* (*om.*
ACGLS+LaRV):
        \et ideo factum predicatoris trahitur in exemplum. Ideo apostolus ait castigo
        corpus meum etc./; B continues: et in seruitute redigo ne alias, etc.' [1 Cor
        9:27]. Propter quod dicitur de Cristo capite nostro Actuum 1[:1], 'Cepit Iesus
        facere et docere'.
277 subtilitate] sublimitate A   278 proprie] *om.* L   279 libro 1] libro 2 *marg.* CD, *om.* L

when one's life and one's vows resist one another. This is the poison of false religious people, who are compared to the salamander. According to Isidore, book 12, this is a little poisonous animal that lives only in fire; nevertheless the flaming of the fire does not burn it; indeed, the salamander extinguishes it. Likewise, evil religious people are in the middle of the fire of grace, just as Ez 28:14 says of their chief, 'Thou hast walked in the midst of stones of fire'. Nevertheless the poison of malice may rule in them, and it extinguishes every effect of grace, not only in them because of their evil life, but in others because of their evil teaching. Pliny says of this little animal in book 4 that it never appears outside its oven, except when it rains. A salamander's touch is as cold as ice so that it may put out a fire, and from its mouth it spews out milky pus that infects the heat of a body when it touches it. So he says. Thus a false religious person appears during the rain of carnality and through his bad example, extinguishes in others the gift of grace. This exemplar of a depraved life puts forth the milky yet poisonous pus of his teaching that afterwards more infects than converts his hearers. Isidore shows how harmful this poison is; he says that the poison of other snakes infects individuals. But the salamander kills many at the same time, so that if it has crept into a tree, it infects its fruits and kills all who eat them. If it falls into a well, it infects all those who drink from it. Thus an evil preacher, according to 'Anselm' in the *Book of likenesses*, although he instructs well in the manner of a physician, takes up a poisoned plant and infects both himself and others with it afterwards.

[277] The poison of pride rises up from the subtlety of wisdom and the craftiness of cunning, because that is properly the nature of a snake which, according to Pliny in *On animals* 1, is naturally cunning, just as

280   dicitur Genesis 3, 'Serpens erat callidior cunctis animantibus'.
Hoc uenenum + inficit omnes sapientes mundi, quorum
sapientiam d[escri]bit beatus Gregorius, 3 *Moralium* 10, 'Sapientia',
inquit, 'mundi est cor machinationibus tegere, sensum uerbis
uelare, que falsa sunt uera ostendere, que uera sunt falsa
285   demonstrare. Hanc qui sciunt, ceteros despiciunt; qui nesciunt,
subiecti et timidi in aliis mirantur [quod ipsi nesciunt]'. Tales
principem suum imitantur, qui de scientia superbiuit; qui,
secundum beatum Augustinum, *De ciuitate Dei*, capitulo 22,
'Dicitur *demon* Grece, a magnitudine scientie Latine, quia de
290   scientia superbiuit. Scientia enim que charitate non informatur
inflat in superbiam uanissime u[ent]ositatis'. Hec ille.

Attendere ergo debent falsi iudices et garruli aduocati, quia
scientia eorum sine charitate non est nisi uenenum et angelice
ruine occasio. Gregorius, libro *Moralium* 32, 'Cum', inquit 'Lucifer
295   ceteros claritate nature et subtilitate scientie excesserit, contra
Deum + elatus fuit, et ideo cecidit'. Attendant etiam quod hec
scientia terrena et diabolica + conceditur iis qui iudicio diuino
sunt magis contemptibiles in ecclesia Dei. Ad Corintiorum 6,
'Contemptibiles qui sunt in ecclesia, [illos] constituite ad
300   iudicandum'. Gregorius, libro *Moralium* 26, 'Qui minoris meriti
sunt et nullis magnorum donorum uirtutibus pollent, ipsi de
terrenis negociis iudicent'. ℂ

Superbie uirus intumescit ex lingue subtilitate et eloquentie
suauitate, et hoc est proprium serpenti, quia secundum Isidorum,
305   libro 12, nullum animal mouet ita cito linguam sicut serpens.
Ita enim subito mouetur ut una lingua uideatur tres lingue.

---

281 uenenum] *add* iam Sp • mundi] *om.* S   282 describit] distribuit p
282–83 sapientia … mundi] *om.* A   283 sensum] propositum G   284 uelare]
celare uel uelare CDL   286 subiecti et timidi] subici tumidi A • quod ipsi
nesciunt] *om.* AGSp   287 qui²] Tales enim demon qui L   289 Grece] *om.* A
290–91 Scientia … uentositatis] *after* 287 superbiuit L   291 uentositatis]
uiciositatis Sp
292 Attendere] Attendant G • debent falsi iudices et] debunt CDL, falsi iudices
et G   293 angelice] etiam CD, *om.* L   294 occasio] *om.* G   295 ceteros]
om. CDGL • nature et] seu A • scientie] *om.* L   296 elatus] eleuatus p
• Attendant] Attende ACDL   297 diabolica] *add* animalis Sp   299 ecclesia]
add Dei CGL (*a corr.* C) • illos] *om.* Sp   301 et nullis] *om.* CDLS
• magnorum] maiorum A • donorum] dominorum (?) L
305 animal] *om.* S   306 subito] cito et subito AL • mouetur] *add* lingua
serpentis AG • mouetur … lingue] mouet quod uidetur habere tres linguas.
Hoc Ysidorus ibi (*om.* L) CDL

it says in Gn 3:1, 'The serpent was more subtle than any of the beasts'. This poison infects all who are worldly wise, whose wisdom Gregory describes in *Morals* 3.10, where he says, 'The wisdom of this world is to cover one's heart in stratagems, to shroud the plain sense in verbiage, to show that false things are true, to prove that true things are false. Those adept in this wisdom despise others; those who don't know it, their fearful subjects, marvel at what they do not know, when it is displayed by others'. Such people mimic their chief, who became proud because of his knowledge; according to blessed Augustine, *On the city of God* 22, he is called *demon* in Greek, from 'the breadth of knowledge' in Latin, because he grew proud because of his knowledge. But that knowledge that is not informed by love is puffed up most vainly in pride about being emptily windy'. So he says.

[292] False judges and gabbing lawyers ought to pay attention to this, because their knowledge is only poison and the cause of the angel's fall, unless it shows love. Gregory, *Morals* 32, says, 'When Lucifer exceeded others in the brightness of his nature and the subtlety of his knowledge, he raised himself up against God, and therefore he fell'. They should also notice that this worldly and devilish knowledge is granted to those who in God's judgement are most to be despised in His church. 1 Cor. 6:4 says, 'Set them to judge who are the most despised in the church'. Gregory, *Morals* 26, says, 'Those who are lesser in merit and who are strong in none of those virtues that come from great gifts should judge about worldly transactions'. ℂ

[303] The poison of pride swells up from subtlety of the tongue and the pleasantness of eloquence, and this is appropriate for a snake, since as Isidore says in book 12, no animal moves its tongue as swiftly as a snake does. For it is moved so quickly that one tongue appears as if it were three.

Gloriari ergo de eo quod conceditur serpenti est imitari serpentem,
et hoc est uenenum ualde perniciosum in iis qui linguam uendunt.
Unde Tullius, libro 2 *De officiis*, 'Quid tam inhumanum quam

310   eloquentiam, a natura ad salutem homini datam, ad bonorum
perniciem pestemque conuertere'? Quere plus de ueneno lingue
infra, capitulo de inuidia et de detraccione. +

De triplici remedio contra superbiam.
Capitulum IIII.

Remedium [et tyriaca] superbie est humilitas, et sicut
uenenum [basilisci est difficilimum ad curandum, ita uenenum]

315   superbie, cui comparatur uenenum illius, et eius remedium est
ualde rarum, quia secundum Augustinum, 'Superbia est primum
uicium in accedendo et ultimum in recedendo'. Ideo notandum
quod contra uenenum basilisci est triplex remedium. Primum
+ est quod animal illud, quod occidit omne uenen[o], a sola

320   mustela uincitur, quia secundum Isidorum, libro 12, 'Ille conditor
rerum nihil nociuum sine remedio reliquit'. Unde secundum
Plinium, libro 8, mustella ducitur ad cauernam basilisci et
istam bestiam uenenatam timens, redit et rutam comedit, et ex
succo eius se perlinit et basiliscum inuadit et occidit. Item dicit

325   Isidorus, libro 12, quod mustela est mus longus. Unde nota hic:
mus significat humilem [uirum] qui uirtute herbe amare, id
est passionis dominice, expellit uirus superbie, quia secundum

---

307 imitari] mutari in G   308 iis] *add* maxime CDL   310 bonorum] horum S
311 plus] *om.* A   311–12 Quere … capitulo] De hac materia quere ubi agitur CD,
whole sentence om. L   312 infra capitulo] *om.* A   • detraccione] (?) dracone A;
pGS+BLaV *add (om.* ACDL+R):
     Quere de ueneno diuiciarum (*adds* infra in S) capitulo (infra p) de auaritia.

heading] Remedium contra superbiam A, Humilitas est remedium superbie CD,
     om. GS, Remedium contra uenenum superbie L
313 et tyriaca] *om.* Sp   314 uenenum … uenenum] uenenum Sp   316 primum] *add*
     et principale Gp   318–19 quod … sola] quod a ACDL   319 ueneno] uenenum p
     320 uincitur] *add* et occiditur ACDL   • conditor] doctor A   321 reliquit]
     condidit A   322 cauernam] cameram CD   • basilisci] *add* siue reguli ACDGL
     324 succo] sicco S   325 12] *adds* et dicit A, *add* et dicit ulterius CDL
     325–26 Unde … mus] *om.* G   326 mus mustela S   • humilem uirum qui]
     humilem uitam que CDL, humilem S, humilitatem qui p

To be glorified by something that is granted to a snake is to imitate a snake, and this is a very perverse poison in those who sell their tongues. For this reason, Cicero, *On duties* 2, says, 'What is more inhuman than to transform eloquence, given by nature for man's salvation, into a plague and the destruction of good things?' Look for more about the poison of the tongue below, in the chapter on envy and backbiting.

On the threefold remedy against pride.
Chapter 4.

[313] The remedy for and antidote to pride is humility. Just as the poison of a basilisk is most difficult to cure, so is the poison of pride, which is compared to its poison. Its remedy is quite rare, because, according to Augustine, 'Pride is the first vice that comes and the last to go away'. Therefore one should notice that there is a threefold remedy against the basilisk's poison. The first is that this animal that kills everything with its poison is conquered only by the weasel (mongoose). According to Isidore, book 12, 'The creator of all things left nothing harmful without a cure'. For this reason, according to Pliny, book 8, a mongoose is led to the basilisk's cave, and because it fears this poisonous beast, it goes back and eats some rue, and it smears itself with some rue-juice and attacks and kills the basilisk. Also Isidore says in book 12 that a mongoose is a long mouse. And thus notice: this mouse stands for a meek person who drives out the poison of pride through the power of a sour plant, that is of the Lord's passion. For according to

Augustinum, libro *De trinitate*, capitulo 4, 'Remedium elationis
est contuitus dominice crucis'. +

330   Secundum remedium est quod basiliscus seipsum uidendo
occidit. Dicit enim glossa super illud psalmi, 'Qui timent te
uidebunt me, etc.', 'Magna uirtus in oculis quod in naturalibus
apparet'. Basiliscus si prius uidet, occidit; si prius uidetur,
occiditur. Quod intellige a seipso, sicut narratur de Alexandro

335   quod quandam ciuitatem obsidens, amisit sine aliquo uulnere
multos milites. Et cum de hoc miraretur, responderunt
philosophi quod basiliscus erat super murum, cuius aspectu illi
interierunt. Tunc arte philosophorum speculum fuit eleuatum
et muro oppositum, et intuitus uenenosi animalis reflexus fuit

340   in seipsum et sic interiit. In hunc modum, summum remedium
elationis est consideratio proprie uanitatis, quia si queratur
quare homo superbit, bene respondetur, quia pondere uirtutis
deficit. +

Tertium remedium est quod, licet basiliscus sit

345   irremediabiliter uenenosus, tamen combustus et in cinerem
edactus, ueneni malitiam perdit. Immo cinis eius ad multa
ualet, et specialiter ad artem alquimie. In hunc modum,
superbus igne contriccionis [ad]ustus, se putredinem et futurum
cinerem recognoscens, uincit elationem. Hoc est ergo triplex

350   remedium superbie, scilicet con[sideratio] dominice passionis,
cuius peccator reus est; et consideratio proprie uanitatis,

---

329 contuitus] commemoratio L • crucis] passionis uel crucis A, passionis
CDL; pGS+V *add* **(following G)** (*om.* ACDL+LaR, *an expansiue analogous
explanation* B):
    Nota de aspectu serpentis enei, supra capitulo 2°
330 remedium] *add* contra basilisci uenenum CDL   **331** occidit] interficit CDL
    • psalmi] *om.* A   **333** Basiliscus] *add* namque CL (*a corr.* C)
333–34 si² … occiditur] *om.* D   **335** uulnere] ictu G   **336** responderunt]
dixerunt CDL   **337** murum] portam uel murum G • illi] *om.* A, milites ADL
339 et muro oppositum] et impositum curru ponebatur in oppositum basilisci
CDL, mouetur in oppositum et G   **340** et sic interiit] sicque sui intuitu se
occidit CDL, sicque sui intuitu G   **341** elationis] proprie elacionis ACD
proprie] *a corr.* CD)   **342** pondere] racio A, pondus CDL   **343** deficit]
GSp+BLaR *add* **(GV** *illeg.*; *om.* ACDL [A *at page-bound*]):
    Considerando (Confitendo S) ergo propriam (suam B) uanitatem recurrit
    (recurrere S) ad suam fragilitatem, et defectum suum percipiens repellit (p.r.]
    sic expellit B) elacionem (*adds* suam B).
344 remedium] *add* contra uenenum basilisci CGL (*a corr.* C)   **348** adustus]
combustus Gp   **351** consideratio] contuitus p   **351** proprie] *om.* A

Augustine, *On the trinity*, chapter 4, 'The cure for raising yourself unduly high is meditation on the Lord's passion'.

[330] The second cure is that the basilisk, when it sees itself, dies. Also the gloss on Ps 118:74, 'They that fear thee shall see me', says, 'There is great strength in the eyes, as appears in natural things'. A basilisk, if it sees first, it kills; if it sees itself first, it is killed. And you should understand this about yourself, just as the history tells about Alexander. When he was besieging a certain city, he lost many of his soldiers, and they were not apparently wounded. When he wondered about this, his philosophers answered that there was a basilisk on the town wall, through whose gaze they died. Then, following learned science, a mirror was raised up and placed opposite the wall, and the gaze of the poisonous beast was reflected on itself and thus it died. In this way, the best cure for being raised up is thought on one's own vanity, for if it were asked why a man gets puffed up, one might properly answer that it is because he lacks the weight of virtues [and floats away].

[344] The third cure is that, although the basilisk is incurably poisonous, nevertheless when it is burned and turned to ashes, it loses the virulence of its poison. For this reason, its ashes are constructive in many ways, particularly in the science of alchemy. In this way, a proud man, burned in the fire of contrition, and recognising his own rottenness and that he will become ashes [at his death], conquers his vanity. This is thus the triple remedy for pride, namely consideration of the Lord's passion, for which a sinner is guilty; and the consideration of one's own vanity,

quia ideo peccator superbit, quia omni uirtute est uacuus. Tertia
consideracio est scilicet sue uilis resolutionis siue mortis, quia
nullum animal habet tam uilem et horribilem mortem. Ideo
355   dicitur Ecclesiastici 10, 'Quid superbis, terra et cinis, etc.'? Hec
ergo tria contra omnes species superbie +.

Remedium contra uenenum salamandre, id est mali religiosi,
est incendium religionis admittere et uitam suam ad radium
superne gratie et illustracionis diuine conuertere. Unde Dionysius
360   ad Timotheum, 'Uerte te ad radium', scilicet superne gratie. Nota ad
hoc quod genus salamandre est, cuius pellis est uillosa et pilosa sicut
uituli marini, de qua cingulum in usus regum fit, quod postquam
diu est in usu iterum in ignem proiiciatur. Et tunc penitus per
ignem renouatur, et de hoc potest fieri [lychinus] in lampadibus et
365   lucernis, et nunquam corrumpitur. Sic + religiosus, ad disciplinam
religionis conuersus, fit lucerna incorruptibilis in ecclesia Dei.

De ueneno inuidie.
Capitulum U.

Uenenum inuidie sequitur uirus superbie, quia secundum
Augustinum, *De ciuitate Dei*, 'Per hoc quod quis est superbus,
fit inuidus'. Hoc uenenum comparatur aspidi, quia serpens
370   perniciossisimus aspergendo diffundit uenena. 'Ysos enim

352 quia ideo] quare CL (*a corr*; ? *further marg. corr. suggests* quia C), quare
non D, quanto ideo G, qua … ideo S • superbit] *om.* S • omni] eciam L
• Tertia consideracio est] Tercium est c. A, consideracioque CDGL
354 mortem] *add* Bene deberet reducere hominem de monte superbie ad
uallem humilitatis uere CDL   **356** tria] ibi A, *add* ualent CDL • superbie]
adds nota A; *add* GSp (*om.* ACDL)
    adepta triplici modo quo uincitur uenenum basilisci.
358 est] *adds* animi A • uitam] mentem S   **359** diuine] anime D, dominice L
360 ad Timotheum] *om.* ACDL, ad Ti. p   **361** salamandre] serpentis CDL
• sicut] *adds* pellis L   **362** in usus regum] regis S   **363** iterum] iterum
expunged C, *om.* L   **364** lychinus] lichini CL, lithini D, ellychnium p
365 religiosus] bonus religiosus GS, malus religiosus p   **366** religionis] *om.*
ACDL • lucerna] lucis A • incorruptibilis] *om.* S • Dei] *add* si in bono
fuerit perseuerans CDL

heading] De inuidia A, Uenenum inuidie CD, *om.* GS, De ueneno inuidie L
367 uirus] uenenum CDL, uirum G   **369** fit] est CDL, sit G   **370** perniciossimus]
perniciosus qui A • diffundit] fundit ACD • uenena] uenenum suum A
• Ysos] Yos ACDL

since a sinner grows proud only because he is empty of all virtues. And the third consideration is this, thinking about one's disgusting dissolution or death, for no other animal has so disgusting or terrifying a death. Therefore it says in Sir 10:9, 'Why is earth and ashes proud?' Thus, these three work against every kind of pride.

[357] The cure for the poison of the salamander, that is of the evil religious person, is to admit the fire of religion and to conform one's life to the beam of the highest grace and of divine illumination. For this reason, Dionysius wrote to Timothy, 'Turn to the light', that is of the highest grace. In this regard, notice that there is one kind of salamander whose skin is hairy and furry like a seacow's, and out of it is made a belt for kings to use. After it has been used for a long time, it is thrown back into the fire, and then it is completely renewed by the fire. From it, one can make a wick for lamps and lanterns, and it never wears out. Thus a religious person, when he is converted to the discipline of his order, is made an incorruptible light in God's church.

On the poison of envy.
Chapter 5.

[367] The poison of envy follows that of pride, because, as Augustine says, *On the city of God*, 'Whoever is proud will be envious as well'. This poison is compared to the asp, because it is a snake, most harmful in pouring out its poisons by casting them about. For *isos* in

Grece uenenum dicitur Latine', secundum Isidorum, libro 12;
unde dicitur aspis quasi 'aspergens uenenum'. Secundum Plinium,
libro 8, huic serpenti est hebes sensus uisus, quia oculos habet in
temporibus, non in fronte; et ideo non u[al]et aduersarium
375   directe set oblique [uidere]. Unde persequitur eum auditu et
olfactu. Talis est inuidus, qui nunquam potest uidere bonum
alicuius directe, set solo auditu uel olfactu unius infamie
persequitur bonorum famam.

Nota ergo quod Gregorius, libro *Moralium* 31, dicit quod
380   uenenum inuidie habet species quinque. Et secundum hoc,
inueniuntur diuerse species aspidis que diuersa habent uenena.
Primum uirus inuidie est, secundum Gregorium, latens odium,
cui respondet species aspidis que dicitur *hypnalis*, serpens
scilicet qui somno necat. Huius uenenum Cleopatra filia regis
385   Egypti, uxor Antonii imperatoris, post mortem mariti et stragem
suorum, ex odio presentis uite sibi apposuit et [somno] mortua
fuit. Similiter faciunt quibus prosperitas huius uite non succedit.
Unde seipsos perimere + coguntur, quid est crudelius quam
alium occidere. Uenenum ergo quod somno, scilicet interiori
390   studio sine nocumento alterius, necat est odium latens. Ideo
dicitur prime Ioannis 3, 'Qui odit fratrem suum homicida est',
scilicet sui [ipsius].

Secundum uirus inuidie, secundum Gregorium, est
susurracio, id est quedam eructacio malitie interioris, que
395   appetens bonum quod uidet in altero et non adi[pisc]ens, uisum
intendit interficere siue fascinare. Unde super illud ad Galatas 2,
'O insensati Galate quis uos fascinauit, etc.'; glossa: 'Fascinatio
uulgo dicitur corruptio oculorum que infantibus nocet.

---

372 Plinium] *corr. from* philosophum C, philosophum DS   373 uisus] *om.* S
(*at line end*)   374 fronte] fron A   • ualet] uidet (*and om.* uidere) AGSp
375 directe ... uidere] nisi oblique A   • directe] *adds* set oblique uidere potest L
377 uel olfactu] *om.* CDL   • unius] et cupidus A   378 bonorum] ualde false
(u.f.] *om.* A) uitam bonorum et ACDL   • famam] *add* quantum potest CDL
380 quinque] *om.* A   381 diuerse] quinque S   382 odium] *adds* in corde L
383 respondet] correspondet A   • species] *a corr.* C, *om.* D (*with* \aspis/ ille)
• serpens] *om.* A, *a corr.* CD   384 Huius] *add* aspidis ACDL   385 Antonii]
Antonini ACL   386 somno] *om.* ASp   388 coguntur] noscuntur C (*read as*
cognos-?), dicuntur | siue coguntur Sp   389 alium] *om.* L   390 studio] *add* in
corde CDL   • studio sine] scilicet studio uel A   392 ipsius] *om.* Sp
394 eructacio] eructuacio A   395 adipiscens] adhibens p   • uisum] nisum p
396 interficere] inficere A   397 Fascinatio] *adds* proprie siue A, *add* est proprie
sicut CDL

Greek means 'poison' in Latin; for this reason, it is called an asp, as if it were casting about (*aspergens*) its poison. According to Pliny, book 8, this snake has a weak sense of sight, because it has eyes in its temples, not in its forehead; therefore, it lacks the power to see its enemy head-on, but sees him only obliquely. For this reason, it pursues its victim by hearing and smell. An envious person is just like this: he can never see the good anyone does directly, but he pursues the fame of good men by the hearing and smell of slander alone.

[379] Therefore notice that Gregory, in *Morals* 31, says that the poison of envy has five species. And in accord with his view, there are diverse species of asp that have diverse poisons. The first poison of envy, according to Gregory, is hidden hatred; this corresponds to a species of asp that is called *hypnalis*, a snake that kills by putting its victim to sleep. Cleopatra, the daughter of the king of Egypt and wife of the emperor Antony, after the death of her husband and their overthrow, out of hatred for this present life put its poison on herself and died through sleep. Others act similarly who think no good times lie ahead in this life. For this reason, they feel compelled to kill themselves, an act more savage than killing another person. Therefore this poison that kills by sleep, that is by an inner anxiousness without harming anyone else, is hidden hatred. Therefore 1 Io 2:11 says, 'He that hateth his brother [is in darkness]' and a murderer, that is of himself.

[393] According to Gregory, the second poison of envy is insinuation, a certain belching forth of inner malice. Desiring the good he sees in some-one else but not attaining it himself, he intends to kill or bewitch the thing he has seen. For this reason, the gloss on Gal 3:1, 'O senseless Galatians, who hath bewitched you [that you should not obey the truth]', says, 'A disease of the eyes that harms infants is commonly called "bewitchment".

Similiter inuidia, tanquam fascinatio, bonum proximi urit'.

400   Hec ibi. Tanta est enim malitia in corde hominis ut radius
oculorum inde exiens bonum quod uidet in altero inficit, ita
quod creatura uirtutem et pulchritudinem amittat. Dicit enim
Auicenna quod oculus fascinantis camelum proicit in foueam.
Cui concordat scriptura, Sapientie 4, 'Fascinatio malignitatis

405   obscurat bona', quia eneruat bona naturalia et diminuit per
detraccionem et uenenosam e[mulat]ionem bona gratuita. Cui
respondet quiddam genus aspidis que dicitur *dipsas*, que Latine
dicitur situla, quia quem momorderit siti p[erim]it +. Sic inuidia
in corde fascinantis siti bonitatis [ui]se interimit inuidendo.

410   Ecclesiastici 13, 'Nequam est oculus inuidi'. Unde dicitur in
Polycratico, libro primo, capitulo 4, 'Secundum Plinium, quod
in [Illy]ricis quidam homines nascuntur qui solo uisu interimunt,
quos diutius irati uident'. Et hoc habetur in glosa super illud
psalmi, 'Qui t[i]ment te uidebunt me, etc.', ubi dicitur quod radii

415   exeunt per oculos usque ad rem uisam, que uel a iusto conferunt
rei uise uel ab iniusto inficiunt.

Tertium uirus inuidie est exultatio in aduersis proximi, scilicet
quando patitur, applaudendo suis aduersitatibus ut plus patiatur,
quam Iob excludens a se dicit, 'Si gauisus est ad ruinam proximi',

420   Iob 31. Istud uirus comparatur aspidi que dicitur *hemorrhois*,
sic dicta quia illius sanguinem [sugit quem mordet. Sic inuidus
sanguinem illius sugit] cuius bonitatem extinguere intendit. Sed
quando non preualet +, magis sibi nocet. Unde narratur in historia
Alexandri Magni quod Permeneon, magister militie Alexandri,

---

399 inuidia] in malicia S   **400** hominis] *add* mali CDL   • radius] *adds* in
corde L   **401** oculorum] occulte S   **405** obscurat] *adds* uel obfuscat (*an int.
corr.*) C, obfuscat L   • quia] que fascinacio scilicet inuidia CDL   • et] et dirimit
et CDL   • diminuit] d+fiue minims+t G   **406** et uenenosam emulationem]
om. S, et uenenosam euulsiooonem [*sic*] p   **407** respondet] corespondet CD
• dicitur] uocatur ACDL   • dipsas] *add* Grece ACDL   **408** perimit] perimit
et occidit GS, punit et occidit p   **409** uise] in se ADGL, se p   • inuidendo]
inuidum A   **412** in Illiricis] in hililicis A, in Illirico G, *om.* L, in Hibernicis S,
in hildricis p   **413** in glosa] *om.* L   **414** timent] tement p   **415** uel] nichil G
416 rei uise] *om.* S
418 quando patitur] quando inuidus non compatitur CDL   • patiatur]
placeatur A   **419** quam] *add* exultacionem CDG   • Iob] *a corr.* C, *om.* D
420 aspidi] *om.* A   **421** sic dicta] *om.* A   **421–22** sugit … sugit] *om.* Sp
421 sugit] scitit A, *a corr.* C, fugit D   • mordet] *adds* aspis emeroys A
422 illius] *om.* A, suum DL   • sugit] scitit A, sitit DGLSp   **423** preualet] *adds*
alii G, *adds* aliquando S, *adds* alium ledere p   **424** militie] *om.* CDL

Similarly, envy, as if it were a bewitchment, burns up one's neighbour's goods'. For there is so much malice in a man's heart that the visual ray going forth from the eyes infects the good that one sees in someone else so that that creature loses both virtue and beauty. Also Avicenna says that a bewitching conjurer's eye throws a camel into a pit. He agrees with scripture, since Sap 4:12 says, 'The bewitching of vanity obscureth good things', because it weakens natural goods and diminishes those that come from grace through detraction and poisonous rivalry. This corresponds to a specific species of asp, one called *dipsas* (and *situla* in Latin), because it kills the person it has bitten with thirst (*siti*). Likewise, envy in a bewitching heart in its envying kills by its thirsty desire for the good it has seen. Sir 14:8, 'The eye of the envious is wicked'. For this reason, it says in *Polycraticus* 1.4, 'According to Pliny, there are some men born among the Illyrians who kill with their sight alone, because in their wrath they can see very far'. And in the gloss on Ps 118:74, 'They that fear thee shall see me', it says that rays pass out from the eyes so far as the thing seen, and these, if they come from a just person, strengthen the thing seen, and if from an evil person, infect it.

[417] The third poison of envy is rejoicing in bad things befalling one's neighbour, for instance, when he suffers, in applauding his ill fortune so that he suffers more. Job refuses to do this, when he says (31:29), 'If I have been glad at the downfall of my neighbour'. This poison is compared to the asp that is called *hemorrhois*; it is called this because it sucks out the blood of the person whom it bites. Likewise the envious person sucks out the blood of the person whose goodness he wishes to extinguish. But when he does not prevail, he hurts himself more. For this reason, the history of Alexander the Great tells that Parmeneon, the master of Alexander's host,

425   [Philippo] physico illius inuidens propter familiaritatem regis, tempore quo sibi ministrabat pocula recupande salutis, epistolam [talem] scripsit regi quod physicus ob fauorem Darii intendebat eum intoxicare. Sed Alexander, epistola posita ad caput lecti, poculum sumpsit et postmodum epistolam legendam physico

430   tradidit. Cum ergo Alexander sanitatem recuperasset, physicus de inuido et mendace iusticiam petiit. Unde rex Permeneonem pena capitis puniri iussit. Sic inuidus qui querit proximo aduersitatem incurrit eandem. Hec est inuidia fratrum Ioseph que fecit eos eidem seruire.

435   Quartum uirus inuidie, secundum Gregorium, est affliccio in prosperis proximi, cum blasphemia et iniuria creatoris qui tales exaltat. Cui respondet aspis que dicitur *prester*, horribilis ualde, quia secundum Papiam et Isidorum, libro 12, semper ore patente et uirus euaporante incedit. Sic inuidus nunquam bene potest

440   loqui, nec Deo regratiari propter bonum proximi. Et de hoc dicit Seneca, 'Utinam oculus inuidi esset in qualibet ciuitate ut propter bonum, scilicet cuiuslibet, torqueretur?' Unde poeta, 'Inuidus alterius rebus marcessit optimis'. Talis est linx, animal scilicet lupo simile, cuius urina, secundum Plinium, libro 8, conuertitur

445   in gemmam preciosam que ligurius uocatur. Unde bestia illa, hoc sciens et inuidens quod urina sua in usum hominum deueniat, quando mingit, sub arena urinam suam abscondit. Sed ibi cicius consolidatur [in gemmam preciosam], secundum Plinium, ubi supra, capitulo 29 et Isidorum, libro 12, sed bestia de hoc

450   torquetur. Sic inuidus, Iob 5, 'Paruulum occidit inuidia', ubi Gregorius ponit signa sui doloris, que sunt hec: 'Color pallore afficitur, oculi deprimuntur, mens accenditur, membra frigescunt,

---

425 Philippo] *om.* Ap, philosopho CDLS • regis] *add* qui regi CDGL
426 sibi] *add* phisicus suus CD • recuperande salutis] causa (*a corr.* D) recuperande sanitatis (salutis L) CDL   **427** talem] statu <…> G, *om.* p
428 posita] apposita CDG   **429** poculum] potum A • epistolam] *om.* S • physico] *om.* A   **431** mendace] *adds* animose G   **432** querit] *add* malum aduersum CDL   **434** eidem] *a corr.* C, eisdem L; *add* postea CDL
436 cum] *om.* CDL   **437** *prester*] priscus G   **439** bene] bona A, uerum CDL
440 propter] nec audire CDL • dicit] *om.* CDL   **443** rebus, optimis] opimus G, opimis S • Talis] Inuidus autem talis CDL, Et uidet illius prospera cum lacrimis talis G   **445** preciosam] preciosissimam G • ligurius] ligurinus A
• uocatur] nominatur ACDL   **447** quando mingit] *om.* D   **448** in gemmam preciosam] *om.* AGSp, et fit gemma ut predicitur preciosa L   **449** sed] et addit CL, et addidit D • bestia] *om.* D   **450** Gregorius] glossa A • Color] uirtus et color L

envied Alexander's physician Philip because of his close relations with the king. So at a time when he gave Alexander a drink to restore his health, Parmeneon wrote the king a letter to the effect that the physician intended to poison him in order to gain Darius's good will. But Alexander placed the letter at the head of his bed and took the drink; afterwards, he gave the physician the letter to read. Therefore when Alexander had regained his health, the physician sought justice for this deceitful envy, and the king ordered Parmeneon to be beheaded as a punishment. Likewise, the envious person who seeks ill-fortune for his neighbour receives the same thing. This is the envy of Joseph's brothers, which caused them to become his servants (Gn 37:3–11).

[435] According to Gregory, the fourth poison of envy is distress at the good things that befall one's neighbour. This is accompanied by blasphemy and an injury to God, who has raised up these people. This corresponds to the truly terrifying species of asp called *prester*; according to Papias and Isidore in book 12, it always goes about with its mouth open and steaming poison. Likewise, an envious person can never speak well of others, nor thank God for any good thing that happens to his neighbour. Seneca says of this, 'Shouldn't an envious person's eye be in every city so that it may be tormented by everyone else's good fortune?' And the poet Horace says, 'Envy pines at the very good things that befall someone else'. An envious person is like the lynx, an animal resembling the wolf, whose urine, according to Pliny, book 8, is changed into a precious gem that is called *ligurius*. For this reason, this beast, aware of the outcome and being envious because its urine might become useful to men, when it pisses, it hides its urine under sand. But there it hardens into a gem very quickly, according to Pliny, in the same place, chapter 29, and Isidore in book 12, and the beast is further tormented by this. An envious person is like that; Iob 5:2 says, 'Envy slayeth the little one'. In his discussion of that passage, Gregory gives the signs of the envious person's sorrow: 'His complexion becomes pale, and his eyes are cast down; his mind is inflamed, and his limbs grow cold.

fit in cogitatione rabies, in dentibus stridor, dolor in corde, que
faciunt cecitatem in mente'.

455   Quintum uirus inuidie, secundum Gregorium, est detractio.
Cui respondet aspis que dicitur *seps*, serpens ualde uenenosus qui
cum hominem momoderit, statim eum destruit et consummit ita
ut in ore eius totaliter liquefiat. Nec solum corpus set etiam ossa
ueneno suo dissipat. Talis est detractor, in cuius ore lique[sc]it et
460   adnichilatur omnis uirtus proximi. Et secundum Plinium, libro 8,
hic aspis supra modum diligit comparem suum, quia detractor
defendit et diligit detractorem. Et de talibus dicit psalmus,
'Uenenum aspidum sub labiis eorum'. [Detractor etiam aspidi
comparatur, de quo in psalmo, 'Sicut aspidi surde obturantis
465   aures', scilicet ibi dicit] glossa, 'Recte aspidi comparatur, qui non
uult audire preceptum legis', illud scilicet Deuteronomii 19,
'Surdo, id est absenti, non maledices'.

       Et nota quod lingua detractoris est serpentina, quia
secundum philosophum, lingua serpentis est liuida et nigra et ad
470   mouendum uelocissima, et hoc propter fu[rio]sitatem uenenosam
que non permittit eam quiescere. Sic lingua detractoris, propter
uenenum inuidie agitantis, nunquam potest a detractione
quiescere. Iacobi 3, 'Lingua est plena ueneno mortifero'. Et ut
dicit Isidorus, libro 12, ui ueneni ita agitatur ut serpens, qui non
475   habet nisi unam linguam, uidetur habere tres +. Sic detractor tres
uidetur habere linguas, quando simul, secundum [Bernardum],
tres occidit, [ipsum scilicet qui loquitur, et de quo loquitur, et
etiam cui loquitur]. Ideo detractor recte [compar]atur serpens.

---

453 fit] sit CG • cogitacione] cogitante (*a corr.*), C, cogitantes L
456 respondet] corespondet ACDL • aspis] serpens ACDL • seps] aspis ACD
• serpens ualde uenenosus] qui ualde uenenosus est AL, *om.* CD
457 destruit] detrahit A • et consumit] *om.* S   **458** liquefiat] lu|crificat S
• corpus] carnem corporis CDL   **459** liquescit] liquefit \uel liquescit/ (*an int.
corr.*) C, liquefit DGp   **460** omnis] *om.* A   **462** et diligit] *om.* GS
463–65 Detractor ... dicit] *om.* AGSp   **466** audire] *om.* A • preceptum] uerba,
and add preceptum *after* scilicet ACDL
468 est] *adds* lingua A   **469** mouendum] modum S   **470** et] *a corr.* C, *om.* D
• furiositatem] ferocitatem ACDL, fumositatem GS, feruositatem p
472 nunquam] unquam C   **473** est] eius CDGL • ueneno] *adds* eciam,
expunged C, *adds* eciam D   **474** 12] *add* lingua serpentis CDGL • ut] *add*
quasi CDL   **475** tres] *add* linguas Ap   **476** quando] quia CGS • Bernardum]
illam Sp   **477–78** ipsum ... loquitur] *om.* ASp • et de quo ... loquitur] et
eciam audientem L   **477** recte] non immerito CDGL • comparatur] uocatur Sp

His thoughts become furious; he gnashes his teeth and is sad at heart – all of which render him mentally blind'.

[455] According to Gregory, the fifth poison of envy is backbiting. This corresponds to the species of asp that is called *seps*, an extremely poisonous snake that, when it has bitten a man, it immediately destroys him and consumes him to such a degree that he melts completely in the snake's mouth. With its poison, it wastes not just the body but even the bones. A backbiter is just like this: in his mouth every virtue of his neighbour melts and is reduced to nothing. According to Pliny in book 8, this kind of asp loves his mate excessively, because one backbiter loves and defends another one. Ps 13:3 says of such people, 'The poison of asps is under their lips'. Also the backbiter is compared with an asp, as Ps 57:5 says, 'Like the deaf asp that stoppeth her ears'. The gloss on the verse says, 'The person who doesn't wish to hear the command of the law is properly compared to an asp', which is referring to Lv 19:14, 'Thou shalt not speak evil of the deaf'[, that is of a person who is absent].

[468] And notice that a backbiter's tongue is snakelike, because according to Aristotle, a snake's tongue is 'black and blue' and exceedingly swift in its movement; that is because of the poisonous fury that does not allow it to be still. Likewise, a backbiter's tongue can never rest in its backbiting because of the envious poison that agitates it. Iac 3:8 says, 'The tongue is full of deadly poison'. And as Isidore says in book 12, the snake is so stirred by the strength of its poison that it appears to have three tongues, although it really has only one. Likewise, a backbiter appears to have three tongues, since, according to Bernard, he can kill three people at the same time, namely the speaker himself, the person he speaks about, and the hearer to whom he speaks. Therefore a backbiter is properly compared to a snake.

Ecclesiastes 8, 'Si momorderit serpens in + silentio, nihil minus
480   eo habet qui [occulte] detrahit'. + Et nota quod Auicenna, libro
De uenenis, dicit quod uenenum masculi acucius percutit, sed
femina plures habet dentes, quia secundum philosophum,
De animalibus, femina est magis inuida.

Secundo, dicit Auicenna quod uenenum senum peius est
485   quam iuuenum, quia inueterata malitia est in senibus. [Unde seni
malo dicit] Danielis 3, ['Inueterate dierum malorum']. Tertio,
dicitur quod + acutius est uenenum habitantium in montibus et in
syluis quam in pratis, ut intelligas quod acutius pungunt solitarii
et religiosi quam seculares actiui. Quarto, dicitur quod peius est
490   uenenum quod infunditur a ieiunis et uacuis quam repletis, ut
intelligas quod magis et lethaliter pungunt hypocrite abstinentes
quam [uiri] sociales.

479 8] *add* ubi dicitur CDG   •   in] in occulto siue in Sp   **480** occulte] *om.* Gp
•   detrahit] *add* Sp+B (*om.* ACDGL+LaRV):
Unde uersus (U.u.] *om.* S+B), 'Qui mel in ore gerit et me retro (tergo B)
pungere querit / Eius (Ei B) amicitiam nolo michi sociam'
481 masculi] masculinum CDL   •   acucius] non acucius A   •   percutit]
penetrat CDL   •   sed] *om.* A, quam feminum CDL, licet G   **482** femina] *add*
serpens CDL
484 Secundo dicit] Dicit eciam LS (*the first of a series of variants involving the
numbered points of the paragraph, here ignored*)   **485** senibus] serpentis S
485–86 Unde … dicit] *om.* Gp   •   Unde … malorum] Daniel A, *om.* S
486 dicit Danielis] \dicit/ Daniel dicitur C (*the inserted '3' has been misplaced
after* Danielem *in the subsequent addition, but* L *there reads* inuidia, Danielis
iii), Danielis [ ] dicitur D (*and has blank after* Danielis, *with* \3/)   •   malorum]
add nota de inuidia (iudicibus A) contra Danielem ACDL   **487** acutius]
actiuius p   •   uenenum] *adds* serpentum, *a corr.* C   •   habitantium] serpentis
qui habitat L   **488** quam] *add* habitancium ACDL   •   pratis] *add* uel in planis
CDL   •   quod] quando CDG, quod quando L   •   acucius] *om.* L   •   pungunt]
add uiri ACDL   •   solitarii] *add* qui deberent esse contemplatiui CDL, *adds
further* magis letaliter pungunt per inuidiam L   **489** seculares] *add* et ACDL
490 et uacuis] *om.* S   **491** lethaliter] letanter A, latenter G   **491** uiri] *om.* Sp
•   sociales] sodales G

Ecl 10:11 says, 'If a serpent bite in silence, he is nothing better that backbiteth secretly'. Notice that Avicenna, in his book *On poisons*, says that the male snake's poisons penetrate more sharply, but female snakes have more teeth, because Aristotle in *On animals* says that females are more envious.

[484] Second, Avicenna says that the poison of old snakes is worse than that of young ones, because the old have practised malice for a long time. For this reason, in Dn 13:52, he says to the wicked old man, 'Thou that art grown old in evil days'. Third, Avicenna says that the poison of snakes that live in mountains or in woods is more penetrating than that of those who live in meadows. From this, you should understand that solitaries and other religious people pierce more sharply than do people active in worldly affairs. Fourth, he says that the poison poured out by fasting and empty snakes is worse than that from full ones so that you should understand that fasting hypocrites pierce more deeply and harmfully than do people socially engaged.

De triplici remedio contra inuidiam et quibus inuidia comparetur et quanta mala ex ea sunt orta.
Capitulum UI.

Remedium et tyriaca ueneni inuidie est caritas, que considerat
in [homine] identitatem diuine imaginis et expellit omne uirus
495   iniquitatis. Unde Martianus narrat quod aspis non nocet Afris
et Mauris; immo pueros sibi natos, si habent eos suspectos quod
sunt de adulterio nati, exponunt aspidi, et si non sunt sui, statim
perimuntur; alioquin nihil mali senciunt. Dicit etiam Plinius,
libro 8, quod 'anguis siue serpens circa Eufratem terre incolis non
500   nocent, nec infestant eos dormientes; alios autem cuiuscumque
gentis homines cruciant. Et dicit ibidem quod aspis compari suo
interfecto, zelo ultionis persequitur interfectorem ut perimat;
[permeat] omnes difficultates terrarum et aquarum, [et illum
solum in medio agmine nosc]ens, nititur de morte comparis
505   uindicari'. Hec ille. Crudelior ergo et malignior est omni serpente,
quod hominem diuina imagine insignitum et eodem commercio,
scilicet Cristi precioso sanguine, redemptum persequitur
per inuidiam.
Secundum remedium contra inuidiam est zelus mystici
510   corporis et odium iniquitatis. Ad quod nota quod lingua
aspidis, quamuis in corpore uiuentis serpentis plena sit ueneno
mortifero, separata tamen a corpore et desiccata, uenenum
perdit – immo ad uenenum, si presens fuerit, [prodit, quia] in

heading] *om.* AGS, Remedium inuidie est caritas CD, Remedium contra
inuidiam L
493 considerat] consistit CDL   **494** in homine] *add* per CDL, primo in GSp
• identitatem] *adds* uel ueritatem (*int. corr.*) C   **495** iniquitatis] uanitatis A,
a corr. C, iniquitans L   **496** pueros sibi] *om.* G • sibi] ibi A   **498** alioquin]
aliter AL   **499** circa] contra CS   **500** nocent] ledent A, ledit CDGL   **501** gentis
homines] generis sunt ACDL • compari] cum pare L   **502–3** ut perimat
permeat] permeat ACDGL, ut perimat Sp   **503** et aquarum] *om.* S
503–4 et illum … noscens] paruipendens Sp   **504** agmine noscens] agmine
(?angmine A) cognoscens AG, agit nocens L   **506** insignitum] signatum A
507 precioso] *om.* ACDL • persequitur] perdet G   **508** per inuidiam]
corporaliter uel spiritualiter ut occidat CDL
511 quamuis] *om.* GS • uiuentis] *om.* A • serpentis] *om.* ACDL   **512** mortifero]
om. S   **513** perdit] amittit ACDL • immo ad] immo et A, nec solum hoc set
et aliud CDL, immo aliud G • prodit] perdit A • prodit quia] *om.* Sp, *add* in
presencia ueneni ACDGL, *adds further* si serpens fuerit G

On the triple remedy against envy and with what envy should be
compared and of the many evils that have their roots there.
Chapter 6.

[493] The remedy and antidote to the poison of envy is charity. It
considers our common identity as humans with the divine image, and
thus it expels every sinful poison. For this reason, Martianus tells that the
asp does not harm either Africans or Moors; indeed, if they suspect that
their newborn children have been born from an adulterous relationship,
they expose them to the asp, and if they are not their own, they die
immediately; otherwise, they do not consider them evil. Also Pliny says in
book 8 that worms and snakes that live near the Euphrates do not harm
the inhabitants of that country nor attack them while they are sleeping;
but they torment other men, whatever their nation. He also says there that
if its mate has been killed, the asp, in its eagerness for vengeance, pursues
the killer so that he can kill him; it passes through all difficulties thrown
up by earth or water, and recognising the killer alone, even if he is in the
middle of a crowd, it attempts to be avenged for its mate's death. So he
says. Therefore an envious person is crueler and more evil than any snake,
because in his envy he pursues a person who is marked with the divine
image and redeemed by the same exchange as himself, that is by the
precious blood of Christ.

[509] The second remedy against envy is zeal for the mystical
body and the hatred of sin. In this regard, notice that an asp's tongue,
although when it is in the living body of the snake is full of deadly poison,
nevertheless when it is separated from the body and dried, it loses its
poison – indeed, it is beneficial, because in the presence of venom, it

sudorem prorumpere consueuit. Tamen quamuis prius sit
515   uenenosa, ita tamen post fit preciosa quod inter thesauros regi[o]s
computetur. Et per hoc nota quod, cum omnes nascantur filii
ire, illi qui per gratiam Christi sunt conuersi et per penitenciam
desiccati nullum debent habere uenenum inuidie; immo ex
amore intimo cordis et compassione, debent compati omnium
520   aliene miserie.
    Tertium remedium est consideratio humane fragilitatis,
tam scilicet aliene in peccando. Unde Gregorius, 'Excusa, si
potes, intentionem; si non potes, excusa factum; puta casum,
puta ignorantiam, puta surreptionem, quam etiam proprie
525   [fragilitatis] in male iudicando'. Unde dicit Plinius, ubi supra,
quod natura aspidi dedit sensum uisus hebetem et quod oculos
dedit ei in temporibus, non in fronte. Et ideo non potest uidere
aduersarium directe, sed oblique. Hec ille. Sic est de homine
inuido, eo quod nullam uirtutem [proximi] iudicat + recte,
530   sed sicut Iudei Christum, 'speciosum [forma] (ad literam)
pre filiis hominum', reputabant leprosum. Et + debet inuidus
imputare suo malo iudicio, si uidet defectum in proximo. Hec
est ergo tyriaca inuidie charitas, que considerat identitatem
imaginis, utilitatem et indigentiam mystici corporis +, et proprie
535   fragilitatis considerationem.
    Nota quod ad uenenum aspidis qui dicitur *spuens*, qui
scilicet sputo inficit, nullum remedium ualet, nisi combustio uel

514 Tamen … prius] Unde quamuis primo A, quia cum prius CDL, Quia
quam|uis G   **515** ita … fit] postea tamen fuit A   •   regios] regum CDL, regis Sp,
add cum haberi poterit CDL   **516** cum] quamuis A   •   nascantur] nascimur
ACDL, *adds* natura A   **518** habere] *om. and add* in se pati manere *after* inuidie
CDL   **519** et] *add* uera CDL   •   compassione] contricione L   •   debent] *a corr.* C,
om. D

521 remedium] *adds* contra inuidiam L   **522** scilicet] *adds* sue quam G
   523 intentionem] temptacionem G   •   puta casum] *om.* S   **524** etiam] *adds*
habet G   **525** fragilitatis] *om.* Sp   •   dicit] *a corr.* C, *om.* D   **526** dedit] *adds*
quantum ad *and later reads* sensum proprium G   •   uisus] *om.* S   •   hebetem]
ebes A, ebetudinem CD, ebetem uisum L, hebetes S   **526–27** quod … ideo]
om. L   **527** dedit] Dei S   **528** homine] *om.* S   **529** proximi] Christi p, C
a corr.   •   recte] directe AGLSp   **530** forma] *om.* Sp   •   ad literam] *om.* S
   531 reputabant] iudicauerunt CDL   •   Et] *add* ideo AG, *adds* non Lp
   533 charitas] *om.* L   •   considerat] considerare debet unionem humane nature
cum diuina quod est considerare G   **534** corporis] *adds* communionem Sp
   •   et proprie] *both corrs.* C, *both om.* D   •   proprie] humane G
   535 considerationem] miseriam humane A, condicionem G
536 *spuens*] serpens spuens G

customarily breaks into a sweat. Although it is first poisonous, it later becomes precious so that it may be accounted among royal treasures. In this regard notice that although all are born as children of wrath, those who are converted through Christ's grace and dried out through penance should have no poison of envy; indeed, out of the deepest love of their heart and out of their compassion, they ought to share the sufferings of all other people in a wretchedness not properly their own.

[521] The third remedy is the consideration of human frailty, especially that of others in their sinfulness. For this reason, Gregory says, 'If you are able, excuse the intention; if you are not able, at least excuse the deed. Imagine the circumstance, imagine the ignorance, imagine the trickery, not to mention your own weakness in judging poorly'. For this reason, Pliny, as cited above, says that nature has given the asp a weak sense of sight and that she has given it eyes in its temples, not its forehead. Therefore it cannot see its enemy directly but obliquely. So he says. The envious person is similar, because he judges no virtue of his neighbour properly but judges just like the Jews who accounted Christ a leper [alluding to Isa 53:4], rather than, as the text says (Ps 44:3), 'beautiful above the sons of men'. And an envious person, if he sees a defect in his neighbour, ought to impute it to his bad judgement. Therefore charity is the antidote to envy, since it considers our identity with the divine image, the usefulness and our need for the mystical body, and the consideration of our own weakness.

[536] Notice that no remedy avails against the poison of the asp called *spuens*, the one that infects with its saliva, except for burning or

precisio membri infecti. Ita enim ui[o]lentem est illud uenenum
quod interficit omne uiuum quod tangit. Sic nullum remedium
540   est contra uenenum detractionis, nisi amputatio membri
inficientis corpus mysticum Christi. ₡

De ueneno ire.
Capitulum UII.

Uenenum ire recte est appropriatum uermi qui dicitur buffo,
quod est genus rane perniciosissimum, quia ira humane nature
inter omnia uitia est magis contrarium. Unde Seneca, libro 1
545   *De ira*, 'Hominis natura nihil mitius, ira nihil crudelius; homine
nihil amantius, ira nihil infestius'. Et nota, secundum Gregorium,
libro 31 *Moralium*, '[Differentie] ire sunt tumor mentis, indignatio,
contumelia, rixa, clamor, blasphemia'. Nota ergo quod tumor
mentis est primus effectus ire. Similiter buffo inter omnes
550   serpentes magis intumescit, quia ad omnem tactum, et quanto
plus tangitur, tanto magis intumescit. Sic est de irato: [quanto
plus sibi respondetur, tanto plus se consumit]. Et ideo secundum
Seneca, libro 3 *De ira*, 'Ira est miserabilior omni uicio, nam
auaricia acquirit unde quis melior sit, sed ira i[mp]endit.

538 precisio] incisio S • uiolentem] uirulentem Ap 539 interficit] inficit
CDGS 540 membri] *adds* infecti uel G 541 Christi] *adds* Similiter est de
ueneno illius quidam serpens (for *seps*?) A, *adds* Similiter dicit de ueneno illius
qui dicitur *and expunged* C, *adds* Similiter dic de ueneno illius qui dicitur *and*
cancelled D, *adds* Similiter dicitur de ueneno illius qui dicitur seps G

heading] *om.* AGS 542 recte] *om.* ACDL • dicitur] uocatur CDGL
543 perniciossimum] *add* et humane nature ualde contrarium (u. c.]
contrariosissimum L). Qui buffo (*a corr.* C, *om.* D) bene comparatur uitio ire
CDL 545 ira] *adds* in A, *adds* libro 1 S • mitius] uiciosius A 546 amantius]
amabilius CDL • nota] est notandum C (*a corr.*), *om.* DG 547 Differencie ire
sunt] Diuerse sunt species ire (*a corr.*) C, diuerse \fiunt/ species \ire/ D, effectus
ire sunt GSp, differencie siue || species ire sunt L • tumor] timor D (also 548)
549 Similiter] Ira enim ut predicetur buffoni comparatur quia ADL;
adds eciam, *expunged* C; *adds* eciam D • omnes] *a corr.* C, *om.* G
550 intumescit] *corr. from* tumescit C, tumescit DG • tactum] *adds*
intumescit G, tractatum L 551 irato] *add* homine (*om.* L) seu iracundo CL
(*a corr.* C), iracundo DG 551, 552 plus] magis ... magis G 551–52 quanto ...
consumit] *om.* Sp 554 acquirit] querit L • sed ira impendit] *om. here* CDL
• impendit] incendit AGSp

cutting off the infected limb. Its poison is so virulent that it kills anything alive that it touches. Likewise, there is no remedy against the poison of backbiting except to cut off the infecting limb from the mystical body of Christ. ₡

On the poison of wrath,
Chapter 7.

[542] The poison of wrath is properly associated with that vermin called a toad, a most harmful kind of frog, because among all the vices, wrath is most contrary to human nature. For this reason, Seneca, *On anger* 1, says, 'There is nothing meeker than human nature, and nothing more savage than wrath; nothing more loving in a person, and nothing more aggressive than wrath'. And notice that, according to Gregory, *Morals* 31, 'Wrath is distinguished as swelling of the mind, indignation, scornful words, quarrelling, outcry, and blasphemy'. Therefore you should notice that swelling of the mind is the first effect of wrath. Similarly, the toad swells up more than all other snakes, and it does so whenever it is touched, because the more it is touched, the more it swells up. And so it is with an angry person: the more anyone responds to him, the more he consumes himself. And therefore, according to Seneca, *On anger* 3, 'Wrath is more wretched than any other vice, because avarice acquires things through which an avaricious person may appear better, but wrath just wastes its resources.

555   Luxuria sua uoluptate fruitur; hec autem, scilicet ira, alieno
malo gaudet'. ₡

Item secundus effectus ire est indignacio. Gregorius super
illud Iob 'Uirum stultum etc.', 'Ire sue stimulis cor accensum
palpitat, corpus tremit, lingua se prepedit, facies ignescit,
560   exasperantur oculi, et nequaquam cognoscuntur amici'. Et addit
quod '[Tunc] non differ[un]t iratus et phreneticus'. Similiter
buffonis conditio est quod oculos habet igneos et lucentes,
et est tanto perniciosior, quanto aspectus eius est ardentior.
Non multum ergo differunt iratus et buffo. Unde secundum
565   Gregorium, ubi supra, 'Cum mansuetudo per iram amittitur,
diuine imaginis similitudo uiciatur'. Unde sequitur quod sit non
homo; secundum Boetium, libro *Consolacionis*, 'Induit formam
bestie cuius mores imitatur'.

Tertius effectus ire est contumelia, que extinguit lumen
570   ueritatis in homine. Unde secundum Gregorium, ubi supra, 'Dum
perturbata mens iudicium sue rationis exasperat, quicquid furor
sibi suggerit, rectum putat'. Unde tunc nihil bone [ratione] uite
uel fame inuenit in proximo quod non maculet. Et hec est una
conditio buffonis, secundum Plynium, libro 8, quod licet habeat
575   clar[os oculos], solem tamen odit, et loca fetida diligit, in paludibus
habitat, et odorifera fugit, quia irato nihil de proximo redolet.

Quartus ire effectus est rixa, que in homine irato et illo
irascitur, extinguit omnem ardorem charitatis et deuocionis. Unde
Gregorius, ubi supra, 'Per iram penitus gratia socialis uite amittitur'.
580   Et tunc + iratus buffoni comparatur. Refert enim Plynius, ubi supra,

---

555 hec … ira] set ira proprium subiectum incendit et CDL   **556** gaudet] *add*
Unde Iob 5 uirum stultum interficit (occidit L) iracundia CDL
557 ire] *a corr.*, est *expunged* D   **558** Uirum stultum etc.] predictum G
• accensum] *om.* S   **559** corpus tremit] cor cremat L   • se prepedit] prepeditur
ACDGL   • ignescit] nigrescit A   **560** cognoscuntur amici] recognoscuntur |
noti S   • addit] *add* ibidem Gregorius dicens CL (*int. corr.* C), quod S
561 Tunc] Totum id est totaliter p   • differunt] differt ALSp   **562** igneos]
ignitos ACDL   • lucentes] succensos S   **563** tanto] *om.* D   **564** multum] *adds*
tunc G, *om.* S   **565** amittitur] admittatur L, dimittitur S   **566** sequitur]
dicitur G   **567** Consolacionis] *add* iratus CDL   **568** mores] morem ACDL
571 per-] *om.* L   • furor] *om.* D   **572** bone] *om.* A, boni CDL   • ratione] *om.* GSp
• uite] *om.* L   **573** maculet] uacillat A   • una] uera L   **575** claros oculos]
clarum aspectum GSp   **575-76** loca … fugit] *om.* S (*at line end*)   • loca] *om.* G
576 quia] sic irato nichil, *corr. from* Hic iratus C, hic iratus D, nichil S
578 et deuoccionis] *om.* S   **579** penitus] *om.* S   **579-80** Gregorius … Plinius] *om.* G
580 tunc] *adds* similiter S, *adds* recte p   • Refert] dicit CDL

Lechery enjoys its pleasure, but wrath only rejoices in doing harm to others'. ₡

[557] The second effect of wrath is indignation. Gregory says of Iob 5:2, '[Anger indeed killeth] the foolish', 'Through the stimuli of wrath the heated heart pulsates, the body trembles, the tongue impedes itself, the face grows red, the eyes show irritation, and a wrathful man never even recognises his friends'. And he adds, 'Then there is no difference between a wrathful man and an insane one'. Likewise, a toad has fiery and shining eyes, and the more fiery his look, the more deadly he is. Therefore a wrathful person and a toad do not differ much. For this reason, Gregory, as cited above, says, 'When meekness is lost through wrath, our likeness to the divine image is dissipated'. For this reason, it follows that the wrathful is not a human being at all; according to Boethius in the *Consolation*, 'The person who imitates bestial behaviours clothes himself in that beast's shape'.

[569] The third effect of wrath is scornful words, which extinguish the light of truth in a person. For this reason, as Gregory says in the same place, 'So long as the mind in its troubled state roughens its capacity to judge, it thinks proper whatever its rage has suggested to it'. For this reason, at that time, it finds through reason nothing good in its neighbour, whether it concerns his behaviour or his reputation, that it may not sully. This is a further property of a toad, according to Pliny, book 8, that although it has shining eyes, it nevertheless hates the sun and loves filthy places, lives in marshes, and flees sweet-smelling things, because for a wrathful person, nothing associated with his neighbour smells good.

[577] The fourth effect of wrath is quarrelling, which, in both an angry person and one who has angered him, extinguishes completely the heat of love and of devotion. For this reason, Gregory continues, 'Through wrath, the grace of social life is completely lost'. And then the wrathful person is appropriately compared with a toad. Pliny tells, as cited above,

quod in latere buffonis dextro est os paruum, quod proiectum in
aquam feruentem, subito facit eam frigefieri, nec postea potest
feruere. Et illo osse utuntur magi ad odium concitandum. Hec ille.
Sic rabies et furor et iracundia excitat odium et extinguit feruorem
585   dileccionis proximi. Ideo dicitur in Prouerbiorum 22, 'Noli esse
a[micus] ho[mini] iracundo'.

Et nota secundum Senecam, libro *De ira*, quod hoc uicium
cauendum est iudici pre omnibus uiciis. Unde refert quod
quidam iudex condemnauit quendam militem accusatum de
590   morte commilitonis, eo quod essent duo in uia, et unus rediit
sine altero. Unde putabatur quod iste occidisset alterum, et cum
centurio, post sentenciam latam, duceret militem ad supplicium,
uidens illum militem pro quo fuit adiudicatus, ambos reduxit ad
iudicem. Iudex uero iratus primo dixit, 'Iubeo te interfici, quia
595   damnatus es'. Secundo dixit, 'Et te similiter, quia causa mortis
commilitonis fuisti'. Tertio dixit, 'Similiter iubeo te interfici,
quia iussus occidere militem, non obedisti'. Unde Seneca,
'Quam sollers est iracundia ad fingendas causas furoris! Tres
enim hic iudex puniuit propter unius innocentiam'. Fugienda
600   est igitur iudicis ira, quia u[era es]t + sentencia Gregorii, ubi
supra, 'Quicquid furor suggerit, rectum putat'. Unde potestas et
auctoritas iracundi fingit sibi causam + iustam.

Quintus effectus ire est clamor contra proximum et
blasphemia contra Deum, et tunc in iracundo inueteratum
605   generat odium. Et tunc, secundum [Bernardum, 'Ira est odium
inueteratum', et tunc secundum] Gregorium, ubi supra,

---

581 in] *add* dorso CDL   582 feruentem] bullientem ACDL   • subito] *om.* S
• postea] *om.* G   583 magi] ira S   585 Prouerbiorum] *a corr.* C   586 amicus]
assiduus ACDGSp, *om.* L   • homini] cum homine DGLS, hoc p
587–88 quod ... est] hoc uicium cauendum AG, docet hoc uicium multum esse
cauendum CDL   588 omnibus] *add* iudicat AG   589 iudex] miles S
591 alterum] socium ACDL   592 duceret ... uidens] uideret A   • supplicium]
iudicium G   593 militem] *add* uiuum CDL   • fuit] innoxius fuit morti CDL
• adiudicatus] *add* rediit et ACDL   595 mortis] *om.* L   596 dixit] *om.* S (*at line
end*)   • iubeo interfici] *om.* LS   597 iussus] *om.* A   598 ad] *adds* iudicandum
et ad G   598–99 Tres ... innocentiam] *om.* ACDL   599 puniuit] *om.* G
600 uera ... Gregorii] secundum Gregorium CD, uariat superiorum
sentenciam Gregorii p   • Gregorii] superior G   601 Unde potestas] *om.* L
602 auctoritas] *add* iudicis CDL; *and further adds* eciam, *expunged* C; *and
further adds* eciam D   • iustam] iusticiam p
605 generat] est L   • Bernardum] Gregorium 21 A   605–6 secundum ...
secundum] secundum Sp   606 supra] *adds* tunc A

that a toad has a little bone in its right side, and this, thrown into boiling water, immediately makes it grow cold, nor can it boil again afterwards. Magicians use this bone in order to foment hatred. So he says. Thus fury and rage and wrath provoke hatred, and they extinguish the heat of love of one's neighbour. Therefore Prv 22:24 says, 'Be not a friend to an angry man'.

[587] And notice that Seneca says in his book *On anger* that a judge should avoid this vice above all others. For this reason, he tells that a certain judge condemned a soldier who was accused of the death of one of his fellows, simply because they were travelling together, and one returned without the other. For this reason, it was thought that this soldier had killed the other one. And after he had delivered his sentence, when the centurion who was taking the soldier to execution saw the soldier for whom he had been condemned, he led them both back to the judge. The angry judge said to the first, 'I command you to be killed, because you have been condemned'. And to the second, 'And you likewise, because you have been the cause of your comrade's death'. And to the third, 'I likewise order you to be killed; you were commanded to kill the soldier, and you have not obeyed'. Seneca concludes, 'How ingenious wrath is at making up causes for its rage! This judge punished three, because of a single man's innocence'. Therefore one should flee a judge's wrath, because Gregory's opinion is true: 'Whatever rage has suggested, he thinks proper'. For this reason, angered power and authority present themselves as if they were a just cause.

[603] The fifth effect of wrath is outcry against one's neighbour and blasphemy against God, and then it gives rise to deep-seated hatred in a wrathful person. And then, according to Bernard, 'Wrath is an engrained hatred'; and according to Gregory, as cited above,

Spiritus Sanctus a corde excluditur. 'Cum', inquit, 'ira menti
quietem subtrahit, suam Spiritu Sancto habitationem claudit'.
Hec ille. Tunc hominem replet uenenum buffonis, quod
610   secundum Plynium, ubi supra, est frigidissimum inter omnia
uenena, quia omne membrum quod percutit facit insensibile et
[quasi] congelatum. Sic nichil remanet in corde irati, nisi rancor
et odium inueteratum.
        Nota quod hoc uenenum nunc regnat in dominis terrenis,
615   cum quibus pre ira et impaciencia uix homo potest loqui +.
Unde dicitur de buffone antiquo quod in capite eius generatur
lapis, et tunc, propter elacionem, duobus pedibus anterioribus
non tangit terram sed erectus incedit. Et [spiritual]iter hic lapis
est in mitra superborum prelatorum, quos cum pauper semel
620   offenderit, nunquam + quousque se uindicent [placabuntur].
Unde uenenum talium est simile ueneno rabidi canis, quod est
ualde periculosum. Quia secundum Constantinum, in homine
quem mordet aliquando usque ad anni reuolucionem uenenum
[lat]et quod non nocet, et tunc eadem hora qua percussit,
625   ascendit ad caput, et hominem facit esse freneticum. Sic est de
odio talium reseruato usque ad tempus uindicte. Multi tamen
+ canes regnant hodie. Unde refert Plynius, libro 6, quod

607 excluditur] expellitur \uel excluditur/ C, expellitur D, expellitur et excluditur L
• ira] *om.* S   608 Sancto] *the phrs. a corr.* C, (s.= ?) scilicet D   609 uenenum]
ueneno ACG (*corr. from* uenenum C) • quod] *add* uenenum CDL
612 quasi congelatum] congelatum AGSp, et quasi glaciem congelat (*corr. to*
congelat C, congelatur D, congelatum L) CDL, *with further corrs.*: quasi] *adds*
diabolica, *then cancelled* C; *adds* diabolica D (*and* glaciem *expunged*) • irati]
iracundi CDL, irato G
614 quod hoc uenenum] *a corr.* C, quod istud uicium D • nunc] *om.* ACDL
615 homo] aliquis CDL • loqui] *adds* aut prosequi p   618 spiritualiter] *add*
autem intelligendo (*om.* A) ACDL, specialiter S, ueraciter p   619 in mitra]
mitra CDL, in curiis S   620 uindicent placabuntur] cessant (cessent Ap;
after nunquam) … uindicent ASp, uindicauerint p. DL, pacificantur (*after*
nunquam) … uindicent G; **p** *adds* (*om.* ACDGLS+BLaRV):
    explorando maliciose scilicet tempus uindicte.
621 quod] *add* uenenum ACL (*a corr.* C)   622 periculosum] perniciosum
siue periculosum S   623 aliquando] *om.* ACDL • anni] annium C • anni
reuolucionem] reuolutum CDL   624 latet] iacet Sp, *add* et toto illo tempore
CDL • et tunc] set in fine anni CDL • percussit] percutit AGS, hominem
canis momordit per uenas CDL   625 caput] *adds* hominis A, *add* percussi CDL
626 odio] ira A • odio talium reseruato] rabido odio talium prelatorum *and*
add miserabiliter reseruato *after* • uindicte CDL • tamen] *add* rabidi Sp
627 hodie] in mundo A, *a corr.* C

wrath shuts the Holy Ghost out of the heart. He says, 'When wrath withdraws peace from the mind, it closes the Holy Ghost off from his lodging'. So he says. Then the toad's poison fills a person up, because according to Pliny, in the same place, it is the coldest poison of all, and it makes every limb that it strikes lose sensation and become, as it were, frozen. Thus nothing remains in the heart of a wrathful person except rancour and deep-seated hatred.

[614] Notice that this poison now rules in worldly lords; one can scarcely speak with them on account of their wrath and impatience. For this reason, an aged toad is said to grow a stone on his head and then, because of his pride, he does not touch the ground with his two forefeet but walks upright. In spiritual terms, this stone sits in the mitre of proud prelates; when a poor man has offended them just once, they will never be pleased until they may avenge themselves. For this reason, the poison of such men is like the poison of a mad dog, and it is very dangerous. According to Constantine the African, sometimes its poison lies inert in a person whom it has bitten for a full year so that it does no harm, and then at the same hour the person was attacked, it rises to his head, and makes the person mad. That is like the hatred of those people that is stored up until there is an opportunity for vengeance. Nevertheless, many dogs rule things today. For this reason, Pliny, book 6, tells that

sunt quidam Ethiopes qui canem habent pro rege, cuius motu
augurantur. Sic Ethiopes nigri uita, nunc ponunt canes rabidos
630   pro prelatis in ecclesia [Dei]. ₡

Remedium ire.
Capitulum UIII.

Remedium et tyriaca contra iram est patiencia. Circa quam
considera[nda est] causam motiuam; secundum Gregorium,
'Ira et impatiencia habent uel ex uicio esse uel ex zelo. Prima
est culpabilis, secunda meritoria'. Patiencia ergo habenda est
635   semper ad personam uel naturam. Et ad hoc potest adaptari
uerbum Plynii, libro 8, quod dicit quod buffo habet duplex iecur,
unum quod est summe uenenosum et aliud quod est contra
uenenum antidotum. Que sic cognoscuntur: utrumque projicitur
in nido formicarum, et illud iecur uenenosum fugiunt; aliud
640   uero amplectuntur et appetunt. Et illud homines reseruant
contra uenenum, et de iis tradunt mira doctores'. Hec Plynius.
In hunc modum ira ex uicio contra naturam et Dei imaginem
est uenenum. ₡
Etiam ut dicit Gregorius, ubi supra, scilicet in principio, 'Irasci
645   ex zelo contra culpam est magni meriti', secundum glossa super

628 quidam] *adds* homines quasi A   628–29 qui ... Ethiopes] habent *and* cuius
motu augustiantur *corrs.* C; *added marg.* D, *and after* 630 Dei, *adds* et qui
canem habent pro rege cuius motu augustiantur, *marked* ua ... cat D
  629 augurantur] auguantur AG, augustiantur CDL, auguriantur S • Sic] *add*
prodolor est hodie CDL (hodie *a corr.* C) • nigri uita] nigri in uita A, qui
nigri sunt uita peccatorum dico nigredine deturpati CDL, inuidi nigri uita G
  630 Dei] *om.* Sp

heading] *om.* AGS, *adds* est paciencia C, Remedium contra iram L
631 Remedium] Circa remedium (*with adjustment of cases and later* quod est) L
  • iram] uirus ire CDL • Circa quam] Primo igitur CDL (\Pri/mo \igitur/ *a
corr.* C, igitur *a corr.* D), Circa quod G   632 consideranda est] consideranda G,
consideracionem S, considera p • causam motiuam] necessariam S
  633 Ira et impatiencia] Uel de ira uel <im- *erased*> paciencia S • et] quia D
  • impaciencia] paciencia CDLS   634 culpabilis] culpa G • secunda] *add* est
ACS (*a corr.* C), die L   635 adaptari] aptari S   637 uenenosum] uenenum ACDS
  638 antidotum] *om.* S   639 et illud iecur] formice S • illud] *adds* formice L
  641 et ... doctores] *om.* ACDLS   642 ira] irasci AC • contra] *add* humanam CDL
644 Etiam ... principio] Set CDL

there are some Ethiopians who have a dog as their king, and using his movements, they foretell the future. Just like the Ethiopians, of black life, mad dogs now get appointed as prelates in God's church. ₡

The remedy for wrath.
Chapter 8.

[631] Patience is the remedy and antidote against wrath. On this point, one should consider the motivating cause, for, according to Gregory, 'One can have wrath or impatience either from vice or from zeal. The first is sinful, but the second meritorious'. Therefore patience should always be preserved, either toward the person or toward nature. On this point one may adopt Pliny's words in book 8, where he says that the toad has a double liver, one that is extremely poisonous and the other that is an antidote against poison. These can be easily recognised: if one throws each of them into an anthill, the ants flee the poisonous liver, but they embrace and desire the other one. People save that second one as a remedy against poison, and learned men say of them that they are wonders. So Pliny says. In this way, the vicious wrath is a poison attacking both nature and God's image. ₡

[644] Also, as Gregory says, at the beginning of the same passage, 'To become angry from zeal against sin is an act of great merit'; this follows from the gloss

illud Psalmi, 'Irascimini, et nolite peccare, etc.', nam [talis ira]
procedit ex amore. Ecclesiastici 20, 'Quam bonum est arguere
quam irasci'. Unde quia iecur buffonis cogit amare +, hec ira
attribuitur illi iecori salutifere. [Aliud remedium contra iram
650   tradit Gregorius super illud Iob, 'Uirum stultum etc.', *Moralium*,
dicens 'Duplex est remedium contra iram. Primum est munire se
exemplo Christi et sanctorum'; unde iracundi sunt serpentes igniti,
contra quos precepit Dominus respicere serpentem eneum, id est
Christum, in cruce pendentem. Nota supra, capitulo 2.] Secundum
655   remedium est considerare culpas nostras commissas contra Deum.
Unde Gregorius, ubi supra, 'Quasi ex aqua ignis extinguitur, dum
surgente furore anime ad mentem culpa reuocatur'.

Aliud remedium, secundum Senecam, contra iram est
consideratio iniuriantis persone, quia 'Contendere cum pare
660   anceps gladius est; cum superiore, furiosum; cum inferiore,
sordidum'. Et [ita nulli est irascendum. Et] addit, 'Amicus
offendit? fecit quod uoluit; inimicus, fecit quod debuit. Stultiori
remittamus; prudentiori cedamus'. Item dicit ibidem quod
'Consideranda est natura irascentis, quia', dicit 'mundi pars
665   superior nec in nubem cogitur, in tempestatem non pellitur,
nec uersatur in turbedinem; omni tumultu caret, sed in[f]erior
pars fulminat et tonat. Sic sublimis animus quietus semper est
et in loco tranquillo collocatur, omnia intra se premens.

---

646 talis ira] *om.* AGp, talis ira scilicet ex zelo CD, ira que ex zelo est L
647 Quam] *om.* S (*a caret, but no reading supplied*)   647–48 Ecclesiastici …
irasci] *om.* G   648 amare] *add* recte Sp   649–54 Aliud … capitulo 2]
paraphrased p+B:
  Sequitur de remedio contra iram propriam, quorum primum est consideratio
  dominice passionis. Unde legitur quod filii Israel respicientes serpentem in
  pallo a morsu serpentis sanabantur. Nota de hoc supra, capitulo 1.
649 Aliud] ? Ad A • contra iram] *om.* AGS 650–51 Gregorius … munire]
uidelicet minuere S   652 Cristi] *om.* S • et sanctorum] *om.* A • iracundi]
ire condiciones G • serpentes] semper S   654 Nota … 2] *om.* GL
654–57 Secundum … reuocatur] *om.* CDL
658 secundum Senecam] *om.* CD • contra iram] *om.* G   659 consideratio]
consimile (?) G • iniuriantis] eminencioris CDL, murmurantis G
660 est] *om.* D • furiosum] *add* est ACGL (*a corr.* C)   661 Et … Et] Et p
• irascendum] *a corr.* C, iracundum D • addit] *add* Seneca ACDGL
662 inimicus] *add* offendit CDGL   663 cedamus] concedamus S • Item] Idem
CDL   665 nec[1]] *om.* C, non DL • nubem] *a corr.* in nubem \uel imbrem/ C,
imbrem D   666 omni] cum S • inferior] interior p   667 sublimis] -is *a corr.*
CD • animus] ?cuius A, amicus *an int. corr.* C, *om.* S   668 omnia] *om.* A

on Ps 4:5, 'Be ye angry and sin not', for this wrath grows out of love. Sir 20:1, 'How much better is it to reprove than to be angry?' For this reason, because the toad's liver compels one to love, this anger is attributed to the healing liver. Gregory puts forward another remedy in his discussion of Iob 5:2, '[Anger indeed killeth] the foolish', where he says that there is a twofold cure for wrath. The first is to arm oneself in accord with the example of Christ and holy people; thus the wrathful are the fiery serpents, against whom the Lord commanded that one look at the brazen serpent, that is Christ, hanging on the cross. See chapter 2 above for this. The second cure is to think about the sins we have committed against God. For this reason, hence Gregory says, in the same passage, 'So long as you recall your sin, with its surging rage in your soul, it will be extinguished, just as fire is by water'.

[658] According to Seneca, another remedy against wrath is to consider the person who is injuring you, because 'To contend with your equal is a double-edged sword; against your superior, madness; against your inferior, demeaning'. And thus one should not be angry at anyone. He adds, 'Has your friend offended you? He has done what he wished; an enemy, what he should. We should forgive in a foolish man what we allow in a prudent one'. He also says there that 'One should consider the nature of a person who is growing angry, for the higher parts of the world are not compelled to be cloudy, nor are they shaken by a storm, nor whirled about in turbulence; while they lack all trouble, the lower parts thunder and resound. Thus, a lofty spirit is always at peace and resides in a calm place; it represses everything in itself.

[Cui]us ira [intra se] contrahitur, modestus et uenerabilis est,
670   quorum nihil inuenies in irato'. Hec ille.

Multum ergo cauenda est ira Christiano et maxime iudici uel
prelato. Unde Seneca, libro 2 *De clementia*, 'Rex apum aculeum
non habet, quia natura eum sibi negauit et inermem eum
reliquit'. Philosophus tamen dicit, libro 17 *De animalibus*, quod
675   habet [aculeum], et soluitur per uerba, libro 10, Plynii, qui dicit
quod 'si habet aculeum, usum tamen feriendi natura sibi negauit.
Noluit natura ipsum seuum esse, nec concito petere ultionem.
Ideo telum ei subtraxit, scilicet quoad usum, sed mai[es]tate eum
armauit'. Hec ille. Sufficit ergo iudici uel prelato auctoritas uel
680   dignitas. ℭ

De ueneno accidie.
Capitulum IX.

Uenenum accidie est ualde perniciosum, quia secundum
Gregorium, *Moralium* 31, 'Accidia est tristicia anime' que non
inuenit in se nec in alio bonum quo gaudeat. Unde sibi nihil
spirituale sapit, sed tristis et frigida torpet. Et propter hoc accidia
685   potest comparari omni ueneno, quia secundum Ysidorum, libro 12,
'Omne uenenum est frigidum et humane [natur]e contrarium'.
Accidiosus ergo bene comparatur serpenti, qui in omni frigore
torpet et in hyeme tota in cauernis latens, in nidos se uoluit, ac in

669 Cuius … contrahitur] cuius ira contrahitur A, quibus ira trahitur
(contrahitur p) Sp

671 cauenda] timenda S • ira] *add* homini ACDG, *add* omni L • iudici] *adds* uel
principi S   **673** eum[1]] eam A, aculeum CDGL   **675** aculeum] *om.* Gp
• et soluitur] set hoc soluitur (hoc *a corr.* C) CDL, set soluitur G, *adds*
contrarietas p   **676** si] *add* apis CD, *adds* apex L • feriendi] *adds* non habet S
677 Noluit] uoluit ACG • seuum] *blank left* CD • esse … concito] *om.* L
678 telum] celus L • maiestate] mansuetudine G, maioritate Sp   **679** prelato]
add sine armis CDL   **680** dignitas] *add* iudicialis uel eciam pastoralis CDL

heading] *om.* AGS
684 spirituale] *om.* S • sapit] placet uel sapit CL (*int. corr.* C)   **685–86** Ysidorum …
et] Plinium libro xj. frigidum est A   **686** Omne uenenum] *om.* GS • nature]
uite Gp   **687** comparatur] *add* omni ACDLS • qui] *a corr.* C, quia D
688 latens] iacens et latens L; *add* totaliter ACDL

The person who restrains his wrath internally is calm and stately, and you may discover none of these attributes in a wrathful person'. So he says.

[671] Therefore a Christian, and especially a judge or prelate, should particularly avoid wrath. For this reason, Seneca says, *On mercy* 2, 'The king of the bees does not carry a sting because nature has denied it to him and left him unarmed'. However, Aristotle says, *On animals* 17, that he does have a sting, and Pliny, in book 10, resolves this disagreement and says that 'even if he has a sting, nature has denied him the power to use it to attack others. Nature has not wished the king to be fierce, nor to seek vengeance in a headlong fashion. Therefore nature has withdrawn his power to use his javelin, but has armed him as sign of his majesty'. So he says. Therefore authority or dignity is quite sufficient for a judge or prelate. ₵

Concerning the poison of sloth.
Chapter 9.

[681] The poison of sloth is very harmful, for according to Gregory, *Morals* 31: 'Sloth is a sorrow of the spirit' that finds no good in itself or elsewhere in which it may rejoice. For this reason, it understands nothing of a spiritual nature about itself, but it sits inertly, sorrowful and cold. Because of this, sloth may be compared to all poisons, because Isidore, *Etymologies* 12, says, 'All poison is cold and is opposed to human nature'. Therefore the slothful person is properly compared to a snake, which becomes sluggish whenever it is cold and hiding in caves for the whole winter, winds itself up into knots, and

690   noctis algore non repit. Sic piger in frigore semper quiescere
appetit, Prouerbiorum 20: 'Propter frigus piger arare noluit;
mendicabit ergo in estate et non dabitur ei'. Et nota secundum
Gregorium, ubi supra, 'De accidia oriuntur torpor mentis circa
diuina, euagatio circa illicita, desperatio, pusillanimitas, rancor,
malitia'.

695   Et inter animalia uenenosa, accidia comparatur eruce, que
secundum Plinium, libro 8, est uermis uillosus in summitatibus
arborum corrodens frondes, uiroremque consummens. Et texit
de suis uisceribus quasdam telas more aranearum, quibus se
inuoluens per totam hyemem, custodit semen suum pestiferum.

700   Ecce: torpor et euagatio circa illicita. Nam eruca ab erodendo
dicta est, et membrum quod tangit eius cutem urit et pustulas
[fac]it. Et secundum Isidorum, libro 12, '[Ex erucis] papiliones,
auicule abundantes in fructibus malue, efficiuntur, et iterum ex
papilion[um] stercoribus super folia derelictis eruce generantur.'

705   Et dicit Papias quod papiliones sunt uolatilia que de nocte, igne
uel candela accensis, [circumuolita]nt et ignem uel lumen alis
extinguere nituntur. Sed ipsi in corpore proprio puniuntur, quia
igne uruntur. Nota ergo quod papilio, uolans sed nihil utile
operans, est accidiosus religiosus, qui tunc inutilis et maliciosus

710   + probatur, quando ignem gratie, quem in se non inuenit, in alio
per infamiam exinguere intendit. Sed penam non euadit, quia
seipsum, sicut papilio ign[i exponens, dum lucem extinguere
nititur, ab eodem igne iuste incineratur.] ₡

689 algore] frigore Ap, fulgore G • in] *a corr.* C, *om.* D 694 malicia] *om.* A
695 Et … uenenosa] *om.* ACDL • animalia] alia S 697 corrodens] rodens A
• consummens] *add* et flores ACGL 702 facit] ibi derelinquit GSp
• Ex erucis] *om.* Sp 703 abundantes] habentes S 704 papilionum] -onibus p
• folia] *add* malue ACD 706 circumuolitant] querunt A, conueniunt GLSp
• lumen] *add* accensum CD • alis] *add* suis ACD, *om.* GL, aliis S
707-8 Sed … uruntur] *om.* ADCL 709 operans] faciens CD • inutilis] *om.* G
710 probatur] comprobatur Sp 712-13 igni … incineratur] igne iudicii (iudicis
Sp) exponit ASp, sicut … nititur *int. corr.* C, igne iudicis exponens G
713 incineratur] incrematur uel (i.u.] *om.* L) incineratur CDL (uel incineratur]
a corr. C, *om.* D)

does not crawl about in the night-time chill. Thus a sluggard always seeks to rest when it is cold, as Prv 20:4 says, 'Because of the cold the sluggard would not plough; he shall beg therefore in the summer, and it shall not be given him'. Notice what Gregory says, in the same place, 'From sloth spring forth inertness of mind about divine things, waveryness about what is illicit, despair, cowardice, testiness, and malice'.

[695] Among poisonous animals, sloth is compared to the caterpillar which, according to Pliny, book 8, is a furry worm that sits in the tree-tops, gnawing at the shoots and eating the green leaves. It spins out of its guts, like spiders, webs, and wrapping itself in these for the whole winter, it preserves its venomous seed. See: this is inertness and waveryness about what is illicit. A caterpillar (*eruca*) is called that because of its gnawing (*erodendo*), and it burns any limb that touches its skin and leaves blisters there. And, according to Isidore, *Etymologies* 12, 'Caterpillars produce many moths, small flying beasts, in the fruits of mallow, and in turn, caterpillars are bred from the moths' shit that is left on the leaves. Papias says that moths are flying things that at night, once a fire or a candle has been lit, fly in circles around it and try to extinguish the fire or the light with their wings. But they are punished in their own bodies because they are burnt up by the fire. Therefore notice that a slothful religious person is a flying moth that is not doing any useful work. Such a person is plainly shown to be useless and malicious. For he intends to extinguish through detraction that fire of grace in others that he has not found in himself. But he does not avoid punishment for this, for, just like a moth that exposes itself to the fire, so long as he tries to extinguish the light, he will justly be burned up by that same fire. ℂ

De remediis acidie.
Capitulum X.

715   Remedium etiam contra uenenum acidie est prudentia, que
est exemplorum inspectrix. Primo, laboris et fatigationis Christi
a pueritia usque ad supplicium crucis. Secundo, debet esse
inspectrix omnium sanctorum. Unde dicit philosophus, libro 7
De animalibus, quod in sepulchris antiquorum regum inuenitur
lapis preciosus, qui cum uino datus, curat morsum serpentis.
720   Hic lapis potest dici margarita illa que 'inuenta uendit homo
omnia' et comparat eam, Matthei 11. Que margarita, secundum
Gregorium, est 'dulcedo regni celestis, propter quam inardescit
animus in celestibus', ita quod omnes [sancti], spretis terrenis,
exponebant se laboribus et suppliciis. Deberet ergo acidiosus
725   torporem sue pigritie excutere et dulcedinem istam cum sanctis
gustare, et sic non tederet eum in presenti peregrinatione +
laborare semper.
Tertio, debet esse inspectrix prudentie naturalium animalium.
Dicit enim philosophus, libro 11, quod inter apes null[us debet
730   esse ociosus], et officia diuersa habent. Nam quedam domos
construunt, alie poliunt, alie cibos parant, et senes earum + intus
operantur et iuuenes exeunt. Et dicit Auicenna quod apes iuu[en]es
et uirgines faciunt mel melius quam seniores, supple quia plus
habent de uigore. Apes etiam puniunt morte operari nolentes.

heading] *om.* AGS, Remedium accidie est prudencia C, Prudencia D, Remedium
contra uenenum accidie L
715 est exemplorum inspectrix] primo debet esse conspectrix exemplorum S
• exemplorum] eorum L • Primo] *add* exemplorum CDL • et fatigationis]
om. ACDGL   716 ad] *adds* passionem uel G   716–17 esse inspectrix] inspicere
exempla CD (exempla *a corr.* CD), inspectrix G, esse conspectrix S   719 uino]
humo A • datus] *add* percusso a serpente CDL • morsum] morbum G
720–21 margarita … margarita] margarita L   722–23 inardescit … quod] *om.* G
723 sancti] statim p • terrenis] *om.* S (*at line-break*)   724–27 Deberet …
semper] *om.* S   724 acidiosus] *add* a se CDL   726 tederet] tedebit C[S?] (*a corr.*
C), tetebit L • perigrinatione] *adds* exemplo sanctorum p
728 Tertio] *add* qui uult uitare uenenum accidie CDL (u.a.] *int. corr.* C, hanc D
• inspectrix] inspector ACDL • naturalium] *om.* S   729–30 nullus … ociosus]
nulli licet (libet A) ocio uacare AGSp, *add* et quod CDL   730 et] et hunc A,
quia G • diuersa] *adds* uel diuisa, *int. corr.* C   731 parant] portant G • intus]
interius CLp (*a corr.* C)   732 iuuenes] et non A • apes] *om.* CDGL • iuuenes]
a corr. C, innubes p   733 seniores] senes A, *a corr.* C   734 puniunt] premunt A
• morte] *om.* GS

Concerning the remedies for sloth.
Chapter 10.

[714] Also the remedy against the poison of sloth is prudence, the inspector of examples. First, the example of Christ's labour and exhausting work, from his boyhood all the way to his suffering on the cross. Second, prudence should be the inspector of the labour of all holy people. For this reason, Aristotle, *On animals 7*, says that there is a precious stone, found in the tombs of ancient kings, that given with wine, cures snakebite. This stone may be identified as the pearl that, 'having found it, the merchant sold all that he had' and bought it, Mt 13:46. According to Gregory, the pearl 'is the sweetness of the heavenly kingdom, on whose account the soul burns in longing for heavenly things', so that all the saints, having despised earthly things, exposed themselves to labours and torments for it. Therefore a slothful person ought to drive away from himself lazy slothfulness and long to taste this sweetness, as the saints do, and thus he should not be irritated to always labour in this pilgrimage.

[728] Third, one should be the inspector of the prudence of Nature's animals. For Aristotle says, *On animals* 11, that among the bees, none should be at leisure, and they all have various duties. For some of them build their hives, others polish, others prepare food, and the old ones work indoors and the young go forth. And Avicenna says that young virginal bees make honey better than the old ones, because they are more vigorous. Moreover, the bees punish those who do not want to work with death.

735   Contra ergo naturam uiuit qui ocio uacat; de labore aliorum
cibum sumit. Unde bene beatus Franciscus talem fratrem non
apem argumentosam sed muscam uilem uel uespam uocauit.
Dicit enim Plynius, ubi supra, quod formicarum maiora
sunt onera quam corpora, et de re publica est eis cura, ratio,
740   et memoria; de quibus, queritur plus capitulo de auaritia. Bene
ergo dicitur acidioso, Prouerbiorum 6, 'Uade ad formicam, o
piger, et disce ab ea prudentiam, [que cum non habeat ducem
nec preceptorem, congregat cibum in estate' quem comedat in
hyeme]. Dicit etiam Dioscorides quod serpentes postquam per
745   hyemem latitant in cauernis, uerno tempore caliginem oculorum
tunc contractam tunc disponunt. Et pro remedio querunt radicem
feniculi, cuius pastu contractam, cecitatem deponunt. Miser
ergo peccator [est qui sic torpet per ignauiam, quod per aliquam
predicatorum prudentiam a se non excutit pigritiam. Sed torpens
750   in uiciis, non emendatur saltem instinctu] naturalis sollertie qui
uiget in bestiis. Ideo 'bestialior est omnibus bestiis', secundum
Augustinum, 'qui ratione non utitur'.

735 qui ocio uacat] uacans (uagans L) ocio ACDGL; *add* et AGS, *add* quia (qui
D) semper ociosus CDL (quia semper *a corr.* C)   736–37 Unde … uocauit] *om.* S
737 argumentosam] augmentosam L
738–39 maiora sunt onera] *corrs.* (maiora *only* D) CD   739 de] *a corr.* CD
• cura ratio] curacio A, cura CDLS, causa racio G   740 et memoria] *om.* S
• queritur plus] quere \plus/ C, que\re/ D   • plus … auaricia] plenius in
capitulo S   742 que] *a corr.* C, quia D   742–44 que cum … hyeme] *om.* AGSp
742 habeat] *a corr.* C, habet D   745 tempore] *a corr.* CD   746 remedio] *add*
uisus CDL   746–47 disponunt … deponunt] deponunt L   747 pastu] *a corr.* CD
• contractam] *add* in latitando CDL (*a corr.* C)   748–50 est … instinctu] per
ignauiam impugnat instinctum AGSp   750 naturalis] uel L   751 uiget] *a corr.* C,
est L   • Ideo] *add* homo CL (*a corr.* C)   751–52 bestialior … ratione] *om.* A
752 qui] *add* ratione preditus CDL   • utitur] *add* CDL+V (*om.* AGSp+BLaR):
set ut asinus infatuatur. Unde in psalmo 'Homo cum in honore esset, etc.'
CDL (cum] *a corr.* C, *om.* D)

Therefore the person who lazes about in leisure leads an unnatural life; he takes his food from the labour of others. For this reason, the blessed Francis called such a friar, not a busy bee, but a vile fly or a wasp.

[738] Also Pliny says, as cited above, that ants carry loads larger than their own bodies and that their care, rationale, and memory are for the common good; about the ants, see further the chapter on avarice. The slothful person is properly addressed in Prv 6:6–8, 'Go to the ant, O sluggard, and consider her ways and learn wisdom; which, although she hath no guide nor master nor captain, provideth her meat for herself in the summer', which she eats in the winter. Also Dioscorides says that after snakes have been lurking all winter in caves, they contract cloudy sight, and they remove this in the spring, when they seek fennel-root to restore their vision. Having eaten this, they cast off their blindness. Therefore the sinner who lazes about through cowardice is wretched, because he does not cast off from himself his sluggishness through the prudence enjoined on him by preachers. But lazing about in his vices, he is not immediately improved by that instinct of natural wisdom that rules in beasts. Therefore Augustine says, 'The person who doesn't use his reason is more beastlike than all the animals'.

De auaritie ueneno.
Capitulum XI.

Uenenum auaritie ebibit homo a serpente quando appetiit scire bonum et malum, quia secundum Gregorium, 'Auaritia non tantum
755   est pecunie, sed sciencie'. Notandum quod inter omnia uenena, auaritia comparatur ueneno aranee. Unde diues, auarus circa diuitias congregandas, aranee in uenando comparatur propter consimiles, hinc inde, proprietatibus repertas. Prima proprietas eorum est labor consimilis in acquirendo, qui labor est triplex. Primo est continuus;
760   Isidorus, libro 12: 'Aranea semper tele intenta, nunquam de[sin]it a labore'. Et secundum philosophum, libro 4 *De animalibus*, contra occasum solis maxime laborat. Sic auarus, licet omnibus diebus uite sue diuitiis acquirendis estuet, c[ontr]a mortem tamen [maxime] amore diuitiarum exce[catur]. Secundo, labor eius est curiosus.
765   Unde dicit Auicenna et Plynius, libro 9, quia ex uisceribus aranee quodam mirando artificio et subtilissima compositione tela contexitur, more rethis componitur, et filis subtilissimis connectitur, ne a muscis et aliis bestiolis quibus tenditur propter + grossiciem uideatur. Hunc in modum, auarus curiositatem studii circa
770   temporalia acquirenda omnia intima sua proicit. Ecclesiastici 10, 'Auaro nihil est scelestius. Hic animam uenalem habet, etc.'. Tertio est labor anxius et periculosus, quia in tele superficie [immobi]liter se suspendit. Psalmus, 'Tabescere fecisti sicut araneam, etc.'; glossa, Augustinus, 'Texit inanes telas' ut dolo capiat muscas.
775   Sic auarus in studio suo nullum habet fructum, nisi capere muscas temporalium, ad quas, ut dicit Augustinus, 'Non uolat caritas'.

---

heading] *om.* AGS
753 ebibit homo] homini ... infusum est L   754 Auaricia] *om.* G   756 auaricia]
om. G, *add* magis proprie CD (magis *a corr.* C)   757 comparatur] appropriatur
et eciam comparatur L   759 consimilis] *om.* ACDL   •   labor] *after* Primo CDL
760 desinit] deficit p   761 *animalibus*] *add* aranea CDL   762 licet] *om.* G
763 contra] circa Ap   •   maxime] *om.* Sp   764 excecatur] excecat A, diuiciarum
multiplicandarum anxius elaborat cum tamen cui eas congreget penitus
ignoret CDL, excedit p   766 mirando] miro CDL   767 connectitur] contexitur
uel connectitur CD, contexitur conuertitur G, contexitur L   768 grossiciem]
grossitudinem Ap, suam gracilitatem CDGL   770 intima] interiora CDL
771 scelestius] celestius G, scelerius L   772 Tertio est labor] Tercio labor aranee
est omni labore CDL (aranee, labore *corrs.* C)   •   anxius et periculosus]
grauior et periculosior CDL, grauis et periculosus G   773 immobiliter]
mortaliter Sp   775 Sic auarus] Auarus itaque CD, Auaricia inquid L   •   capere]
add si potest DL   •   muscas] *add* rerum CDL

On the poison of avarice.
Chapter 11.

[753] A person drinks the poison of avarice from a snake when he longs to know good and evil. For as Gregory says, 'Avarice is not just about money, but knowledge as well'. One should notice that, among all the poisons, avarice is compared to a spider's poison. For this reason, a rich man, grasping about gathering together wealth, is compared with a hunting spider on account of the similarities on either side that one can discover in their characteristics. Their first characteristic is a similar labour in acquiring things, and it is threefold. First, it is continuous. Isidore in book 12 says, 'A spider, always intent on its web, never stops working'. And according to Aristotle, *On animals 4*, it works hardest in anticipation of sunset. Likewise, the avaricious person, although he burns in acquiring riches every day of his life, nevertheless he is most blinded by his love of riches as he approaches death. Second, a spider's labour is fastidious. For this reason, Avicenna and Pliny, in book 9, say that the spider weaves a web out of its guts with a wondrous art and in the most delicate form, so that it is put together as if it were a net and joined with the very finest threads so that it may not be seen in some gross form by the flies and the other vermin for whom it is stretched out. In the same way, an avaricious person tosses out all his deepest self in a fastidious study of how to acquire worldly goods. Sir 10:9–10 says, 'Nothing is more wicked than the covetous man. Such a one setteth even his own soul to sale[, because while he liveth he hath cast away his bowels]'. Third, a spider's labour is anxious and danger-filled, because it hangs itself in the surface of its web and does not move. Ps 38:12 says, 'Thou hast made his soul to waste away like a spider', and Augustine says in the gloss, 'It has weaved empty webs' so that it may catch flies deceitfully. Likewise, an avaricious person derives no profit from his study, unless it is in catching the flies of temporal goods. And Augustine says about these, 'Charity never flies away'.

Secunda proprietas est quod inest utrique + timor in
possidendo. Tela [e]nim aranee, secundum Plynium, ubi supra,
cum labore miro modo texitur, sed miro modo f[acil]iter
780   dissipatur. Ignem non sustinet, flatum uenti timet, et si parua
animalia capiat, a maioribus tamen rumpitur. Sic auarus timet
pro suis diuitiis quemcunque uidet. Seneca: 'Uidet diuitem,
estimat predonem; uidet pauperem, suspicatur furem'. Et
secundum Ambrosium in *Hexameron*, 'More piscis, et si deuorat
785   inferiorem, a ualidiore tamen deuoratur'.

Tertia proprietas est consimilis dolor qui inest utrique in
amittendo. Quicquam enim tangit telam, cum sit de uisceribus
aranee, tangit [arane]am. Sic qui tangit diuitias tangit intima
diuitis. Unde super illud psalmi, 'Tabescere fecisti sicut
790   araneam, etc.', glossa, 'Aranea, egestione uiscerum unde telam
texit, moritur; ita homo, dum [ex]trahit + a se iniquitatem,
moritur'. Cupiditas uel auaritia contra proximum autonomatice
est iniquitas, secundum illud 1 Timothei 6, 'Radix omnium
[malorum] est cupiditas'.
795   Quarta proprietas est infructuositas in remunerando.
Aranea enim, secundum philosophum, humore muscarum dum
uiuit pascitur, sed pro labore suo plus non recipit. Sic auarus
in uita presenti suis bonis non satiatur, et in futuro omni spe +
defraudatur. Iob 4, 'Sicut tela aranearum fiducia eius', id est auari.

777 est quod inest] que inest AL, inherens C, *om.* D • utrique] *add* consimilis Sp
778 enim] omni p • enim aranee] *om.* S   779 modo texitur] contexitur AL,
modo *a corr.* C • sed] *add* non ACDL • faciliter] feliciter p   781 auarus]
add in studio suo nullum habet fructum CDGL   782 pro suis diuiciis] *int.
corr.* C, *om.* D   783 suspicatur] estimat A   784 *Hexameron*] *add* Diues raptor
CDL

786 proprietas] *add* eorum scilicet aranee et auari CL (*int. corr.* C), *adds* eorum D
• qui … utrique] *om.* CDL • inest] est A • utrique] in utroque AG
788 aranee] eius • tangit … tangit] tangit S • araneam] ipsam Sp
• diuitias] intima diuitis *and add* scilicet substanciam suam temporalem tangit
animam suam CDL   789 psalmi] *om.* AG   791 dum] de se S • extrahit a]
trahit a CDL, contrahens ad S, contrahit ad p   792 contra proximum] *a corr.* C,
om. D • autonomatice] -mastice CL, caan/cono (?) G   793 est] dicitur CDL
794 malorum] *om.* p

795 proprietas] *add* eorum (*om.* L) scilicet aranee et auari L • infructuositas]
infructuosus A, infructuosus labor (\sap/or L) CDL   797 plus] *om.* A, toto
plus CDL   798 futuro] *adds* eciam D, *expunged* C   799 defraudatur]
defraudabitur p • Sicut] *om.* ACDGL

[777] Their second common characteristic is that both of them are afraid when they possess things. According to Pliny, as cited above, the spider weaves its web in a wondrous way with great labour, but it's equally wondrous that the web can easily be torn apart. A web does not stand up to fire; it fears a puff of wind, and even if it captures small animals, it is still broken apart by bigger ones. Likewise, an avaricious person, whomever he sees, he fears for his goods. Seneca says, 'He sees another rich man, and assumes he is a robber; he sees a poor man, and imagines him a thief'. According to Ambrose, in his *Hexameron*, 'He is just like a fish: even if it gobbles up a smaller one, it is eaten by a stronger one'.

[786] Their third common characteristic is that both have a similar sorrow about losing their things. For whoever touches a spider's web, since it comes from the spider's guts, touches them as well. Likewise, whoever touches riches touches the innermost parts of the rich man. For this reason, the gloss on Ps 38:12, 'Thou hast made his soul to waste away like a spider', says, 'A spider through emptying out of its guts until it has woven a web, dies; likewise, a person dies, so long as he draws evil out of himself'. Desire or avarice exercised against one's neighbour is automatically evil, according to 1 Tim 6:10, 'The desire of money is the root of all evils'.

[795] Their fourth common characteristic is the lack of profit in return for their efforts. For according to Aristotle, a spider, so long as it lives, is fed by the moisture of flies, but receives nothing more for its labour. Likewise, an avaricious person is not fulfilled by his goods in this life, and in the world to come, he will be defrauded of all hope. Iob 8:14 says of an avaricious person, 'His trust shall be like the spider's web'.

800   Gregorius, 'Uanis fauoribus populi decipietur et non stabit'.
       [Item Gregorius, 'Qui labenti innititur, necesse est ut cadat cum
       labente, uel eciam ut labatur et non stabit]', id est non consurget,
       'scilicet ad gratiam in presenti uel gloriam in futuro'. Nota
       quod omnia predicta possunt aptari de auaricia mercatorum
805   [et] usura[rariorum], conuertendo tamen ea ad auariciam
       dominorum mundi.
          Peccatum auaritie mercatorum comparatur ueneno draconis.
       Qui secundum Solinum, uenenum habet in lingua et in felle. Et
       secundum Plynium, libro 8, ui ueneni semper erigitur eius lingua;
810   hec est subdola et mendax lingua mercatorum. In felle uero notatur
       fraudulentia et malitia. Dicit enim Plynius, ubi supra, quod super
       omnia desiderat et sitit sanguinem elephantis. Draco enim est
       animal sitibundum quod ui ueneni et caloris non potest dormire,
       sed quasi semper uigilat et siti estuat. Unde super illud Hieremie 24,
815   'Attraxerunt uentum sicut dracones', dicit Hieronimus quod
       draco est animal ualde sitibundum, in tantum quod uix potest
       in aqua saciari. Hic est auarus, qui nunquam satiatur pecunia;
       [Ecclesiastes, 'Auarus non implebitur pecunia']. Et sanguinem
       elephantis, quod est animal temperatum, frigidum, et manusetum,
820   sitit, quia substantiam pauperis et innocentis semper iste sitit. Dicit
       enim Plynius, ubi supra, quod solent u. dracones caudis mutuo
       se complecti et erectis capitibus uelificare per mare et flumina ad
       pascua meliora. ₡ Hec + est coniuncta societas mercatorum, que
       omnia pericula paruipendunt in hiando lucris mundanis.

800-1 Gregorius … Gregorius] Gregorius L   800 Uanis] *om.* D, bonis G
800-2 stabit … stabit] *om.* Sp   801 cadat] labatur, *and om.* uel … labatur G
803 ad gratiam] *om. at column bound* L   804 omnia predicta] hec omnia CDL
• possunt aptari] pertinent (*later in sentence*) L   • aptari] conuerti CD,
adaptari G   • mercatorum] merca|toro C   805 et usurariorum] et naurariorum
L, siue auaricia et usura S, siue usura p   • conuertendo … mundi] *om.* L
806 dominorum] adds huius A, hominum huius CD
807-38 *appear after* 958 G+V   807 Peccatum] *prec. by rubric* De auaricia
mercatorum C, Auaricia D   • Peccatum auaritie mercatorum] Peccatum
auaricie in mercatoribus AS, Mercatorum auaricia CDL   810 In] *adds* ore in L
811 quod] *add* draco CDGL   • super] dicitur eo quod \super/ L   813 caloris]
calore CDGL, doloris S, *add* nimio estuans uix CDL   817-18 pecunia … pecunia]
pecunia GSp   818 Ecclesiastes] sicud dicitur Ecclesiastes \capitulo 5/ A, *blank
left* C   • Et] *add* draco iste CDL   821 u.] decem ACDGL, quatuor S   • mutuo]
iunctis S   822 capitibus] ceruicibus uel capitibus A   823 Hec] *adds* similitudo p
• coniuncta] *add* cupida CDL   paruipendunt] -pendunt *a corr.* C, paruipendit DL
824 mundanis] *add* maris uel fluminis et cuiuscumque suspecti itineris CDL

Gregory says, 'He will be deceived by the empty graces of the people and not stand firm'. Gregory also says, 'The person who leans on something that is slipping necessarily falls with the slipping thing, or at least he will slip and not stand', that is, he will not rise up, 'to grace in the present life or glory in the world to come'. Notice that all the things I have said previously may be adapted from applying to the avarice of merchants or of people engaged in usury by converting them to address the avarice of the lords of this world.

[807] The sin of mercantile avarice is compared to a dragon's poison. Solinus says the dragon has poison in its tongue and in its bile, and according to Pliny, book 8, its tongue is always raised up because of the strength of its poison; this represents merchants' deceitful and lying tongue. Fraud and malice are indicated by the bile. Pliny also says, in the same place, that above everything else a dragon desires and thirsts after an elephant's blood. And this very thirsty animal may not sleep because of the strength and the heat of its poison, but it's as if it were always wakeful and burning with thirst. For this reason, Jerome says concerning Ier 14:6, 'They snuffed up the wind like dragons', that a dragon is a beast so very thirsty that it may scarcely be satiated by water. This is the avaricious person, never satisfied with the money he has; Ecl 5:9, 'A covetous man shall not be satisfied with money'. The dragon thirsts for the blood of an elephant, a temperate animal, cool and meek, just as an avaricious person always thirsts for the substance of the poor and innocent. Pliny also says, in the same place, that five dragons are accustomed to wind their tails together and, with their heads erect, to sail through the sea and rivers to better pasture. ¢ This represents the company of merchants who disdain all dangers in their gaping after worldly profits.

825   Unde fabulose depingitur Mercurius [mercator], habens
uirgam serpentibus innexam et pennas + ad talos, cui datur galea
in capite et gallus in tutelam. Et sic deus furti uocatur. Fulgencius
in libro *Mythologiarum* sic exponit: 'Mercurius dicitur quasi
"mercium curius", id est deus. Sic est mercator omnis; uirgam
830 serpentinam fert, quia uulnus dat serpentinum siue uenenatum.
Pennas autem habet [ad] talos, quia pedes sui sunt pennati
uolantes ubique; galea abscondit caput, quia eius intentio semper
est abscon[s]a. Gallus ei datur, quia quasi semper uigilat, uel
quia galli cantu semper surgit ad peragenda negocia. Deum uero
835 furti esse ac presulem dicunt, eo quod nihil sit inter negociantis
rapinam atque eius periurium et furis operationem et raptum'.
Hec Fulgencius.

        Nota quod aranee, secundum Plynium, libro 29, tres sunt
species. Una, que *sphalangia* appellatur, formata ad modum
840 formice sed longe maior corpore, rufum habens caput, reliquum
uero corporis nigri coloris, respersum quibusdam guttis albis;
et hec uiuit maxime iuxta furnos. Morsus huius ueneni longe
acerbior est quam uipere. Hec ar[a]nea, re[quies]cens [iuxta]
furnos et coquinam, significat diuites, predones et exactores,
845 quorum studium uenenosum est pauperes spoliare et uentres
suos replere. Alia species aranee [dicitur] *lanuginosa*, cum grosse
capite, et dolor ueneni eius sicut scorpionis, ex cuius morsu genua
labefactantur. Hec aranea significat mediocres, scilicet sequaces

825 mercator] mercatorum deus G, *om.* Sp • habens] *a corr.* C, *om.* D
  826 innexam] *a corr.* C, innixam D, *om.* S • et pennas] \et pennas habens/
(*marg., Herbert*) A, *om.* CDL • ad] usque ad ACDGLSp 827 uocatur] *add* et
dicitur ACD 829 curius] cirrus \kirios/ (*marg., Herbert*) A, currus CDLS,
carus G 829–30 uirgam serpentinam fert] *om.* ACDL 830 uenenatum]
uenenatorum L 831 habet] *om.* L • ad] usque ad CDGL, in p 832 uolantes]
add quia quasi CD, *adds* quia sunt L, *adds* et S 833 absconsa] abscondita p
• datur] *add* in tutelam ACDL • quasi] *om.* AS 834 Deum] Ipsum autem
deum ACDL 836 operationem et raptum] *om.* A
  839 appellatur] uocatur ASL • formata] formica S 840 longe] longior ac L
• rufum] rubeum S 841 corporis] corpus ACDL 842–44 furnos … furnos]
furnos S 842 ueneni] aranee CDL 843 aranea] arena p • requiescens iuxta]
respiciens AGp, *add* et uiuens CDL 844 diuites] *om.* S • et] *add* pauperum
CDL 845 et] *add* in pigricia uiuentes CDL 846 suos] *add* de rapinis
pauperum CDL • replere] adimplere CDL, implere S • Alia] *adds rubric*
Contra diuites predones A • dicitur] est p 848 labefactantur] labescantur A,
labefacit S

[825] For this reason, in fables Mercury is depicted as a merchant, having a staff with snakes wound around it and wings on his heels, and he is also given a helmet on his head and a cockerel as a guardian. And thus, he is called the god of theft. Fulgentius in his *Mythographies* explains it, 'He is called Mercury as if he were the *kyrios* 'master', that is the god, of payments (*merces*). Every merchant is like this: he carries a snaky staff because he gives a snakelike or poisoned wound. He has wings on his heels because his feet are winged so that he can fly everywhere, and a helmet hides his head, because his intention is always hidden. He is given a cockerel, because he is almost always wakeful, or because he always rises at cock-crow to pursue his deals. They truly call him god or bishop of theft because there is no difference between the theft associated with business deals or a merchant's misrepresentations and a thief's work and his seizures. So Fulgentius says.

[838] Notice that, according to Pliny, book 29, there are three species of spider. The first of these is called *sphalangia*, and it is shaped like an ant, but with an extended and larger body; it has a red head and the remainder of its body is black and sprinkled with some white drops, and this species lives mostly around ovens. The poison from its sting is much sharper than a viper's. This spider, lounging about near ovens and the kitchen, indicates rich men, thieves and taxing officials, whose poisonous study is to despoil the poor and to fill their own bellies. The second kind of spider is called *lanuginosa*. It has a big head, and the pain from its poison is like that of the scorpion, whose sting weakens one's knees. This spider indicates people of middling station, the

850   predonum, qui complacent eis per adulationem, et de hoc uide in
fine huius capituli.

Tertia species [aranee] dicitur *myrmicoleon* uel *formicoleon*,
quod idem est, sic dicta quia 'formicarum leo'. Formice similis
est in corpore, al[b]um in capite, corpus habens nigrum, cuius
morsus est ut uesparum. Uenatur ergo formicas ut leo et earum
855   sugit humiditatem, sed a passeribus deuoratur. Sicut *formic[oleon*
leo est formicis], passer quidem est quasi leo respectu ipsius.
Hec aranea significat balliuos siue officiales mundi, qui leones
sunt respectu pauperum et innocentium, sed postea fiunt preda
superiorum. Iob 4, 'Tigris periit, eo quod non haberet predam';
860   litera 70. interpretum habet '*myrmicoleon*'. Glossa: 'Paruum
scilicet animal quod est ut leo respectu formicarum, quia latens
in puluere eas comedit, sed postea [a uolatilibus deuoratur. Per
quod animal significatur crudelis balliuus, qui est ut leo respectu
pauperum, sed postea] preda fit dominorum'.

865   Nota quod Creta nobilis insula Grecie, a centum [nobilibus]
ciuitatibus, '[cent]opolis' quondam dicta, secundum Isidorum,
libro 15 et Plynium, libro 4. Terra est ita munda quod nullum
animal gignit uenenosum, nec serpens, nec aliquid simile
ibi inuenitur – immo si illuc aliunde ad terram transferatur,
870   statim moritur. Tamen *sphalangia* aranea uenenosa ibi abundat,
secundum Isidorum, ubi supra. Huic insule Grecie conformis
est Maior Scotia, scilicet Hibernia. ₵ Scotia enim est uocabulum
Grecum, secundum philosophum, libro *De animalibus* 16. Etiam
Hibernici sunt Greci origine. Sed ultra Cretam Deus dedit ei

---

849 predonum] pre|dictorum S • adulationem] *adds* et participant predam
unde dicuntur similes scorpioni propter adulacionem G • uide] quere CDL
851 aranee] *om.* Sp 852 quod idem est] *int. corr.* C, *om.* D, quod est ideo L
• quia] quasi GS 853 album] albo S, altum p 854 ut leo] *om.* G sugit]
fugit D 855 sugit humiditatem] uenatur humorem S 855–56 formicoleon …
formicis] formica Ap, *add* sic eciam ipsi formicaleoni CDL, formica ab ea S
857 mundi] *a corr.* C, *om.* D 858 et innocentium] *om.* S 859 non] *om.* S
860 interpretum habet] *om.* G • habet] ponunt CDL 862–64 postea …
postea] postea LSp 863 animal] *a corr.* C, *om.* AG 864 sed … dominorum]
corr. D

865 a centum] pre S • nobilibus] *om.* Ap, aliis S 866 centopolis] metropolis Sp
868 animal] *om.* S • nec[1]] quia nec CDGL • aliquid] aliud A, aliquid
\aliud/ CD (*a corr.* CD), a[i]d L (*also a corr.*) 869 ibi inuenitur] ibi *a corr.* C,
om. L • illuc] *om.* CDL, illud S 870 sphalangia] *add* que dicitur CDGL
• aranea] *om.* A 871 Grecie] *add* quantum ad hoc CDL • conformis]
consimilis S 872 Maior] *om.* CDL 874 Hibernici] Hibernia L

followers of thieves, who please them through their flattery; about them, see further at the end of this chapter.

[851] The third kind of spider is called *myrmicoleon* or *formicoleon*, terms that refer to the same thing, and it is called *formicoleon* as if it were an ant (*formica*)-lion. Its body is similar to an ant's, but it has a white head, a black body, and a sting like that of wasps. It hunts ants like a lion does and sucks out their moisture, but it is eaten by sparrows. Just as the *formicoleon* behaves like a lion with the ants, so the sparrow is like a lion in comparison to it. This spider indicates bailiffs or worldly officials, who are lions in their treatment of the poor and innocent, but afterwards they become the prey of their superiors. Iob 4:11 says, 'The tiger hath perished for want of prey'; the Septuagint version has the word *myrmicoleon*. The gloss here says, 'It is a small animal that behaves like a lion with respect to ants, because it hides in the dust and eats them, but afterwards it is eaten by birds. This animal indicates a cruel bailiff, who is a lion with respect to the poor, but afterwards becomes the prey of lords'.

[865] Notice that Crete is a noble island of Greece and from its hundred noble cities was once known as *centopolis*, according to Isidore, book 15; and Pliny, book 4. The land is so pure that it produces no poisonous animal, nor is a snake or anything like it found there – indeed, such a creature transported to that land from elsewhere dies immediately. Nevertheless the poisonous spider *sphalangia* abounds there, according to Isidore, in the same place. Greater Scotland, that is Ireland, is similar to this Greek island. ℂ For Scotland is a Greek word, according to Aristotle, *On animals* 16. Also the Irish are of Greek origin. But God granted Ireland this virtue, surpassing that of Crete, that it

875   uirtutem, ut nullum uenenum admitteret, nec in aranea, nec in
       aliquo animali. Et ut credo, salua meliori op[in]ione, quod est
       proprietas consequens terram, quod patet per hoc, quod terra
       eius portata ad alias re[gione]s repellit uenenum, sicut dicit Beda,
       De gestis Anglorum, et alii historiographi.
880   Sed prothdolor! uenenum quod negauit ei Deus in aranea
       bestiali, [u]t in [C]reta, permisit regnare in humana natura, nam
       ultra omnes terras abundat in triplici aranea superius dicta,
       spiritualiter tamen intellecta. Habet enim *sphalangiam*, id est
       predones, quia omnes fere terre natiui sunt tales. Et ut dicit
885   philosophus, libro uiii. *De animalibus*, femina aranee ponit oua
       primo, ex quibus postea modice aranee formantur, que subito
       formate, informantur ad [uenan]dum et ad texendum telas,
       que subito operantur ac si in utero materno fuissent inst[ru]cte
       ad uenandum. Ita est de pueris natis in terra illa, quasi studio
890   paterno et materno fuissent instructi [ad predandum], sic fiunt
       comuniter predones. Hinc est quod raro in dicta terra inueniuntur
       aliqui diuites, sicut in aliis regionibus, quia non permittit Deus
       predones fieri diuites. Prouerbiorum 12, 'Sunt qui rapiunt non sua
       et semper in egestate sunt'. Naturam enim habent milui, cuius
895   quoddam genus est quod in pri[ncipi]o aues rapit, post e[scus]
       animalium comedit, tandem uix muscas et uermiculos capit, et
       in fine fame moritur. Sic Dei ultione, quia tales in principio uite
       innocentibus reddunt se crudeles, in fine uite sibi fiunt inutiles.

---

875 uirtutem] talem uirtutem CDL • uenenum] uenenosum S • admitteret]
admittat CDGL   876 aliquo] adds alio A • animali] similis A • credo]
secundo L • salua … opinione] saluo … iudicio CDL, salua … oppositione p
877 consequens] conueniens A, quasi sequens CD   878 eius] illa ACDG, illius L
• portata] apportata A • regiones] terras Sp, *adds* non A   879 historiographi]
historie A
880 ei … aranea] inde S   881 bestiali] uel in alio genere animalis dico brutalis
(a.d.b.] animalium brutalium L) CDL, natura bestiali S • ut in Creta] et in
terra Sp, *add* similiter in Ybernia CDL • regnare] *add* supra modum CDL
882 ultra] *om.* S • abundat] regnat G • dicta] memorata S   884 terre] *add*
illius ACDGL • natiui] nati S   886 que] unde quasi A • subito] sepius L
887 uenandam] formandum p   888 materno] matris S • instructe] instincte p
889 uenandum] *add* et ad texendum CDL • illa] dicta ACDGL (*again in* S *at*
891 dicta)   890 materno] *add* in utero CDL • ad predandum] *om.* Sp
• fiunt] *add* pueri et senes CDL   892 aliqui] *om.* S   893 non sua] aliena ACDL
894 cuius] *adds* naturam sumunt G   895 principio] primo Sp • post] p. deinde
ACDGL, et postea S • escus] exta CDLSp   898 innocentibus … sibi] *a corr.* C,
marked for corr., but not supplied (?) D, *om.* L

would admit no poison, neither that of a spider nor of any other animal. As I believe – although I would bow to a more informed opinion – this is a characteristic instinct in Irish soil, as is evident from the fact that Irish soil carried to other lands drives away poison. Bede says this, in *On the deeds of the English*, and other historians agree.

[880] But alas! The poison that God withheld from Ireland, as he did from Crete, in the spider, a beast, he allowed to rule there in human nature. For more than all other lands, Ireland abounds in the triple spider discussed above, here understood in a spiritual sense. Ireland has the *sphalangia*, that is robbers, for nearly everyone native to the land is such. As Aristotle says, *On animals* 8, the female spider first lays her eggs and later small spiders are formed from them, and these, just as soon as they are hatched, know how to hunt and weave webs, for they instantly behave as if they had been taught to hunt in their mother's womb. It is the same with children born in Ireland, as if they had been instructed in their father and mother's craft of pillage, for they routinely become thieves. For this reason it is rare that any rich people are found in Ireland, as they are in other lands, because God does not permit thieves to become rich men. Prv 11:24 says, 'Some take away what is not their own, and are always in want'. They have a kite's nature; it is a kind of bird that at the start preys on other birds, later eats the carrion left by other animals, next can scarcely catch flies and little worms, and at the end of its life dies of hunger. And so by God's vengeance, because such people in the beginning of their life behave cruelly to the innocent, at the end of their life they are made powerless to help themselves.

900 Et quod uolunt uiuere de aliena substantia, postea moriuntur
inedia. Prouerbiorum 3, 'Egestas a Domino in domo impii'.

Habet etiam insula illa araneam *lanuginosam*, id est
histriones et adulatores, quorum maledicta laude predicti
predones in superbiam elati, nunquam possunt ad bonum
conuerti. Et nota secundum philosophum, libro 8 *De animalibus*,
905 quod coruus est amicus uulpis et pugnat cum eo contra taxum,
quorum societas bene eis conuenit. Uulpes enim est animal rapax
et fraudulentum et decept[or]ium; quando enim non habet cibum,
fingit se mortuam, et tunc aues descendentes super se rapit et
deuorat, secundum Isidorum, libro 2. Semper etiam claudicat,
910 quia crura partis dextre sunt breuiora aliis, cui naturale odium
est contra taxum siue melum. + Hic est predo uorax, periurus,
et mendax, qui fingit se mori et non posse familiam sust[enta]re
uel patriam regere, nisi possit bona pauperum tollere. Unde
partem dextram, scilicet electorum, nunquam habet dispositam,
915 cui quasi naturale odium est contra taxum, animal ualde
mundum, scilicet pauperem mundum et innocentem.

Coruus uero est auis [garula] et quasi per adulationem,
semper tempus futurum pro[phe]tans. Habet enim secundum
Fulgentium, libro *Mythologiarum*, solus inter aues 74. uocis
920 significationes; unde dicitur habere uim diuinationis. Et
secundum Isidorum, libro 12, pullos non pascit quousque
conformentur sibi in nigredine pennarum, et etiam immunda
auis est, quia cadaueribus insidet. Est etiam auis dolosa, res
furtiue subtrahens et abscondens. Sic est adulator omnia prospera

---

899 moriuntur] *adds* afflicti uel affecti (*a corr.*) C, afflicti D, affecti … et afflicti L
901 insula illa] Ybernia CDL   **65** elati] et elacionem prorupti L   **904** conuenit]
conueit C   **907** deceptorium] deceptiuum Sp   •   cibum] *add* iacens in terra
rubra CDL (*a corr.* CD)   **909–10** et deuorat] uel deuorat (*a corr.*) C, *om.* DG
910 aliis] cruribus partis eius alterius CDL   •   naturale] mere habet G
911 siue melum] animal sine malicia   •   Hic] Spiritualiter hic p
912 et mendax] *om.* S   •   sustentare] sustinere p   **913** uel patriam] uel domum
suam CL (*a corr.* C), *om.* D   •   pauperum] aliorum … et maxime pauperum
hominum suorum CDL   **914** habet dispositam] *blank left* A, recuperabit CDL,
habet bene dispositam S   **915** quasi] *om.* AG, ut predicitur CL (*a corr.* C), ut
dicitur D   **916** scilicet … innocentem] et innocens CDL   pauperem] *om.* G
917 garula] *om.* Sp   **918** futurum] *om.* CDLS   •   prophetans] procrastinans
ACDGLSp   **920** significationes] mutaciones CDGL   •   unde] *add* secundum
fabulas CDL   **921** pascit] *adds* ad plenum S   **923** auis] *om.* AG   •   res] *add*
quas attrahere poterit uel asportare (portare L) CDL   **924–27** Sic … societatem]
om. S

Because they wish to live on other people's goods, they afterwards die in need. Prv 3:33 says, 'Want is from the Lord in the house of the wicked'.

[901] This island also has the spider *lanuginosa*, that is actors and flatterers, through whose cursed praise these thieves have become puffed up in pride and may never be converted to good. Notice that, according to Aristotle, *On animals* 8, the crow is the fox's friend and fights with him against the badger, and this companionship accords well with them both. For the fox is a greedy, tricky, and deceitful animal; when it lacks food, it pretends to be dead, and then it seizes birds that descend on it and eats them, according to Isidore, book 2. It also always limps, because the thighs on its right side are shorter than the other pair, and it has a natural hatred for the badger. The fox is a thief, voracious, perjured, and lying, because he pretends to be dead and not able to support his family or rule his land, unless he can carry off poor peoples' goods. For this reason, it never has a part poised toward the right, that is, the side of the elect, and has a hatred, as it were naturally, for the badger, a very clean beast, representative of the clean and innocent poor.

[917] Truly the crow is a chattering bird and one that is always prophesying about time to come as an act of flattery. For it has, according to Fulgentius, in his book *Mythographies*, alone among the birds, 74 different meanings in its cry; for this reason, it is said to have the power of divination. According to Isidore, book 12, it does not feed its chicks until their colour resembles the blackness of its feathers, and it is also an unclean bird because it frequents corpses. It is also a treacherous bird; it takes things away like a thief and hides them. Likewise a flatterer promises

925   pr[o]mittens, nulli nisi sibi simili in moribus complacens, fedis
       moribus insistens. Sic ergo predo rapax et adulator mendax;
       indiuiduam habent societatem in dicta Hibernia, que bene
       conuenit in conditionibus cum Creta, quia 'Cretenses semper
       mendaces', ad Titum 1.
930   Habet etiam Hibernia tertiam araneam, scilicet *formicoleonem*
       multiplicem, scilicet balliuos et officiales, quibus in dicta terra,
       ut uidetur, innata est astutia uenenata ad destruendum pauperes
       et innocentes. Et ad hoc nota quod dicit Plynius quod tota
       species lupi ita inimicatur oui, ut si chorda facta de intestinis
935   lupi collocetur in cythara iuxta chordam factam de intestinis
       ouis, ipsam totaliter corrodit et consumit. Similiter penna aquile,
       collocata in pharetra iuxta pennas aliarum auium, eas corrodit et
       consumit. Sic in terra dicta, totus numerus balliuorum et
       officialium uidetur quasi naturaliter uenenatus esse contra
940   pauperes et innocentes, et hoc est contra instinctum naturalem,
       scilicet [non] nocere innocenti.
            Narrat enim Iorath, libro suo *De animalibus*, quod delfines
       per odorem sentiunt et cognoscunt si homo mortuus in mari
       unquam comederit de delfine. Quod si, sic ipsum comedunt; si
945   uero non comederit, a morsibus aliorum ipsum saluant et rostris
       suis pellunt eum ad littus. Nec aliquis idiota, nesciens instinctum
       nature in talibus uigere secundum gradum perfectionis sibi
       naturaliter collatum, de hoc admiretur. Sciat, secundum

---

925 promittens] premittens p • nisi] *om.* A • simili] *om.* CDL   926 rapax]
uorax A   927 dicta Hibernia] hac Scocia AG, Hybernia CD, predicta insula
scilicet Hibernia L, dicta Scocia S   928 conditionibus] moribus S
929 ad Titum 1] *adds* uentris pigri C *(extending the citation of Tit 1:12), adds*
sicud dicit apostolus ad Tytum Cretenses semper sunt mendaces uentris pigri D,
adds Similiter sunt semper histriones adulatores mendaces G, *adds* || ad Titum
Cretenses sunt semper mendaces uentris pigri L
930 Habet etiam Hibernia] *om.* • Hibernia] Scocia A, Scocia id est Hibernia G
 • *formicoleon*] mirmicaleon CDL   931 dicta] *om.* (*a corr.*) C, predicta S
934 oui] *om.* S   936 Similiter] Sicut eciam CDGS   937 auium] *om.* D
 • corrodit et] corrodit similiter et CDL, *om.* G   938 consumit] confundit
L • totus] *om.* A, necnon in aliis terris CDL   939 officialium] *add* et eciam
aliorum malorum (ma|lor$\overline{um}$ C, malorum hominum L) uicinorum predonum
scilicet et auarorum CDL   941 non] *om.* Sp
942 Iorath] Socrates L   943 homo mortuus] cadauer hominis mortui sit …
qui CDL   944 unquam] nunquam D   945 saluant et] piscium saluant et ipsum
cadauer CDL • rostris] *a corr.* (*from* restibus D) CD   948 de] quin (*a corr.*) C,
quin (*a corr.*) de D

only good fortune, approves of no one unless they resemble him in their behaviour, and encourages filthy habits. Thus one has both a rapacious thief and a lying flatterer; in Ireland they have a partnership that is unique, although the character of that place well accords with that of Crete, since 'Cretans are always liars', as Tit 1:12 says.

[930] Ireland also has the third kind of spider, multiple examples of the *formicoleon*, that is bailiffs and officials. In that land, it would appear, they have an inborn poisonous cunning they use to destroy the poor and innocent. Notice in this regard that Pliny says that the entire tribe of wolves has such enmity for the sheep that if a string made from wolf-gut is placed in a lyre next to a string made from sheep-gut, the wolf-string gnaws and completely devours the sheep-string. Likewise a feather from an eagle used to guide an arrow and placed in a quiver next to the feathers of other birds gnaws and devours them. Similarly, in Ireland, the whole lot of bailiffs and officials appears naturally envenomed against the poor and innocent, and this desire runs against natural instinct, which is not to harm the innocent.

[942] Also Iorath, in his book *On animals*, tells that dolphins can smell out and recognise whether a man dead in the ocean ever has eaten a dolphin. If he has, then they eat him in turn; but if he has not eaten a dolphin, they save him from being bitten by other fish and drive the body to shore with their beaks. Nor should any fool, not knowing the instinct of nature ruling in such animals – it accords with the level of perfection naturally conferred on them – be amazed about this. He should know

Isidorum, libro 12, capitulo 12, quod delfinus delectatur in
950   symphonia in tantum quod, secundum Augustinum, libro 1
De ciuitate, capitulo 25, '+ Arionem Machinium, nobilissimum
chytharistam, cum esset de naui eiectus, delfinus supra dorsum
suum ad terram ipsum prouehebat', sicut ipse testatur se legisse
in libris philosophorum. Quanta ergo crudelitas est spoliare
955   hominem qui nunquam [alium] spoliauit! Unde Tullius, libro 3
De officiis, 'Detrahere aliquid alteri et hominem [hominis] +
incommodo suum commodum augere, magis est contra naturam
quam mors, quam dolores qui corpori possunt accidere'. +
        Uenenum auaritie prelatorum comparatur formice
960   secundum malas eius conditiones. Dicit enim Solinus et
Plynius, libro 11, quod formice astutiam et prudentiam habent
ad laborandum et in plenilunio de nocte, sed partibus aliis
lunationis quiescunt. Et tunc habent cognitionem de tempore
laboris et fit concur[s]atio et obuiatio atque + collatio. Tunc
965   etiam maiores semitas certas, per quas formice minores
asportando cibum transeunt; et preponunt formicas sapientiores,
ne stulte oberrent. Deinde grana portata abradunt antequam
condant, ne rursus crescant. +
        Nota hic quattuor conditiones prelati mercenarii auari.
970   Nam incremento lune, id est temporalium, + tempore

---

951 Arionem] armonie A, Athimone CL (*corr. from* Atimore C), Atimore D,
Arimonem Sp • nobilissimum] *om.* S   **952** naui] mari L   **954** spoliare] *adds*
et excoriare G   **955** hominem] ipsum L • alium] hominem Sp, *om.* L
956 hominis] detraccione deprauare eiusque Sp (*the prec.* hominem *canc.* C)
958 quam dolores] uel dolor aliquis CDL • corpori] *om.* L • accidere] *add*
GSp+La: (*om.* ACDL+R, *unfound in* V)
    Dico quod tanta (intelligitur p) ut instinctus naturalis qui (ut G) in ceteris
    animalibus uiget extinguatur (exterminatur G).
    an analogous addition B: Cum ergo marine belue naturali instinctu
    uindicant, se de commestoribus piscium sue specie, non immerito Deus
    uindicat se de homine, *with additional material.*
960 conditiones] proprietates C   **960–61** et Plynius] *om.* ACDGL   **962** ad …
nocte] in plenaluno S   **962–63** partibus aliis lunationis] aliis temporibus
lune CDL   **964** concursatio] concursus G, concuruacio Sp • collatio]
collocatio p   **965** maiores] *om.* CDGL • certas] maiores G   **966** preponunt]
ponunt ACDGL   **967** portata] parata L   **967** portata … antequam] atque S
968 condant] commedunt ACDL, condunt S • crescant] *adds* p (*om.*
ACDGLS+BRULa):
    Tandem uenit porcus et totum consumit.
970 temporalium] *om.* S, *adds* id est p

that, according to Isidore 12.12, the dolphin is delighted by music to such a degree that, according to Augustine, *On the city* 1.25, 'When he had been thrown from a ship, a dolphin took Arion the Methymean, the noblest player on the lyre, on his back and carried him to land'. Augustine claims to have read this in the books of the philosophers. Therefore what great savagery it is to despoil a man who has never done the same to any other man! Hence Cicero, *On duties* 3, says, 'To take something away from someone else and to increase one's own advantage by disadvantaging him is more unnatural than death, than all those sorrows that may befall the body'.

[959] The poison of prelates' avarice is compared with that of the ant in accord with its evil behaviours. For Solinus and Pliny in book 11 say that ants work cleverly and prudently, and they do this at night during the full moon, but at other points in the lunar cycle they rest. In the full moon they know it is the time for labour, and they arrange their running about, their meetings, and their gathering things together; also then the bigger ants construct secure paths along which the smaller ants pass carrying food, and they put the wiser ants in front, lest the stupid ones wander off. Then, before it is stored, they scrape the collected grain to stop it from growing.

[969] Notice here four characteristics of a greedy and mercenary prelate. For he works as the moon is growing full, that is of worldly

decimarum congregandarum et aliarum obuentionum, laborat.
Prouerbiorum 7, 'Pecuniam tollit in p[lenilu]nio'; aliis temporibus
dormit. Tempus uero uisitandi, exactiones faciendi omnes prelati
optime obseruant; cursitant, obuiant, et capitula frequentant.

975 Tertio, ponunt formicas, id est uisitatores acutiores, super uias
pauperum, ut eos cum aculeo pungant et merciamenta emungant.
Deinde omnia collecta in modum formicarum, abradunt, ne
rursus germinent, quia de omnibus acquisitis nihil potest sciri,
quia nec in usum rei publice et in elemosynas pauperum, nec in

980 subsidia religiosorum conuertuntur, ac si omnia ponerentur in
saccum pertusum. +

Et [ide]o peior est mercenarius prelatus et rector uagabundus
omni alio mundano qui saltem residet in proprio loco. Solinus
etiam addit quintam condicionem formice, scilicet quod a

985 natura data est ei aqua mordax loco armorum uel ueneni,
quam uulgus, licet falso, uocat urinam eius. Et illam subito non
super tangentes tantum formicas, [sed] super illos quos formice
calcant uenenose spargunt, qui non modicum carnem urit.
Sic nisi fiat omnis uoluntas malorum prelatorum, sententiam

990 uenenosam quasi iniuriosam fulminant ita quod sub manu
talium populus nunquam conualescit, [sed] tam in temporalibus
quam in spiritualibus deficit. Prouerbiorum 30, 'Formice', id
est malo prelato, 'populus infirmus'. Nota quod formica haberet
multum de illa aqua, nimis cruciaret homines. Sic Deus limitauit

995 iurisdictionem talium prelatorum, ne nimis grauarent populum,
et abbreuiauit aliquando uitam.

---

971 laborat, dormit] C *corr. from plurals*; laborant, dormiunt D; laborant,
dormit L   **972** plenilunio] penultimo ACDGLSp   **973** dormit] *adds* uidelicet
tempore hospitalitatis subuentionis et deuocionis G   **974** obseruant] *adds* quia
tunc G   • capitula] capellas G   **975** Tertio] Et CD, Secundo G   • formicas]
add prudenciores CDGL   • uias] uulgus A   **976** aculeo] suis aculeis CDL
• et … emungant] *om.* A   **980** ac] ac set sic sunt ACDG   **981** pertusum] *adds* p
(*om.* ACDGLS+BRULa):
    Tandem uenit porcus, scilicet diabolus, et eos deuorat et collecta dispersit.
982 Et ideo] Hiis S, Sed multo p   • est mercenarius] *om.* A   **983** saltem] solum
CDL   • proprio] uno CD, || *om.* L   **984** quintam] quartam L   **987, 991** sed]
immo Sp   **989** Sic, malorum prelatorum] Similiter est ex parte prelatorum,
eorum CDL   • fiat] *adds* omnis S   • malorum] *om.* G   **990** quasi iniuriosam]
om. S   **991** populus] pauper G, *add* hodie CDL   **991–92** tam … spiritualibus]
omnino S   **993** malo prelato] prelatus malus CD   **994** cruciaret] lederet A
• Sic] Set CDGL   • limitauit iurisdictionem] limitacionem ponit CDL (limitat G)
995 ne] *add* secundum suam maliciam CDL   **996** uitam] *add* eorum CDL

goods. That is the time for gathering together tithes and other sources of income. Prv 7:20, 'He took with him money ... the day of the full moon'; at other times, he sleeps. In truth, all prelates observe most carefully the time for visitation and for making exactions; they bustle about, they have meetings, they attend chapters. Third, they put their ants, that is their shrewdest visitation officials, on the roads travelled by the poor so that they can sting them and swindle fines from them. At last, when everything has been collected in the way that ants do, they scrape it all, lest it should sprout again. For no one can know anything about all that they have acquired, because it is not converted into common public use or into alms for the poor or into support for religious people, but it is as if everything were put into a bag riddled with holes.

[982] Therefore a mercenary prelate and a wandering priest are much worse than any other worldly cleric who always lives in his own place. Solinus adds a fifth characteristic of the ant, namely that nature has given it instead of weapons or poison a caustic fluid that common folk call, although falsely, its piss. And ants spray this poison about immediately, and not just on those who touch them but even on those whom they themselves tread on. And it burns the flesh a great deal. Likewise, unless evil prelates get their way completely, they thunder forth poisonous, that is injurious, sentences, so that under the custody of such men, the people never get well – indeed, they fail in both temporal and spiritual things. Prv 30:25 says, 'The ants', that is with an evil prelate, 'a feeble people'. Notice that if an ant should have a good deal of this water, he would torment people more. Thus God has limited such prelates' jurisdiction, lest they oppress the people too much, and sometimes has shortened their lives.

Uenenum rectorum comparatur amphibene, qui est serpens,
secundum Isidorum, libro 12, habens duo capita, unum in
principio et alterum in cauda. Unde Plynius, libro 8, 'Habet',
1000   inquit, 'amphibena duplex caput, tanquam esset + parum ei
infundere uenenum uno ore'. Et talis est rector uel prebendarius
habens duas ecclesias uel prebendas et [neu]tri satisfaciens. Unde
hic contra legem diuinam et naturalem atque canonicam duas
habet uxores desponsatas; ideo bigamus, et damnandus est cum
1005   Lamech maledicto qui primus introduxit bigamiam, Genesis 4.
    Est aliud uenenum in ecclesia: nepotum, scilicet prelatorum.
Hoc comparatur hydre. Hydras enim, ut dicit Isidorus, libro 12,
est serpens multorum capitum, et dicitur quod uno capite ceso,
tria crescunt. Et hoc si sit in se fabulosum, tamen uerum est
1010   quod pro uno nepote quem estimab[a]tur prelatus habere ante
promotionem, tres nepotes surgunt post cornuum [erectionem,
institutionem, et prebende] assumptionem, ita quod tota patria
uidetur esse de sua parentela. Sed quia 'Breues sunt dies eius',
cito disperguntur, secundum illud psalmi, 'Confregisti capita
1015   draconis', id est nepotes talis prelati; 'dedisti eum escam populis
Ethiopum', id est societati T[artare]orum spirituum.
    Est et aliud graue uenenum quod auget omnia uenena
auaricie et superbie predicta, scilicet adulatorum et histrionum.
Comparatur scorpioni, qui dicitur a *scrope*, quod est [dulce],

---

997 rectorum] prelatorum G • rectorum … amphi-] *blank left, corr. marg.* A
997, 1000 amphiben] amphilen- D (*the readings corr.* C) **999** in] add fine
scilicet in ADL **1000** parum] paruum ACDLSp **1001** uenenum] ueneno A,
a corr. C, *om.* D **1002** uel prebendas] *om.* CDL • neutri] uentri p
1005 Lamech] *adds* homicidia G • bigamiam] *adds* accipiendo duas uxores G
1007 Hoc] *add* uenenum CDGL • hydre] *add* serpenti CL (*a corr.* C)
1008 capitum] *om.* A **1009** crescunt] *adds* capita S **1010** pro uno] *add*
capite CL (*a corr.* C), primo D • nepote] *om.* G • estimabatur] estimabant
ACGL, estimabat L, estimabitur p • prelatus habere] *om.* ACDL
1011–12 erectionem … prebende] ereccionem et A, institucionem et prebende
G, *om.* Sp **1014** cito] *add* dissipantur et Sp; *add* disparent tales nepotes et filios,
et quasi in omnem uentum, secundum sua et progenitorum suorum demerita
CDL **1015** nepotes] filios et nepotes CDL • talis prelati] prelatorum CDGL;
add et sequitur CDGL • escam] *om.* GS **1016** Tartareorum] tyrannorum p
• spirituum] *om.* GS
1017 uenena] *add* uenenum scilicet ACDL **1018** auaricie et superbie] *om.* A
• predicta] superius dicta A, quod aliqualiter predicta est CDL
1019 Comparatur] *add* illud uenenum ueneno scorpionis CDL, Hoc
comparatur S • dulce] blanditie p

[997] The poison of rectors is compared to the *amphibena*, which according to Isidore, book 12, is a snake that has two heads, one at the top and another in its tail. Thus, Pliny, book 8, says, 'The *amphibena* has a double head, as if it were not enough for it to pour out poison from a single mouth'. This snake is just like a rector or prebendary having two churches or prebends and performing satisfactorily in neither. For this reason, against all law – natural, divine, or canon – he is wed to two wives. Therefore he is a bigamist, and should be condemned with the cursed Lamech, who first practised bigamy, as Gn 4:19 says.

[1006] There is a further poison in the church, that of kinsmen, specifically those of prelates. This is compared to the hydra. For as Isidore says in book 12, the hydra is a snake with many heads, and it is said that if one is cut off, three of them grow back. And although the hydra may be a fable, nevertheless it is true that for the single kinsman that people think a prelate has before he is promoted, three kinsmen rise up after he's put on the mitre, been installed, and taken up his prebend, so that the whole country appears to be a part of his lineage. But because 'His days are short' (Iob 14:5), kinsmen like these are quickly scattered, following Ps 73:14, 'Thou hast broken the heads of the dragon', that is, the kinsmen of such a prelate; 'thou hast given him to be meat for the people of the Ethiopians', that is, for the company of Hell's spirits.

[1017] There is another dangerous poison that increases all the poisons of avarice and pride already mentioned, and that is the poison associated with flatterers and actors. This may be likened to the scorpion, which is called that from the word *scrop*, which means 'sweet', and

1020   et *poieo, poieis*, quod est fingere, quia anteriori parte blanditias
        fingit, et in posteriori ferit. Unde Gregorius, *Super Ezechielem*,
        'Palpando incedit, sed cauda ferit'. Et secundum Plynium, libro 11,
        semper cauda eius est parata percutere, nulloque momento cessat
        a lesione, si ei detur occasio ledendi. Sic adulator in presentia
1025   hominis facie blanda semper decipit, sed in absentia, cauda
        percutiendo, semper detrahit. Unde tanto est magis uenenosus
        quanto magis domesticus, quia secundum Hieronimum,
        epistola 14, 'Adulator est blandus inimicus'. + Ideo dicitur in
        Polycraton, libro 3, 'Adulator omnis uirtutis inimicus; eo est
1030   magis cauendus quo sub amantis specie nocere cupit, qui comites
        habet odium, proditionem, fraudem, et notam mendacii. Sequela
        uero seruitutis habet excecationem [proximi] et exterminium
        totius honestatis'. Hec ille. Unde malum est habitare ubi multi
        tales sunt, quia sicut dicitur Apocalipsis 9, 'Cruciatus eorum sunt
1035   cruciatus scorpionis cum percutit homines'.
        Iste cruciatus multum regnat in Hibernia, cuius gens natiua
        histrionibus et adulatoribus carmina mellita sed uenenata
        componentibus omnia sua distribuebant. Et ideo ueneno uane et
        false laudis semper inflati erant. Dicit igitur Alexander Nequam,
1040   libro *De naturis*, 'Uidetur quod adulatio est uenenum mellitum
        aut mel uenenatum'. Unde homines illi non aduertentes uenenum
        false laudis, sed dulcedinem mellitam false adulationis super

---

1020 fingere] fingo fingis CDLG   1022 Palpando] Scorpio palpando A, *adds*
id est plaudendo G   1023 momento] (?) oppm̄tto A   1025 hominis] *om.* ACDL
1025–26 cauda percutiendo] *om.* ACDL, percutiendo G   1026 semper] *a corr.*
C, *om.* D   1027 magis] *om.* A   1026–28 quia … 14] Sp, quia primum Iohannem
epistolam 9 A, quia secundum Ieronimum CDG, ideo L   1028 inimicus] *add*
pGS+BRV (*om.* ACDL+La):
    Unde dicitur in libro qui *Dogma philosophorum* (*adds* dicitur R, *adds*
    appellatur V) scribitur (habetur R, inscribitur S) quod 'Falsi amici pro
    consilio adulacionem (*om.* V) afferunt, et uana (unum G; una SRV, *recte*) est
    eorum contencio quis blandius fallat'.
1030 specie] (?) spem C   1031 proditionem] predacione A, detraccionem CDL
• et] est AL, *om.* CD   1032 proximi] *om.* p • exterminium] eterminium D
1035 cum] qui (que CD) cauda ACDL
1036 regnat] *om.* A, regnum S • natiua] natura ADL   1037–38 carmina …
componentibus] carmina secundum iudicium eorum mellita set secundum
uerum iudicium uenenata componentibus quasi se euiscerantes (*adds* et
nudantes C, *adds* et inuidantes D) CDL   1037 uenenata] uenenosa S
1038–39 uane et false laudis] false laudis et uento uane glorie CDL
1040 Uidetur] *om.* CDL   1041 aut mel uenenatum] *om.* S • homines] *om.* G

from *poieo, poieis*, which means 'to feign'. For a scorpion feigns flattery
with its front part, and with its tail, it strikes. For this reason, Gregory,
On Ezechiel, says, 'A scorpion advances with strokes, but it strikes with its
tail'. According to Pliny, book 11, its tail is always ready to strike a blow,
and it may never hold back from injuring one, if it is given any occasion
to do so. Likewise, a flatterer in a person's presence always deceives him
with an ingratiating face, but in the person's absence always disparages
him, by striking him with his tail. For this reason, the more intimate
he is, the more poisonous, because, according to Jerome, epistle 14,
'A flatterer is an ingratiating enemy'. Therefore it says in *Polycraticus*,
book 3, 'A flatterer is the enemy of every virtue. That person is most
to be avoided who under a loving surface desires to harm; such people
companion with hatred, betrayal, and deceit, and are noteworthy for their
lying. Slavery to such people results in the blinding of one's neighbour
and the death of all virtue'. So he says. For this reason, it is evil to dwell
where there are many such, for as Apc 9:5 says, 'Their torment was as the
torment of a scorpion when he striketh a man'.

[1036] Such tormented people rule widely in Ireland, for the native
race gave away all their goods to actors and flatterers who composed
for them honeyed yet poisonous songs. Therefore they were continually
puffed up by the poison of empty and false praise. Therefore Alexander
Neckam says in his book *On the natures of things*, 'It seems that flattery is
a honeyed poison or a poisoned honey'. For this reason, those people who
are not paying attention to the poison of false praise but to the honeyed
sweetness of false flattery are

statum proprium semper ferebantur. Quia ut dicit Iuuenalis,
'Nihil est quod de se credere non possit, cum laudatur diis equa
1045   potestas'. Unde tales semper percutiuntur illa plaga Egypti quam
intulerunt locuste, Exodi 10, 'Uentus urens leuauit locustas super
totam terram Egypti, et deuastata est herba terre et quicquid
pomorum in arboribus fuit'. Gregorius, libro 31, 'Locuste, id
est lingue adulantium, plus quam cetere plage nocuerunt, quia
1050   quicquid uiriditatis', id est quicquid meriti est in operibus
illorum, 'qui illis a[ssen]ciunt, totaliter eis aufferunt'. Ad hoc nota
exemplum Ambrosii in *Hexameron* de cicada, parua bestiola que
in gutture suo miram format cantilenam et in medio estu quando,
scilicet arbusta amittunt uirorem propter nimium calorem. Unde
1055   a canendo dicitur, quia tunc [quanto] aerem habet [pur]iorem
et spiritum attrahit, [tanto cantu resonat clar]iorem, nec aliquo
calore uincitur, qui[n] etiam de nocte continuet. Perfundatur
tamen paruo oleo, et statim obmutescit – immo moritur, quia pori
clausi non attrahunt aerem, secundum Ambrosium. Sic oleum
1060   adulationis omnem uigorem tollit uirtutis. ₡

De remediis auaritie.
Capitulum XII.

Remedium [et] tyriaca auaritie est restitutio de omnibus male
acquisitis per predas, furta, usuras. Et si queras de quantitate
restitutionis, breuem regulam trado: quod si aliquis talis plus de

---

1043 semper] *om.* CDS   1044 Nihil] Nullus S   •   cum laudatur] cum laudetur A,
om. L   1045 semper] *om.* CD   •   illa] *om.* CL, septima D   1047 deuastata]
deuorata S (*in* ACDGL, *the citation ends at* locustas)   1049–51 quia … aufferunt]
om. supplied as marg. corr. CD   1050 quicquid¹] quia S   •   quicquid … quicquid]
quicquid G   1051 assenciunt] consensiunt D, afficiuntur p   1052 in *Hexameron*]
om. A   •   parua bestiola] auis G   1054 calorem] *add* uiriliter canit CD
1055 quanto] quando AGL, *om.* Sp   •   puriorem] clariorem ACDLSp   1056 et …
clariorem] tanto spiritum attrahit puriorem ACDLSp, tanto cantu resonat
clariorem G   1057 quin] qui p   •   nocte] *add* cantum CDL   •   Perfundatur]
Perfusa CDGL   1058 obmutescit … moritur] *corr. from* obtu|mescit inmoritur C
1060 uirtutis] *add* Cicada est auicula que quodammodo est pennata, Anglice
greshopper (A.g. *om.* A) ACDL

heading] *om.* AS, Remedium auaricie CD
1061 et] *om.* G, in p   •   male] *om.* G   1062 queras] *om.* S   1063 breuem … trado]
respondo quod G

always borne up above their proper state. For as Juvenal says, 'There is nothing that one might not believe about himself, when praise grants him a power equal to that of the gods'. For this reason, such people are always struck by that plague of Egypt that the locusts brought in, Ex 10:13–15, 'The burning wind raised the locusts over the whole land of Egypt, and the grass of the earth was devoured and what fruits soever were on the trees'. Gregory in book 31, 'Locusts, that is the tongues of flatterers, harmed more than the other plagues did; whatever growing thing', that is whatever merit is in their works, 'if they assent to flatterers, the flatterers carry it off completely'. On this point, notice Ambrose's example of the cicada in his *Hexameron*; it is a little beast that produces a marvellous song in its throat, and it does so at midsummer, just as trees lose their growth on account of excessive heat. It is called cicada from its singing (*canendo*) because at this time, the purer the air and the breath it draws, the clearer its song resounds. Nor is it overcome by any heat, but may also continue singing at night. Nevertheless were one to pour a little oil on it, it immediately goes mute; indeed, it dies, because its blocked pores cannot draw in air, as Ambrose says. Thus the oil of flattery carries off all the strength of virtue. ₵

On the remedies for avarice.
Chapter 12.

[1061] The remedy and antidote to avarice is the restitution of all the things one has acquired evilly, whether by exactions, thefts, or usury. And if you ask how much you should give back, I offer you a brief rule: if such a person has received from another more

1065

alieno recepit quam in bonis possidet, totum quod habet reddat, nichil sibi retinens, nisi annonam illius diei naturalis pro se et suis liberis. Alioquin de ueneno uiuit et mortem sibi continue propinat. Nec est remedium quamdiu remanet uenenum, ne per elemosynarum largitionem uel aliquam hospitalitatem + credat saluari.

1070

1075

1080

Meliores enim sunt predones, qui impartiuntur indigentibus de predis, quam illi qui sibi solis omnia retinent. Nam instinctus [nature] hoc docet. Aues rapaces, sicut narrat Plynius de aquila, quod nisi fame attreratur, sola non comedit suam predam, sed auibus insequentibus se illam in communi exponit. portione tamen sua prius recepta. Sed quando sibi preda non sufficit, tanquam rex de republica uiuens, auem sibi proximam arripit et in medio eam ponit. Unde propter hoc multe aues sequuntur eam. Et credo quod hec liberalitas, licet de aliena substantia, multos disponit ad gratiam in Hibernia, ubi fures et predones consueuerunt de rebus alienis esse hospitales. [F]ex enim omnium malorum est tenax predo.

1085

1090

De hiis autem que acquirit auarus mundanus anxio studio, tamen sine actu in lege prohibito, debet fieri distributio pauperibus per elemosynas. Dicit enim Dyoscorides quod tela aranee, licet sit de uisceribus uenenosis, tamen quando inuenitur munda et sine pulueribus, sanguinem restringit a uulnere, prohibet fieri saniem, et sanat plagam recentem ac cohibet fieri flaturam. Tela hec est solicitudo auari circa substantiam temporalem, que si conuersa fuerit in debitam elemosynam, sanat uulnera mentis, cohibet inflaturam elationis, quia iniquitas bene dispensata conuertitur in iustitiam. Et intellige de acquisitis sine actu in lege prohibito.

1064 recepit] recipit AG, *om.* CDL • reddat] reddet CD, reddit L **1065** illius] unius LS • illius … diei] *om.* G **1066** suis liberis] pueris G • ueneno] rapina S • sibi] sic A **1069** credat] credant se (*om.* p) Sp • credat saluari] *om.* G
1071–72 instinctus … rapaces] sicut narrat G **1072** nature] *om.* p • rapaces] rapientes S **1073** atteratur] cruciatur G, moriatur L • sola] *om.* S
1074 illam] predam suam CDL, *om.* S **1079** disponit] *om.* L **1079–80** fures … hospitales] latrones solebant de alieno esse liberales G **1080** hospitales] tales scilicet hospitales A • Fex] fex Rex G, Rex Sp **1081** predo] *add* secundum Senecam CDGL
1083 tamen … prohibito] *om.* L **1084** per elemosynas] *om.* G • licet sit] si sit A, et si sit (*marg. corr. from* eciam fit) C, eciam fit D, que sistit L **1086** saniem] *corr. from* sanguinem C, san|guinem D **1087** cohibet] prohibet AL • flaturam] inflaturam S **1088** conuersa] *om.* G **1090** inflaturam] inflacionem CDL • dispensata] dispensam AL

than the goods he possesses, he should give back all that he has, keeping nothing for himself beyond the supply of grain necessary to himself and his children for a single natural day. Otherwise he is living off poison and continually preparing for his own spiritual death. Nor is this a cure so long as any poison remains in him, nor should he believe he is saved through generosity in almsgiving or some form of hospitality.

[1070] Indeed thieves are better than people who keep everything for their use alone, for the former give away to the needy the results of their plunder. Natural instinct teaches one to do this, as birds of prey show. As Pliny explains about the eagle, unless it is utterly ground down by hunger, it does not eat its prey alone, but exposes it to all the birds that follow it in common – although it takes its own share first. But when its prey is not enough to sustain it, as if he were a king living from goods of the commonwealth, he seizes the bird nearest him and puts it in the middle. For this reason, many birds follow the eagle. I believe that this generosity, even if it is with someone else's goods, makes many people welcome in Ireland, for there thieves and exactors have been accustomed to extend hospitality, using other people's goods. For a grasping thief is the dregs of all evils.

[1082] Moreover, a worldly avaricious person should distribute to the poor through alms those things that he acquires with thoughtful study (yet not those that he has got by some illegal act). For Dioscorides says of a spider-web, that although it comes from the spider's poisonous guts, when one finds a web that is clean and without dirt mixed in, it keeps a wound from bleeding, stops it from becoming infected, heals a recent blow, and prevents it from becoming swollen. This web is the care an avaricious person takes about temporal goods that, if they have been turned into proper almsgiving, heals the mind's wounds and restrains the swelling of pride, because iniquity well disposed of is turned into righteousness. And understand that this refers only to things acquired without an illegal act.

Nota tamen secundum Tullium, libro *De diuinatione*, quod 'Duo sunt genera largorum. Quidam qui in epulis et spectaculis suas profundunt, in eas res quarum memoria non habetur. Alii
1095   qui suis facultatibus aut captos a predonibus redimunt, aut es alienum suscipiunt amicorum causa, aut filios collocant honestate, aut opitulantur in republica augenda'. Primi merentur potius confusionem quam laudem, quia secundum Ambrosium, libro *De officiis*, 'Non est largitas si quod alteri cum impendis alteri
1100   extorqueas, uel dare quod liceat, ut sit iactantie causa magis quam misericordie. Secunda perfecta est [largitas], ubi silentium opus tegit et + necessitatibus singulorum occulte subuenitur, quam laudat os pauperis, non la[bia] propria'. [Matthei: 'Cum facis elemosinam, noli tuba canere ante te, sicut ypocrite faciunt, sed
1105   faciente te elemosinam, nesciat sinistra tua quid faciat dextera'].
      Exemplum narratur quod in Hibernia erat quidam diues et hospitalis et largus ualde. Hic ad mortem propinquans, adiuratus fuit ab amico suo ut sibi reuelaret statum suum [post mortem]. At ille post magnum tempus apparuit amico suo; qui requisitus
1110   de statu, respondit quod damnatus fuit. Et amicus, 'Ubi', inquit 'sunt elemosyne tue multe, pupilli et orphani quos nutristi?' At ille, 'Omnia', inquit, 'propter gloriam mundi et extollentiam iactantie feci, et ideo totum perdidi'.

1092–93 quod duo sunt] quot sunt A   **1093** Quidam … spectaculis] \Quidam/ G
1094 profundit] effundit AG, perfundit CDL   **1095** suis facultatibus] sua
erogant G   •   captos] captiuos (*corr. from* captos) C, aut captos (*with* redim<unt>
over erasure) D, captiuos G   •   a predonibus] *om.* CDGL, predones S
1095–96 es … causa] *om.* G   **1096** alienum] aliorum CDL   •   causa] *om., a corr.* D
•   collocant honestate] parenter educant G   **1097** opitulantur] *om.* G, facultates
suas constituunt S   **1098** secundum] *adds* Gregorium et A   **1099** si] scilicet L
1100 liceat] non licet CD   •   uel … ut] nec dare quod non habeat nec quod A
1101 quam … Secunda] *om.* G   •   Secunda] Secundi merentur et liberalitas S
•   largitas] largicio G, *om.* Sp   **1102** necessitatibus] uite A, necessitantibus p
•   subuenitur] *corr. from* fouentur C, fouentur D   **1103** labia] lingua A, laus CDGL,
os S   **1103–5** Mathei … dextera] *om.* ASp+VLa   **1105** faciente (*corr. from* facite D)
1107 et largus] *om.* G   •   propinquans] appropinquaret (*corr. from* appropinquans)
C, appropinquans || DG   **1108** amico] socio GS   •   post mortem] *om.* Ap, *add* si
quomodo posset CDL (quomodo] *corr. from* quodammodo C, quodammodo D)
1109 post] *a corr.* D   •   post … apparuit] tandem apparens G   **1109–10** qui …
respondit] dixit G   **1110–11** Et … nutristi] Et requisitus quid sibi fecerit omnes
quas facere solebant G   **1111** multe] *om.* CDS   **1112–13** propter … perdidi] anna (?)
super collem iactancie A, sparguntur super collem iactancie CDL   **1112** mundi]
gloriam G   **1112–13** et extollentiam iactantie] *om.* GS   •   totum] ea G, omnia S

[1092] Nevertheless notice that according to Cicero, in his book *On divination*, 'There are two kinds of generous people. There are some people who pour out their goods in banquets and shows, in things that don't last in memory. There are others who use their powers either to ransom captives from pirates, or to take into their protection other people's money for the sake of friendship, or to place their children in virtuous employment, or give their aid to improving the public good. The first group deserves destruction more than praise, for according to Ambrose, in his *On duties*, 'It is not generosity when you extort from one person what you give to another, or to give what is permissible for the sake of boasting, rather than of mercy. A second sort of generosity is perfect; in it, silence cloaks the deed, and support is extended secretly to the needs of individuals. This is a generosity that the mouth of the poor praises, not your own lips'. Mt 6:2–3 says, 'When thou dost an almsdeed, sound not a trumpet before thee, as the hypocrites do, but when thou dost alms, let not thy left hand know what thy right hand doth'.

[1106] There is a story that once in Ireland there was a rich man, welcoming and very generous, and when he was nearing death, he was entreated by a friend to reveal his spiritual state after he was dead. And after a long time, he appeared to this friend and when asked about his state, he replied that he was damned. And the friend said, 'Where are your great alms, all those wards and orphans whom you have raised?' And he said, 'I have done all these things for worldly glory and to be boastfully praised, and therefore I have lost everything'.

1115   Aliud remedium est quod *sphalangia* una, si ostendatur percusso et intoxicato a simili aranea in specie, cito curatur. Et ad hoc reseruantur tales aranee, cum mortue inueniuntur tales. Sic qui recte respicit diuitem auarum mortuum, nihil secum nisi peccata deferentem, et amicos et inimicos eius omnia eius bona distrahentes, habet remedium contra auariciam. Tercium
1120 remedium est quod ualet contra morsus omnium aranearum, scilicet + coagulum agni cum uino potatum. Hic est dolor et paupertas agni immaculati in cruce nudi pendentis, qui cum uino compunctionis sanat uulnera mentis auare, etc. Quartum remedium est quod musce, contrite et posite super morsum,
1125 extrahunt uenenum et mitigant dolorem. Sic desideria auari et studia anxia, nisi fuerit mortificata, nunquam sedatur auaricia. Remedia predicta extrahuntur a Plinio 19.

       Remedium contra uenenum draconis est, secundum Plinium 28, adeps proprius, qui secundum + ipsum, fugat omnia
1130 uenena, quia substantia mercatoris, que est sui cordis adeps, in elemosynam conuersa mundat delicta. Sapientie 4, 'Peccata tua elemosynis redime'. Item dicit Solinus quod si auferatur fel et lingua, que sunt receptacula ueneni, a dracone, caro eius potest comedi, et sanguis eius est remedium contra estum. Sic enim
1135 comedunt e[os] Ethiopes. Psalmus, 'Dedisti eam escam, etc.'.

1114 remedium] *add* contra uenenum (*adds* scilicet L) splangie CDGL (and D *adds, canc.* quod splangie est) • una] Sp, est quod splangia ACDGL   1115 cito] *om.* S   1117 recte] *om.* ACD • mortuum] *corr. from* negocium D   1118 nisi … deferentem] preter peccata portantem CDL   1119 distrahentes] *a corr.* D • habet] habere debet CDL   1120 omnium] *om.* S   1121 coagulum] *corr. from* cogulum CD, coagulatum p   1122 nudi] *om.* CDL   1123 compunctionis] inpugnacionis S   1124 contrite] attrite CDL, trite G • morsum] *add* serpentis CDGL   1126 fuerit] *adds* attrita et L • mortificata] mortiferata G 1127 extrahuntur] excipiuntur CDL

1128 draconis] detraccionis S   1129 (and 1130) adeps] adeptus L • ipsum] secundum philosophum siue ipsum Plynium Sp   1131 delicta] *add* et omnia reddit nitida atque pulcra CDL • Sapientie] Danielis ACDLS   1132 redime] **CDGL+R** *add* (*om.* ASp+LaV):

    et Luce, 'Date elemosinam, et ecce omnia munda sunt uobis'

B *adds*

    Unde dicit Tobias de substancia tua fac elemosinam quia elemosina ab omni peccato liberat etc.

1134 remedium] in r. (in *expunged* C) CD   1135 eos] *om.* G, eam p, *add* scilicet dracones CL (*int. corr.* C) • etc.] *add* Ita ex parte ista CDL, *adds* Sic si G

[1114] A second remedy is if a single *sphalangia* is shown to a person stung and poisoned by the same kind of spider, he is cured at once. And for this reason, if they are found dead, these spiders are preserved. Likewise, a person who properly observes a dead miserly rich person will have a remedy against avarice: the dead man is carrying nothing away with him except his sins, at the same time as both his friends and enemies are dragging off all his goods. A third remedy, and a powerful one against the stings of all spiders, is a lamb's rennet drunk with wine. This is the sorrow and the poverty of the immaculate lamb hanging naked on the cross; and this drunk with the wine of compunction heals the wounds of a greedy soul, etc. A fourth remedy is that ground up flies placed on a bite draw out the poison and relieve the pain. Likewise, unless an avaricious person's desires and his anxious studies are destroyed, avarice will never be laid to rest. These remedies are all drawn from Pliny, book 19.

[1128] According to Pliny, book 28, the remedy against a dragon's poison is its own fat, and he says that it puts all poisons to flight. Similarly, a merchant's possessions, which are the fat of his heart, when they are turned into almsgiving, cleanse his defaults. Sir 3:33 says, 'Alms resisteth sins'. Also Solinus says that if one takes away a dragon's gall and tongue, the places where it stores its poison, its flesh is edible, and its blood is a remedy against heat. For this reason, Ethiopians eat them both. Ps 73:14 says, 'Thou hast given [the dragon] to be meat [for the people of the Ethiopians]'.

Tollantur ergo fraudulentia et mendacia a mercatoribus, et
substantia eorum erit tuta et negociatio toleranda.

    Remedium contra pluralitatem beneficiorum est nullum,
nisi resignatio et de receptis satisfactio, quia omnia fiunt illicita.
1140 Nota quod nemo euadit uenenum amphibene et hydre quamdiu
remanent eius capita. Remedium contra uenenum scorpionis,
quod nunc multum inficit, est ualde necessarium et memoria
dignum. Primum contra adulationem est quod sit ueritas et
soliditas in opere. Unde dicit Isidorus, libro 12, quod scorpio
1145 nunquam in palma manus ferit nec ledit. Unde nota quod ubi
opus est solidum, quod significatur per manus, non timetur
scorpio, scilicet uenenum detractionis et adulationis. Secundum
remedium immunitas carnalitatis. Unde dicit Plynius, ubi supra,
'Nullum animal ledit scorpio carens sanguine', id est carnalitate.
1150 [Nemo ergo adulacioni consentit, nisi ex laudis libidine.]

    Tertium est rigor correptionis. Unde summum remedium
contra morsum scorpionis est oleum in quo ille uermis
submergitur et putrescit. Hoc oleum secundum Augustinum,
super illud psalmi, 'Oleum peccatoris non impinguet caput meum':
1155 'Falsa laus adulatoris et simulata dilectio', que mentes a rigore
ueritatis emollit ad noxia. Quando ergo adulatio percipitur et
adulator uilipenditur et redarguitur, in oleo proprio submergitur

1136 mendacia] *corr. from* mundana C, mundana DG; *add* et periuria CDL
mercatoribus] mercatura A, mercatore CDL, auaris et mercatoribus G
1137 erit tuta] *om.* DCL • tuta] necessaria GS negociatio] mercatura CDL
1138 nullum] possessor nulla G   1139 receptis satisfactio] restitucio de omnibus
bonis S • quia] *add* quamdiu tenet aliquis plura beneficia sine dispensacione
dico (*om.* CD) CDL • quia … illicita] *om.* G   1140 amphibene et] *om.* G
1141 capita] *adds* sic hic A, *add* sic ex parte ista CDGL • contra uenenum] *om.*
S   1142 inficit] interficit AL • ualde] *om.* S   1142–43 quod … sit] id est contra
adulacionem est G • memoria] medicina S   1143 Primum] *add* remedium
ACDLS • ueritas] *adds* in ore S   1146 per] palma CD   1147 detractionis]
om. G • adulationis] *adds* draconis CDL   1148 remedium] *add* contra
uenenum scorpionis est CDL   1150 Nemo … libidine] *om.* p • adulacioni]
adulatori A, *a corr.* C, *om.* D • consentit] -sit S
1151 Tertium] *add* remedium AGS, *add* remedium contra uenenum scorpionis CDL
• correptionis] correccionis G   1153 submergitur] sub- *a corr.* C,
mergitur D   1155 adulatoris] adulationis ALS • dilectio] *add* seductoris CDL
• mentes] *add* non forcium uirorum set effeminatorum CDL   1156 ueritatis]
uirtutis A, uirtutis et ueritatis CDL • adulatio] adulator CDL (*and om. later*
adulator); *add* et perpenditur CL (*int. corr.* C, *om.* D)   1157 uilipenditur]
perpenditur S

Therefore if the fraud and lying of merchants are removed, their substance is safe and should be allowed in business deals.

[1138] There is no remedy against pluralism in benefices, except resignation and restoring all that has been received from them, because it is all unlawful gain. Notice that no one can avoid the poison of the *amphibena* or the hydra so long as any of the heads remain. The remedy against the poison of the scorpion, which now infects many people, is very necessary and worthy of being remembered. The first remedy against flattery is that there be truth and substance in one's works. For this reason, Isidore says in book 12 that 'the scorpion never strikes or harms in the palm of the hand'. For this reason, notice that when one's work is solid, a trait that is indicated by the hand, one need not fear the scorpion, that is the poison of backbiting and flattery. The second remedy is being proof against carnality. For this reason, Pliny says, in the same place, 'The scorpion harms no animal that lacks blood', that is carnality. No one consents to flattery, except from a pleasure in being praised.

[1151] The third remedy is firm rebuke. For this reason, the best remedy against a scorpion's sting is oil in which this vermin has been plunged and left to rot. This oil, according to Augustine on Ps 140:5, 'Let not the oil of the sinner fatten my head', is 'the flatterer's false praise and pretended affection'. These melt minds from the firmness of truth into wrongdoing. Therefore, when one perceives flattery, and then disparages and rebukes the flatterer, he is plunged into his own oil

et moritur, quia confunditur, secundum illud Prouerbiorum 4, 'Remoue a te os prauuum'. Item remedium cicade est quod
1160 perfundatur aceto quod aperit poros. Nota correptionem per aceti acrimoniam.

Quartum remedium est seueritas pun[i]tionis. Nam scorpio occisus et piscatus, si ad proprium uulnus quod infert apponatur, reuertitur uenenum infixum ad corpus unde exiuit, et hoc est
1165 proprium huius pestis. Sic iusti et ueraces principes solebant facere, puniendo adulatores, inferendo eis uulnus quod aliis inferre tentabant. Nota de hoc qualiter Alexander magnus puniuit Permenionem adulatorem suum, supra capitulo de inuidia.

Est et quintum remedium contra adulatores et detractores
1170 quod exhibetur beneficio nature, scilicet utilitas mortis. Refert enim Plynius, ubi supra, quod scorpio parit unde[nos] fetus, quos quandoque occidit et deuorat, sed unus qui magis est sollers scandit supra dorsum matris, ubi tutus a cauda et a morsu eius residet. Hic matrem interficit et fraterne cedis ultor
1175 existit. Et hoc prouide fecit natura, ne uenenata progenies nimis propagetur. Hec ille Plynius. Sic estimo quod Deus in terra ubi adulatores, detractores, et predones multiplicantur, permittit fratricidia, proditiones, et quasi infinita homicidia fieri, ut mala radix extirpetur.

1158 quia confunditur] et consumitur L 1159 remedium] *om.* S, *add* contra uenenum CDL 1159–61 Item … acrimoniam] *om.* G 1160 quod aperit poros] moritur ut supra habetur CDL 1161 acrimoniam] acrimosam A, acrum et mordens notatur correpcionem duram CDL

1162 remedium] *add* contra uenenum serpentis CDL • punitionis] compunccionis G, punctionis Sp 1163 et piscatus] et pulueratus A, *om.* GLS • infert] inflixit ACDL, infigit G 1164 uenenum infixum] *om.* GL • infixum] infusum CD 1164–65 et hoc … pestis] *om.* G 1165 proprium] *adds* remedium S • et ueraces] *om.* G 1166 facere puniendo] punire G • adulatores] *add* et detractores CDL • inferendo eis uulnus] in proprio uulnere G 1167 inferre] *add* iniuste CDL • inferre tentabant] parauerunt G • qualiter] quod G, quomodo L 1168 Permenionem … inuidia] plus adulatores quam latrones G • suum] *add* pro detraccione sua CDL • capitulo de inuidia] *om.* L 1169 contra] *add* uenenum scorpionis scilicet contra CL (*int. corr.* C, *om.* D) • contra … detractores] *om.* D 1170 utilitas] uilitas ADLS 1171 undenos] undecim p 1172 quandoque] quinque ACDLS 1172–73 est sollers] patri et matri est similis reseruatur et CDL 1175–76 natura … quod] *om.* S 1177 et predones] *om.* S • multiplicantur] habundant CDL 1178 fratricidia] paricidia CDGL • proditiones] *om.* S 1179 radix] *add* si fieri poterit CDL

and dies, because he is confounded, according to Prv 4:24, 'Remove from thee a froward mouth'. Also the remedy for the cicada is that it be completely immersed in vinegar, which opens its pores. Notice that rebuke is figured as the sharpness of vinegar.

[1162] The fourth remedy is severe punishment. For a scorpion, once it has been killed and crushed, if it is applied to the wound that it itself has inflicted, the poison that it injected is returned to the body from which it came, and this is a characteristic of this plague. Just and truth-seeking rulers were accustomed to do precisely this, in punishing flatterers by subjecting them to the same wound that they tried to inflict on someone else. Notice in this regard how Alexander the Great punished his flatterer Permenion, in the chapter on envy above.

[1169] There is also a fifth remedy against flatterers and backbiters that is shown through the kindness of nature, that is, the usefulness of death. For Pliny tells, in the same place, that the scorpion gives birth to eleven young that it sometimes kills and eats, but the cleverest one of them climbs on its mother's back, where it sits safe from her tail and her sting. It kills its mother and lives on as the avenger of the slaughter of its siblings. And foresighted nature has done this, lest poisonous offspring be too widely propagated. So Pliny says. Likewise, I suppose that God permits fratricides, treacheries, and almost infinite murders to occur in Ireland, where flatterers, backbiters, and thieves proliferate; in this way, the evil root may be pulled up.

De ueneno gule.
Capitulum XIII.

1180   Uenenum gule propinatum est proprie per serpentem, qui est
animal carnale et gulosum, quod + ostendunt duo. Primum est
status corporis ipsius. Habet enim corpus humidum et uiscosum
et ubicunque repit, terram [uiscositate] inficit. [Sic gulosus et
carnalis: ubicunque comederit, omnes exemplo sue carnalitatis
1185   inficit.] Secundum est modus in incedendo, quia toto nisu corporis
et toto uentre serpens repit. Sic homo carnalis toto uentre tangit
terram et carnalitatem, secundum illud psalmi, 'Adhesit in terra
uenter noster, etc.'. Nota ergo secundum Gregorium, libro 30
Moralium, quod quinque modis peccatur per gulam. Primo,
1190   quando tempus comedendi preuenitur, sicut fecit Ionathas, i.
Regum 14. Ad hoc serpens duxit Euam, ut nature preueniret
appetitum et uiri sui non expectaret consortium uel consilium,
sed sola comederet fructum uetitum, et per hoc intrauit mors
in mundum. Hoc ergo peccatum est mane ient[acul]antium
1195   qui preueniunt et tempus et appetitum, uel prius uadunt ad
tabernam quam ad eclesiam. Et non est dubium quin imitentur
transgressionem primam. Gregorius, ubi supra, 'Mortis quippe
sententiam ore patris Ionathas meruit, quia in gustu mellis
constitutum edendi tempus antecessit'.
1200   Secundo, peccatur quando cibi delectatio[r]es queruntur. Sic
filii Israel, Numerorum 11, 'Esu carnium flagrabant', et hoc est
serpentinum. Dicit enim Auicenna, libro 2, et philosophus, libro 7
De animalibus, quod serpens comedit libenter carnes et sugit

---

heading] *om.* AGL, De gula capitulum D, capitulation *om.* rest
1180 propinatum] appropriatum L • proprie] *om.* S **1181** animal] *om.* G
• ostendunt] euidenter ostendunt GSp **1181–82** duo … ipsius] per hoc quod G
1181 Primum] quorum primus CD **1183** uiscositate] *om.* LSp **1183–84** Sic …
comederit] comederit L, *om.* Sp **1184–85** omnes … inficit] *om.* Sp
1185 Secundum] *add* quod ostendit serpentem animal carnale et gulosum
(animal … gulosum] esse gulosum G) GL • modus] *add* suus CD, *adds* finis L
• in] *om.* ACDGLS **1186** serpens] *om.* CD **1187** et carnalitatem] *om.* GS
1188 etc.] *adds* dicunt gulosi G **1190** comendendi] *om.* G • fecit] *om.* ACDL
1192 appetitum] *corr. from* aspectum L • uel consilium] *om.* A
1194–97 Hoc … primam] *om.* GS **1194** ientaculancium] genrancium (?) A,
comedencium L **1196** imitentur] transgrediuntur A
1200 delicaciores] delicati G, delectationes p **1201** Esu … flagrabant] sicut
superius tactum est G **1202** serpentinum] serpencium A, serpentinum (*corr. to*
serpencium) C, serpenter L **1203** sugit] *om.* G

On the poison of gluttony.
Chapter 13.

[1180] The poison of gluttony is appropriately drunk in through the snake, a carnal and gluttonous animal, as two points show. The first is the state of its body, for it has a moist and slimy body, and wherever it crawls, it infects the earth with slime. Similarly, a gluttonous and carnal person: wherever he eats, he infects everyone through the example of his fleshiness. Second is the way in which it moves, because a snake crawls, putting all its bodily weight, and all its stomach, on the ground. Likewise a carnal man touches the earth with his whole stomach and fleshiness, in accord with Ps 43:25, 'Our belly cleaveth to the earth'. Therefore notice that, according to Gregory, *Morals* 30, one sins through gluttony in five ways. First, when one approaches the proper time for eating too soon, like Jonathan did in 1 Rg 14:27. On this point, the serpent persuaded Eve that she should anticipate the time appropriate to natural appetite and that she should not wait for the company or counsel of her husband but should eat the forbidden fruit alone, and through this act death entered the world. Therefore this is the sin of those who breakfast in the morning and who anticipate the proper time and appetite, or who go to the alehouse before they go to the church. And there can be no doubt whether they are imitating the first sin. Gregory, in the same place, says, 'Truly Jonathan deserved the sentence of death from his father's mouth, because in his taste of honey he anticipated the time set for eating'.

[1200] Second, people sin when they seek more delicious food. Thus, the children of Israel, Nm 21:5, 'yearned to eat flesh', and this is snakelike behaviour. For Avicenna says in book 2, and Aristotle in *On animals* 7, that a snake eats meats with pleasure and that it sucks

humiditatem sicut aranea muscam. Hic serpens inuadit claustrales
1205   qui flagrant esu carnium, non aduertentes quod hec dieta non
conueniebat statui paradisi nec transitui filiorum Israel per uiam
deserti. Et quia irrationabiliter estuabant, cum esce eorum erant in
ore ipsorum, ira Dei [a]scendit super eos.

Tertio peccatur cibos preparatos ac[curat]ius expetendo, sicut
1210   fecerunt filii Heli, primi Regum 2. Et hoc est proprium serpentis,
quia dicit philosophus, libro 7 *De animalibus*, quod serpens diligit
lac ualde et sequitur odorem eius ita quod si intrauit uentrem
alicuius, odore lactis extrahitur. Sic carnalis et gulosus sequitur
dulcedinem carnalitatis, propter quam aliquando infert mortem
1215   et mors ei infertur. Sicut dicit Isidorus, libro 12, quod b[o]as,
serpens magne quantitatis in Italia, persequitur greges uaccarum
et sugit earum ubera et sugendo inficit et occidit animalia. Sic
faciunt moderni predones, et tamen inde sumunt aliquando
mortem propriam, et merito, quia multi eorum se uendunt propter
1220   cibum, nec tamen capiunt exemplum a consimili morte aliorum.

Quo circa narratur in *Apologia* Esopi quod quidam serpens
habitans in quadam cauerna petiit a quodam agricola ut [quolibet]
die portaret sibi parum de lacte, et ipsum ditaret. Quod cum
fecisset, multiplicata est ei proles et possessio et habundauit in
1225   omnibus bonis. Sed ad instinctum uxoris portauit malleum, et
quando serpens, ut solitus erat, caput extendit ut lac lamberet

---

1205 esu] estu G   non] *om.* S   1206 conueniebat] competit CDL
    • transitui] statui … transeuncium ACDL   • uiam deserti] desertum S
    1207 irrationabiliter] *add* carnibus CDL (*a corr.* CD)   • cum] *add* adhuc ACDL
    1208 ascendit] descendit AGLp
1209 preparatos] suos accuracius preparando uel ACDL   • accuratius] *om.* D,
    acrius GLSp   • expetendo] appetendo A, *om.* G   1210 fecerunt] *a corr.* C,
    om. D   • proprium] propositum G   1214 dulcedinem] odorem A   • infert]
    add aliis CDL   1215 et mors ei infertur] *om.* L   276 boas] beas ASp, leas CDL
    1216 magne] in agro parue S   • greges] *adds* eciam (*corr. from* ? ecclesiarum) D
    (eciam *expunged* C)   1217 inficit] interficit S   • animalia] *om.* GS
    1219 propriam] Unde aliis ipsam mortem inferre moliuntur CDL
    1219–20 se … exemplum] exemplum non sumunt G   1220 consimili morte] a
    (de C) consimilibus ACDL
1221 circa] contra GS   • narratur] *adds* de quodam serpente S   1222 cauerna]
    fouea uel cauerna ACD, fouea L   • quolibet die] *om.* CDL, cotidie p
    1223 parum] aliud paruum A, modicum quid CD, modicum L   1224 possessio]
    substancia CDL   1224–25 et² … bonis] *om.* S   1225 omnibus] multum in A,
    multis CDL   1226 ut solitus erat] *om.* CD   • extendit] extenderet CD,
    protenderit L   • lamberet] biberet A, *add* more consueto ACDL, *adds* consueto G

out the moisture, just like a spider does with flies. This snake invades cloisters, where the monks yearn to eat meat, and do not heed the fact that such fare was not appropriate either to the state of paradise or to the passage of the children of Israel along their desert path. And because the Israelites irrationally burned in this way, God's wrath arose against them even as their food was in their mouths.

[1209] Third, people sin in requesting foods more carefully prepared, just as Eli's sons did, 1 Rg 2:12–16. And this is a characteristic of a snake, for Aristotle says, *On animals* 7, that a snake loves milk a great deal, and it follows its smell, so that if a snake has entered someone's belly, it is drawn out with the odour of milk. Likewise a carnal glutton follows the sweetness of his fleshiness, and because of this, he sometimes takes in death, and as a result, he has death inflicted on him. Likewise, Isidore says, book 12, that the boa is a very large snake that in Italy follows herds of cattle and sucks their teats and through its sucking infects and kills them. Modern thieves do the same, and nevertheless from doing this, they sometimes take in their own death – justly so, since many of them sell themselves to gain food, nor do they understand the example provided them by the analogous death of others.

[1221] And on this point, Aesop's fables tell that a snake living in a cave asked a farmer if he would bring him a little milk every day, and, in return, he would make the farmer rich. And when the farmer had done this, his children and his possessions were increased, and he abounded in all good things. But incited by his wife, the farmer returned carrying a mallet, and when the snake, as it was accustomed, stuck out its head to lap up the milk

de lapide consueto, rusticus percussit grandi ictu ad caput
serpentis, set serpens caput retraxit et mallei ictum lapis suscepit.
Credidit enim thesaurum habere in cauerna serpentis qui eum
1230   sic ditauit, sed proditione facta, prolem et omnia bona amisit.
Iterato uxoris consilio, penitens adiuit ostium cauerne serpentis,
ut iniret pacem cum eo et ei seruiret sicut prius. Cui respondit,
'Modo uideo quod tu es stultus, quia non posset esse, quin ictus
ille mallei quem lapis suscepit loco capitis mei mihi ueniret ad
1235   memoriam, tibi etiam occurreret qualiter occidi prolem tuam
et subtraxi possessionem, et sic nulla pax stare posset'. Hec
ergo fabula ostendit eos fatuos qui post homicidia, + incendia,
et [rerum] damna confidunt in pace falsa. [Hec igitur fabula et
consimiles, etsi ex se non sint uere, tamen significant quedam
1240   uera. De fabulis] dicit Augustinus, libro *De mendacio* quod,
[licet in se non habeant ueritatem], faciunt ueritatem pro re
sign[ific]ata, et ideo sunt multum predicabiles.
     Quarto, peccatur quando [a]biecta cibaria cum maiori
auiditate desiderantur, sicut Esau propter edulium lentis +
1245   primogenita amisit, Genesis 25. Et hoc est opus serpentinum, quod
secundum Plynium, libro 8, serpentes quando in cauernis latitant,
lingunt puluerem et sugunt terre humiditatem. Nihilominus
tamen qualitercunque uiliter et parum comedunt, retinent semper
uenenum. Sic est de multis pauperibus, qui propter paupertatem

1227 de lapide] *om.* ACD   1227–28 caput serpentis] serpentem G
1229 thesaurum] *add* magnum CDL   •   serpentis] serpens quieuit S
1231 penitens ... cauerne] petens cauernam adiuit S   •   serpentis] *om.* G
1232 eo] serpente G   •   seruiret] serui (*corr. from* sui|que) C, suisque D
•   respondit] *adds* serpens S   1234 mallei] *om.* CDLS   1235 tibi etiam occurreret]
tu eciam cogitares CDL   1236 possessionem] omnia bona G   •   sic] *adds* iterum
nos L, *add* inter nos CD   •   post] *add* tot DLS (tot *expunged* C)   •   homicidia]
add furta GSp   •   incendia] *om.* A, *add* adulteria CDL   1238 rerum damna] alia
mala perpessa G, rerum damnacio L, damna p   1236–40 Hec ergo fabula ...
uera] *the sentences in reverse order* ACDGL   1238–40 Hec igitur ... De fabulis]
Delicta igitur fabula et de consimilibus A, De hac fabula et consimilibus Sp
1241 licet ... ueritatem] *om.* AGSp   1242 significata] signata ALp   •   et ...
predicabiles] *om.* G   multum] *om.* C
1243 peccatur] *add* gulosi CDL, *adds* homo per gulam G   •   abiecta] oblata A,
obiecta p   •   cibaria] *add* et uilia CDL   1244 desiderantur] desiderant et
summunt ACDL   1245 -genita] -genituram p   •   serpentinum]
serpencium AL, serpentis S   1246 quando, latitant] *om.* A   1248 uiliter]
uiuunt ACD, uiuunt uiliter L   •   parum] paruum ACL   1248–49 uiliter ...
uenenum] *om.* S

from the usual rock, the countryman aimed a great blow at the snake's head. But the snake drew its head back, and the rock took the brunt of the hammer-blow. For the farmer believed that the snake had a treasure in its cave from which it was enriching him, but once he had behaved so treacherously, he lost his offspring and all his goods. In accord with his wife's further advice, the penitent farmer went to the mouth of the snake's cave so that he could make peace with the snake and so that the snake would serve him as it had done before. The snake answered, 'Now I see that you are a fool, because that may not be, should I ever recall that mallet-blow that fell on the stone instead of my head, while it might occur to you how I killed your child and took away your goods; thus, there may be no lasting peace between us'. Thus this fable shows that those who trust in a false peace after murders, arsons, and loss of possessions are stupid. Therefore this fable and others like it, even if they are not true, nevertheless indicate true things. Augustine, in his book *On lying*, says of fables that, although they possess no truth in themselves, they produce a truth through the thing they indicate, and therefore they are eminently useful in sermons.

[1243] Fourth, people sin when they desire despicable food with too great eagerness, just like Esau lost his first birthright for a mess of lentil-pottage, Gn 25:29–34. And this is a snake's work, because according to Pliny, book 8, snakes, when they lurk in their caves, lick up the dust and suck on earthy moisture. Nevertheless, however vilely and however little they eat, they always remain poisonous. That resembles many poor people who think they are going to be saved on account of

1250   uictus et cibi putant saluari. Sed quia retinent uenenum peccati
       et magis aliquando in auiditate sumendi peccant quam diuites,
       penitus decipiuntur. Gregorius, *Moralium* 3, 'Non cibus sed
       appetitus est in uitio, quia lautiores cibos plerumque sine culpa
       sumimus, et abiectiores cum reatu conscientie degustamus. Nam
1255   Esau primatum per lenticulam perdidit, et Helyas in heremo
       uirtutem corporis carnes edendo seruauit. Hinc est quod antiquus
       hostis primum hominem, non carne sed pomo, subdidit, et
       secundum, non carne sed pane, tentauit. Uicium ergo gule
       aliquando committitur, etiam cum abiecta et uilia sumuntur'.
1260   Quinto, peccatur in quantitate, scilicet mensuram refectionis
       excedendo, et hoc est pessimum uenenum, quod prouocauit
       Sodome peccatum; Ezechielis 26, 'Habundantia panis et ocium
       etc.'. Excedere ergo in cibo uel uoraciter comedere est opus
       serpentinum. De quo dicit Auicenna quod transglutit oua
1265   auium et pullos uiuos et reducens ad posteriora, expellit ea, nec
       permittit quod morentur in uentre. Sic gulosus tantum sumit
       quod digerere nequit, et ideo nunquam mente uel corpore est
       sanus. Ecclesiastici 24, 'In multis escis erit infirmitas'.
            Quo c[ontr]a Aristoteles monuit Alexandrum, ut cibum
1270   non caperet quousque alium dige[ssiss]et. Sed gulosus est sicut
       sanguissuga +, qui, secundum Isidorum, libro 12, est uermis
       oblongus et niger, maculis rubeis distinctus, habetque os
       triangulum et [in] ore fistula[m habens, cum qua] sanguinem sugit.
       Et cum nimio cruore uenter repletus fuerit, euomit quod hausit ut
1275   recentiorem sugat. Prouerbiorum 3, 'Sanguissuge sunt due filie, que
       dicunt semper, "affer, affer"', et bis dicit propter excessum gulosi

1250 uictus] uite sue G • et … putant] uel cibi credunt ACD (cibi *a corr.* D),
    credunt L   1252 penitus decipiuntur] qui reficiuntur cotidie delicate CDL
    1255 Helyas] *om.* S   1257 subdidit] substrauit CDL   1258 secundum] *add*
    hominem CDL, Cristum G • carne sed pane] pomo nec carne A • gule]
    culpe CDL   1259 cum] *add* in edendo CDL • uilia] *adds* nimis auide S
1260 peccatur] peccant AG, peccant gulosi CDL, *adds* quando aliquis (*and later*
    excedit) S   1262 Sodome] *om.* A, Sodomiticum CDG • peccatum] ad uicium G
    • ocium] uinum A   1264 serpentinum] serpencium AL • transglutit] *a corr.,*
    with large erasure D   1267 nequit] non potest set aliquando euomit S
1269 contra] circa p   1269–70 cibum non caperet] nuncquam comederet S
    1270 caperet] sumeret CDL • alium] cibum sumptum alium CDL, cibum
    assumptum S • digessissit] digereret Sp, deiecisset D   1271 sanguissuga] *add*
    uermis Sp   1273 in … qua] more fistulan-[tum p • habens] *om.* AGS • qua]
    om. S • sugit] fugit D   1275 sugat] sumat uel sugat CD   1276 semper] *om.* CD
    • excessum] nimium excessum CD • gulosi] gulositatis S

their poor food. But because they retain the poison of sin and because sometimes in their eagerness to eat, they sin more than rich men, they are completely deceived. Gregory, *Morals* 3, says, 'The vice is not in the food, but in the desire for it, because many of us take in more sumptuous foods without sin, and we take a taste of nastier ones with a guilty conscience. For Esau lost his birthright for some lentil pottage, and Elijah in his hermitage preserved his bodily strength – and his virtue – while eating meat. This is why the old enemy conquered the first man, not with meat, but an apple; and tempted the second Adam not with flesh, but with bread. Therefore one can sometimes commit the sin of gluttony even when one takes in despicable and wretched food.

[1260] Fifth, people sin in amount, that is in exceeding moderation in eating, and this is the worst poison, because it excited the sin of Sodom; Ez 16:49 says, '[This was the iniquity of Sodom thy sister, pride,] fullness of bread, and abundance, and her idleness'. Therefore it is a snakelike act to be excessive in food or to eat voraciously. Avicenna says of a snake that it gobbles up birds' eggs, as well as their live chicks, and passing them on to its rear, expels them, and it does not permit them to remain in its belly. Likewise a gluttonous person takes in only what he is unable to digest, and therefore he is not healthy either in mind nor body. Sir 37:33 says, 'In many meats there will be sickness'.

[1269] And Aristotle warned Alexander against this, so that he would not take up food before he digested what he had before. But a gluttonous person is like the horse-leech that, according to Isidore, book 12, is a black oblong worm, marked with red spots; it has a triangular mouth and a pipe in it, with which it sucks up blood. And when its stomach has been filled with overmuch gore, it vomits up what it has drunk so that it can suck more anew. Prv 30:15 says, 'The horse-leech hath two daughters that say always, "Bring, bring"', and the text says 'bring' twice on account of a glutton's excess

tam in cibo quam in potu. Opus enim serpentinum est excedere
in potu sicut in cibo, quia dicit philosophus, libro 7 *De animalibus*,
quod serpentes multum diligunt uinum, et ideo homines uenantur
1280   et capiunt eos cum uino. Sic gulosus capit + diabol[um] per uinum;
immo + ei graue uenenum refundit in uinum. Prouerbiorum 14,
'Ingreditur blande et sicut regulus uenenum refundit'.

Et nota quod docet Constantinus per effectum cognoscere
uenenum materiale cibi et potus, dicens quod 'quando apparet
1285   signum ueneni in digitis et unguibus ex f[um]ositatibus cordis,
et saliua effluit et in lingua ardor fuerit, et oculi obtenebrauerint,
certum est quod uenenum preualuit circa interiora, ex quo se
diffundit circa extrema'. Hec ille. Sic potest cognosci uenenum
spirituale quod ad oculum uidemus, secundum Senecam, quia
1290   'Ex gula et ebrietate incerti fiunt labentium pedes, suffoduntur
oculi, prepeditur ex toto lingua'. Quod accidit ei, secundum
Galenum *Super Aphorismos*, quando cerebrum nimio humore
perfunditur, et ipsa lingua ex nimia humiditate exterius nequit se
dil[at]are. Et quia la[cert]a eius non possunt dil[at]ari nec extendi,
1295   ideo impeditur et fit balbutiens in ebriosis. Quia secundum
Senecam, 'Animus non est in sua potestate, quando est ebrietate
detentus. Et tunc omne uicium ebrietas in[c]endit et detegit,
obstantem malis conatibus uerecundiam ipsam remouet'. Hec ille.
Ue ergo illi qui uidet in se frequenter hec signa exteriora ueneni
1300   interioris et non adhibet remedia, quia secundum Gregorius,
libro 31 *Moralium*, 'Nullus palmam certaminis apprehendit, nisi
qui prius gulam deuicerit'.

1277 serpentinum] serpentis AL, serpentinosum G   1279–80 homines uenantur
et] uenantes S   1280 capit diabolum] capitur diabolus Sp, *add* et gulosos capit
diabolus per uinum CDL   1281 ei] eis AGSp, diabolus gulosis CDL   •   refundit]
infundit GL   1281–82 Prouerbiorum … refundit] *om.* CDL   1282 sicut regulus]
singulis G   •   refundit] diffundit A, regit G
1283 docet] dicit G   1284 materiale] mortale S   1285 fumositatibus] feruositatibus
CLSp, sre|uositatibus D, feruoribus G   1287 quo] *add* sic ACDL   1288 circa]
extra L   •   extrema] exteriora S   1289 spirituale] *add* in excessu potus ACL
(*int. corr.* C)   1290 incerti] infecti G   1291 prepeditur] impeditur G
1292 *Super Aphorismos*] *om.* S   1293 lingua] *om.* CL   1294 dilatare, dilatari]
dilaniare, dilaniari p (dilatari *om.* S)   •   lacerta] latera ACDGLSp
1295 impeditur] prepeditur L   •   fit] *corr. from* fuit CD   1296 Senecam]
Auicennam G   •   quando est] *om.* S   1297 omne uicium] omnis S   •   incendit]
intendit ALp   1297–98 et detegit obstantem] obstinate CDL, *adds* \detenta/ C
1298 obstantem] obstantibus G   •   remouet] remordet AGL   1299 exteriora]
om. S   1300 adhibet] apponit CDL

in both food and drink. This snakelike work exceeds in drink just as much
as in food, for Aristotle says, *On animals*, book 7, that snakes love wine a
great deal, and therefore men hunt and catch them with wine. Likewise
a gluttonous person catches the devil with wine; indeed, the devil pours
back into them, along with the wine, a deadly poison. Prv 23:31–32 says,
'The wine goeth in pleasantly, and will spread abroad poison like a
basilisk'.

[1283] And notice what Constantine teaches about knowing the
physical poison of meat and drink through their effects. He says, 'When
the symptoms of poison arising from vapours from the heart appear in
the fingers and nails, then after saliva has poured out excessively, and
the tongue has felt as if burning, and the eyes have grown dim, it is
certain that poison rules the inner organs, whence it is spreading itself
to the outermost parts'. So he says. Likewise spiritual poison can be
recognised by what we see with our eyes, according to Seneca, because 'as
a result of gluttony and drunkenness, the feet become uncertain to the
point of slipping down, the eyes become sunken, the tongue is hindered
completely'. This happens to a glutton, according to Galen's commentary
on Hippocrates's *Aphorisms*, when the brain is suffused with excessive
moisture, and the tongue, because of this excessive moisture, is unable to
spread itself out. And because its sinews can not be spread or stretched, it
is impeded, and drunks often stammer. For according to Seneca, 'When
someone is held prisoner by drunkenness, his mind lacks its proper
power. And then drunkenness incites and covers over every vice, and for
those attempting evil, it removes even the shame that would oppose it'. So
he says. Therefore woe to him who often sees in himself these outer signs
of inner poison and does not reach out for remedies, for according to
Gregory, *Morals* 31, 'Unless one has first conquered gluttony, one cannot
seize the prize in battle'.

De remediis gule.
Capitulum XIIII.

Remedium contra + gule uenenum est abstinentia.
Quod patet, quia secundum Plynium et philosophum, libro 7
1305   *De animalibus*, sputum hominis ieiuni est uenenum serpenti.
Non tantum ergo a ueneno et morsu diabolico curatur homo per
abstinentiam, [sed etiam per orationem]; Matthei 9, 'Hoc genus
demoniorum non eiicitur, nisi in oratione et ienunio'. Immo
serpens ipse per abstinentiam [re]nouatur, secundum Plynium et
1310   Aristotelem et Auicennam, nam pellem deponit primo usque ad
oculos per abstinentiam, deinde usque ad collum, et postea per
totum corpus quousque pellis deponatur. Hoc etiam tangit glosa
super illud Matthei, 'Estote prudentes, etc.', et Augustinus, libro 2
De doctrina Christiana.
1315   Modus tamen deponendi ualde mirabilis. Traditur et hoc sic
a *Physiologo*: 'Cum', inquit, 'serpens sentit se grauatum + morbo
uel senio, primo diebus pluribus abstinet se a cibo, ut sic pellis
eius a carne laxetur. Secundo, gustata herba amara, prouocatur
ad uomitum et eiicit humorem uirulentum qui fuit causa sue
1320   infirmitatis et defectus. Tertio, ut cutem rigidam temperet et
mollificet, in aqua se balneat et humectat. Et sic rimam petre
alicuius angustam intrat, et cum uiolentia transiens, ab exuuia,
id est sua pelle, se denudat. Quarto, soli expositus, se desiccat et
in carnis superficie nouam tunicam recuperat et tunc sumptis
1325   uiribus, clarius uidet, repit fortius, et comedit auidius quam prius.

---

heading] Remedium gule est abstinencia CD, Remedium contra uenenum gule L,
      De ueneno Incipit remedium contra gulam S (*at the head of a new quire, and the
      first phrase probably a running title*)
1303 Remedium] *adds* et tyriaca G • gule] uicium gule et Sp • uenenum] *om.* S
      1304 Plynium et] *om.* S 1306 homo] *add* solummodo CDL 1307 abstinentiam]
      ieiunium A • sed … orationem] *add* abstinencia coniunctam CD, *adds* cum
      abstinencia iunctam L, *om.* Sp • Matthei] Marci ACDGLS 1309 renouatur]
      nouatur p • Plynium et] *om.* CDL 1310 primo] *om.* ACDGLS
      1313-14 et … Christiana] *om.* GL
1315 deponendi] *add* pellem ACDGL • ualde] *om.* G 1316 *Physiologo*]
      philosopho G • grauatum] *adds* uel infirmum p • morbo] *add* senex CD,
      senex L 1318 amara] *adds* qui uocatur [blank] G, *om.* S 1319 humorem]
      uirorem CDL (*a corr.* D) 1320 et defectus] *om.* S • temperet et] *om.* S
      1321 balneat] baiu|lat C 1322-23 ab exuuia id est sua] a GL 1322 exuuia]
      exuuiis A 1323 expositus] appositus L 1324 tunicam] cutem AG
      1325 repit fortius] *om.* S • quam prius] *om.* S

Concerning remedies for gluttony.
Chapter 14.

[1303] Abstinence is the remedy against the poison of gluttony. This is obvious, because according to Pliny and Aristotle, *On animals* 7, the saliva of a fasting man is poisonous to a snake. But a person is not cured of a demonic bite and its poison by abstinence alone, but also by prayer. Mt 17:20 says, 'This kind [of demon] is not cast out but by prayer and fasting'. Indeed the snake itself is renewed by abstinence, according to Pliny, Aristotle, and Avicenna, for it first casts off its skin up to its eyes by being abstinent, and next as far as its neck, and finally through its whole body until the entire skin has been cast away. This point is also treated in the gloss on Mt 10:16, 'Be wise as serpents', and Augustine, in book 2 of *On Christian teaching*.

[1315] The snake's method of casting off its old skin is quite marvellous. And this is described in the *Physiologus* in this way: 'When a snake feels pained by disease or old age, first it abstains from food for many days so that its skin is loosened from its flesh. Second, having eaten a bitter plant, it is stimulated to vomit, and it spews out the poisonous moisture that was the cause of its sickness and deficiency. Third, it bathes and moistens itself in water so that it may temper and soften its stiff skin. And then it enters a narrow cleft in a rock and passing through it with violence, it strips itself of its clothing, that is its skin. Fourth, it dries itself through exposure to the sun, and it gains a new covering on the surface of its flesh and then, having recovered its strength, it sees more clearly, it crawls more vigorously, and it eats with greater desire than it had done at first.

Si ergo instinctus nature docet serpentem sic renouare statum, quare rationalis creatura non respicit exemplariter quatuor gradus quibus innouatur uita uenenata per gulam? Qui sunt hii, scilicet cibi + subtractio, peccati uomitus et detestatio, scilicet per
1330   contritionem et confessionem. Generale enim remedium contra uenenum in cibis sumptum est uomitus; sic uenenum spirituale, [detestatum per contriccionem], uomitur per confessionem. Gregorius de ulceribus Lazari, 'Quid est', inquit, 'peccator[um] confessio, nisi quedam u[uln]erum ruptio? Quia peccati uirus
1335   salubriter aperitur in confessione quod pestifere latebat in mente'. [Ueterem pellem deponere est ueterem consuetudinem malam relinquere. Unde admonet Dominus per Isaiam: 'Derelinquat impius uiam suam, etc.'. Ad solem desiccatio], ad solem iustitie plena conuersio. [Re]dde hic singula singulis factis serpentis que
1340   supra numerantur, etc.

De ueneno luxurie.
Capitulum XU.

Uenenum luxurie congrue fuit propinatum per serpentem, animal scilicet lubricum et ita libidinosum. Secundum Aristotelem, libro 5, quod serpentes in coitu sic se inuoluunt ut duo uideantur esse unus serpens et duo capita. Et ideo quam cito

1327 quare ... exemplariter] qualiter racionalis creatura non recipit inde exemplum G   1328 innouatur] remouet G   • gulam] *add* et alia peccata CDL
1329 subtraccio] detraccio S, substractio p   1330-32 confessionem ... confessionem] confessionem A   1331 uenenum[1]] *adds* gule S   1332 detestatum per contriccionem] *om.* AGSp (detestatum *corr. from* -tant C, *from* -tatur D)
1333 ulceribus] uulneribus G   • peccatorum] *om.* ACD, peccatoris p
1334 uulnerum] ulcerum p   • uirus] uulnus L   1336-38 Ueterem ... desiccatio] Ueterem consuetudinem siue hominis dereliccio G, Tertium est ueteris consuetudinis siue hominis (siue h.] *om.* S) depositio. Quartum Sp
1337 relinquere] *add* ueteremque uitam malam, eciam uiam (*a corr.* <from uitam?> D) suam CDL   • admonet ... Isaiam] Ysidorus L   • Isaiam] Ieremiam CD, *corr. to* Isaias C   1339 Redde] Adde Gp   • Redde ... etc.] *om.* S   1339-40 factis ... etc.] ad serpentis facta AG, scilicet ueri conuersi hominis ad serpentis facta CDL

heading] *as* p, *but* Capitulum XU *om.* CLS, Uenenum luxurie D, *om.* AG
1341 congrue] proprie [propinatum] et congrue CD, proprie et congrue AL
• propinatum] *adds* \uel procreatum/ C   1344 duo] *om.* ACDL

[1326] Therefore if natural instinct teaches a snake how to renew its state in this way, why does a rational creature not heed as exemplary the four steps by which a life poisoned by gluttony is made new? They are these: the withdrawal of food, the vomiting out and hatred of sin, that is through contrition and confession. Indeed vomiting is a general remedy against poison taken in with one's food; likewise the spiritual poison of sin, hated through contrition, is spewed out in confession. Gregory, discussing Lazarus's sores (Lc 16:20–21) says, 'What is the confession of sins, unless it is a kind of probing of a wound? For the poison of sin, which otherwise hides like a plague in the mind, is healthfully opened in confession'. To cast aside one's old skin is to leave behind one's old bad habits. Thus the Lord warns in Is 55:7, 'Let the wicked forsake his way[, and the unjust man his thoughts]'. Drying before the sun represents a complete turning toward the sun of righteousness. Offer here the individual things that correspond with the individual behaviours of the snake that are numbered above, etc.

On the poison of lechery.
Chapter 15.

[1341] The poison of lechery is appropriately indicated by the snake; it is a slippery animal and thus lecherous. According to Aristotle, book 5, in the sex act, snakes so intertwine themselves that two of them appear to be but a single snake with two heads. And therefore as soon as our

1345   primi parentes annuerunt serpenti, carnis senserunt pruritum
et libidinem; unde coitus ratione libidinis est opus serpentinum.
Notandum tamen quod inter ceteras species serpentis, proprie
comparatur uipere propter proprietates hinc inde conformes.
Primo, quia uipera habet modum generandi similem. Est enim
1350   quoddam genus uipere quod dicitur *tyris*, cuius uenenum est
irremediabile, quia secundum philosophum, libro 3 *De animalibus*,
animalia generat interius; ceteri autem serpentes oua producunt
extra se et ex illis producunt animalia. [Set *tyris* producit
oua interius ex quibus intra uiscera confotis producit interius
1355   animalia]. Et sign[ific]at proprie mehiam cordis; Matthei 5,
'Omnis qui uiderit mulierem ad concupiscendam eam, iam
mehatus est eam in corde suo'.

       Et propter consimilem causam, mechia cordis dicitur aspis
que dicitur *hypnalis*, cuius uenenum occidit in sompno, sicut
1360   dictum est supra, capitulo de inuidia. Sic latens aliquando libido
in corde, etsi nunquam compleatur in opere, inducit tamen
mortem anime. Iob 20 dicitur de peccante solum in cogitatione,
'Caput aspidis sugit'. Gregorius ibidem, 'Initium peccati mortalis
est in cogitatione'. Male ergo dicunt illi qui negant sola operatione
1365   interiori peccatum mortale committi, cum contrarium diceret
filius Dei et textus euangelii. Nec membra peccant exteriora, nisi
quia peccat ipsa anima. Unde Seneca, 'Nihil oculus + peccat, si
non oculus animi imperat'.

       Secundo, conf[o]rm[antu]r propter libidinem consimilem. Dicit
1370   enim Isidorus, libro 12, quod uipera inter omnia genera serpentium

---

1345 parentes] *add* nostri ACDL • annuerunt] consenserunt ACDL
1346 serpentinum] serpentis ALS   1347 serpentis] *add* libido ipse CD, *add*
libido GL • proprie] *om.* S   1348 propter] *add* conformitates conformesque
CL (conformitates *and* -que *corrs.* C), *add* conformes AD • conformes]
om. A, concurrentes CD, repertas et conformes G, currentes L   1349 similem]
singularem ACDGL   1350 est] est quasi CDG   1352–53 animalia … animalia]
animalia Sp   1353 producit] ducit AL   1354 intra] intrat L • interius] *om.* A
1355 significat] signat p
1358 cordis] *om.* ACDL   1359–60 sicut … Sic] sicut G   1362 cogitatione] *add* uel
uoluntate CDL   1364 qui negant] non L, qui dicunt … non S • operatione]
opinione A, cogitacione CDL   1366 et textus euangelii] *om.* G • exteriora]
om. A • nisi] nec L   1367 oculus] animus DL, *adds* carnis p
1367–68 oculus … animi] oculus si oculis anima A, oculus nisi animus oculo
CD (*a corr.* CD), si non oculo animus G   1368 imperat] importat S
1369 conformantur] confirmantur AL, comparatur G, confirmiter p; *and adds* uipera
et luxuria CDL, *adds* ei G   1370 omnia genera serpentium] omnes serpentes CDL

first parents assented to the serpent, they felt the itching and desire of
the flesh; for this reason, sex on account of satisfying desire is a snakelike
deed. One should notice, however, that among the various kinds of snake,
lechery is properly compared to the viper on account of the similar
characteristics they share. First, because the viper has a similar way of
producing young. For there is a certain kind of viper that is called *tyris*,
for whose poison there is no cure. According to Aristotle, *On animals*
3, it produces its young within; but other snakes lay eggs externally and
produce young from them. In contrast, *tyris* produces eggs internally,
from which, having brooded them in its inner organs, it produces
offspring within. This snake properly identifies someone who is adulterous
in his heart. Mt 5:28 says, 'Whosoever shall look on a woman to lust after
her, hath already committed adultery with her in his heart'.

[1358] And for a similar reason adultery in the heart is associated with
that asp that is called *hypnalis*, whose poison kills through sleep, as is
already said above in the chapter on envy. Likewise desire hidden in the
heart sometimes causes the death of the soul, even if it is never completed
by the deed. Iob 20:16 speaks about someone sinning in his thought alone,
'He shall suck the head of asps'. Gregory says of the verse, 'Mortal sin
begins in thought'. Therefore those who deny that one commits mortal sin
simply through an inner operation speak ill, since both God's son and the
gospel text say the contrary. Nor do the outer limbs sin, unless the soul
itself sins. For this reason, Seneca says, 'The fleshly eye would not sin at
all, were it not commanded to do so by the spiritual eye'.

[1369] Second, lechery and the viper agree because of their similar
desire. Isidore says in book 12 that, among all the kinds of snakes, the

est libidinosior, quia 'masculus ore inserto cum in os uipere semen expuit, illa ex uoluptate libidinis in rabiem uersa, caput maris prescindit. Sed cum femine uenter ad partum intumuerit, catuli tempus nature preuenientes, latera eius corrodunt, et sic cum
1375 matris interitu exeunt. Et inde dicitur uipera quasi "ui pariens", et tunc in tali partu uterque parens perit, masculus dum coit et femina dum parit'. In hunc modum tanta libido in actu luxurie est quod uenenum eius non tantum unum occidit, sicut cetera uenena faciunt, set etiam simul multos. Unde intensiue
1380 hec libido est maxima. Est enim mentis extenuatiua. Unde Chrisostomus super Mattheum, omelia 44, 'Nihil ita rescidit, suffodit, et corrumpit mentem sicut luxuria'. Nec mirum, quia secundum Augustinum, *Contra Iulianum*, libro 4, 'ut motus luxurie est maximus, ita immundissimus, cui totus animus et
1385 corpus simul impenduntur'. Sicut dicit glossa super illud prime Corinthiorum 6, 'Qui fornicatur in corpus suum peccat', ibi dicit quod animus in hoc facto absorbetur a corpore.

Tertio, conformantur propter consimilem uexationem. Libido enim uexat uiperam, sicut dicit Ambrosius in *H[e]xameron*, quod
1390 genus nequissimum serpentu[m] est uipera, ex libidine coeundi murene requirit + copulam. Et tunc progrediens ad ripam fluminis, sibilo illam uocat; illa uero statim adest. At uipera reiecto ueneno in terram, cum illa coit; quo completo, resumit uenenum et redit. Et ratio huius habetur ab Isidoro, libro 12, capitulo 6,
1395 quod murena est tantum femin[ini] sexus et non habet masculum, nisi in genere serpentis de quo [coit et] concipit. Idem [sent]it philosophus, libro 2. Unde secundum ipsum, non coit piscis cum pisce alterius generis; unde probatur quod sunt eiusdem generis.

1371 inserto cum] iniecto ACDGL 1372 expuit] exponit D • ex] ex nimia CDL
1373 femine] semine D 1374 tempus] opus G • nature] *om.* L 1375 ui] *om.* S
1379 uenena] *om.* CDL • faciunt] *om.* S 1380 extenuatiua] excecatiua ACDGL,
excessiua S 1385 simul] *om.* G 1387 corpore] carne CDGL
1388 conformantur] *add* uipera et luxuria CDL • consimilem] similitudinem
(*with gen.*) A 1389, 1390 *Hexameron*, serpentem] || hxamcron, serpenten p
1391 murene] murem *or* mureni L • requirit] querit G, *adds* consorcium siue p
1392 fluminis] *om.* G • reiecto] eiecto D 1395 tantum] totum G • feminini
sexus] feminin\ia/ (-inini D) sexus CDG, feminini generis AL, femina siue
femineus sexus Sp • masculum] masculinum AGL 1396 coit et] *om.* GSp
• sentit] dicit Sp 1397 Unde] *add* eciam Ambrosius in Exameron (*adds* omelia
CD, *with large following blank*) dicit quod uipera coit cum ea nam ACDL
1398 generis … generis] generis AGS • sunt eiusdem] murena et uipera sunt
(non sunt D) diuersi CDL

viper is more driven by desire. 'The male spits out his semen into the female's mouth, having inserted his own mouth, but she, her sexual longing become a fury, bites off the male's head. When the female's stomach has swollen up to give birth, her cubs anticipate nature's due time and gnaw through her sides, and thus they come forth by killing their mother. And for this reason the viper has that name, as if it were "giving birth by force" (*vi pariens*), and in that birth both parents die, the male in the sex act and the female in giving birth'. In this way, there is so much desire in the act of lechery that its poison does not kill just one, as other poisons do, but indeed many at the same time. For this reason, this sexual desire is greatest in its inner effects, for it weakens the mind. For this reason, Chrysostom, in homily 44 on Matthew, says, 'Nothing so tears apart, undermines, and corrupts the mind like lechery'. And this is no wonder because, according to Augustine, *Against Julian* 4, 'The force of lechery is greatest because the vice is the most impure, and by it both the whole mind and body are dissipated at the same time'. As the gloss on 1 Cor 6:18, 'He that committeth fornication sinneth against his own body', says, 'In this deed, the soul is consumed by the body'.

[1388] Third, lechery and the viper agree on account of their similar agitation. For as Ambrose says in the *Hexameron*, its desire agitates the viper, because the viper is the most depraved kind of snake and from its desire for sex it seeks to join with the lamprey. And so passing to the shore of a river, the viper calls with its hissing, and the lamprey comes immediately. And the viper, having cast out its poison on the ground, has sex with the lamprey, and having done the deed, it takes up its poison again and leaves. And Isidore 12.6 gives the reason for this, namely that lampreys are only females and have no males, unless they find them among snakes, with whom they have sex and conceive. Aristotle offers the same opinion in book 2. He also says that fish do not have sex with a fish of another species; he thus proves that the viper and the lamprey represent the same species.

1400 Similiter fornicarius uexatur spiritu nequissimo, qui dicitur 'stimulus carnis', secunde Corinthiorum 12, qui non permittit hominem stare intra metas sui uoti uel matrimonii – immo facit eum delectari in actu adulterii.

1405 Nota ergo quod dicit Ambrosius quod uipera non deponit uenenum ad comparem proprium sed ad murenam, quia adulteri mariti magis sunt uenenati ad proprias coniuges quam ad adulteras. Spiritus enim nequam qui eos uexat facit eos magis delectari in adulteris, quibus sunt largiores et blandiores, quam uxoribus propriis. Nota quod mu[ren]a non exit sibilire super uiperam sed [e] conuerso, quia res monstruosa est et contra instinctum nature quod sexus femineus cursitet ad attrahendum uiros ad luxuriam.

1410 Sicut narrat *Physiologus* de sirena, que est monstrum marinum similis pisci in parte [inferiori] et [similis] mulieri in parte [superiori], et cogit nautas pre dulcedine cantus sui dormire et tunc ducit unum ex eis ad locum [sicc]um, quem cogit ad coitum. Et si negat, ipsum occidit et deuorat. Tales sunt monstruose meretrices et uidue quedam, defunctis maritis ueneno diabolico agitate, que circuiendo terras cogunt uiros ad peccandum. [Isaias, 'Sirene in delubris uoluptatis']. Tamen nota dictum Isidori de murena quod tantum est feminei sexus, non habere ueritatem in Hibernia, ubi murena est in utroque sexu. Qui cum sequuntur illam opinionem dicunt quod uno mense anni nulla murena posset inueniri in Hibernia, eo quod oportet eas adire uiperas ultra mare ad concipiendum, sed hoc est falsum. Illud ergo intelligatur dictum spiritualiter, quia adulterium multum ibi regnat et quod est contra naturam murene,

---

1401 uoti] *om.* L   1402 eum] *add* magis ACDL
1404 proprium] suum CD • sed] scilicet AL   suas] proprias CD, *om.* S
1405–6 proprias … adulteras] *trs. nouns* p   1406 adulteras] concubinas S
1407 quibus] *add* et ipsi adulteri CDL, *adds further* magis L   1408 murena]
munera p   1409 e conuerso] e contrario AGL, est e conuerso CD, e contra S,
conuerso p • monstruosa] menstruosa CL   1410 cursitet ad] cursitet AG,
corr. from curritque C, currit D
1412 *Physiologus*] philosophus S   1413 parte inferiori] una parte AGSp
1413–14 similis … superiori] mulieri in parte AGSp   1415 siccum] proprium
ACDGLSp • quem] *add* euigilatum (et euigilatum CD, et *expunged/canc.*
CD) CDL   1417 monstruose] menstruose L   1419 Isaias … uoluptatis] *om.* p
1419–28 peccandum … peccandum] peccandum G
1420 feminei] femini ACDL   1423 nulla] *add* et (*corr. in both*) CD, *om.* L
1423–24 oportet eas adire] adierunt A, illo mense adierunt CDL

Likewise, a fornicator is agitated by a most depraved spirit, called 'a sting of the flesh' in 2 Cor 12:7, and this does not allow a man to remain within the bounds of his vow or of marriage – indeed, it causes him to take delight in the act of adultery.

[1403] Therefore notice that Ambrose says that the viper does not cast aside its poison for its own mate but for the lamprey, because adulterous husbands are more poisonous to their own wives than they are to their concubines. The evil spirit that agitates them makes them take greater delight in their adulterous partners, to whom they are more generous and more pleasant than to their own wives. Notice that the lamprey doesn't come out of the water to hiss at the viper, but the reverse, because it is a monstrous thing and against natural instinct that the female sex should hasten to attract men to lechery.

[1412] The *Physiologus* tells about the mermaid, which is a sea monster, shaped like a fish below and like a woman above; and through the sweetness of her song, she forces sailors to sleep and then leads one of them to a dry place, where she forces him to have sex. If he refuses, she kills and eats him. The sirens are just like monstrous whores and some widows who, stirred up with devilish poison after their husbands' deaths, wander about the countryside and force men to sin. Is 13:22 says, 'Sirens in the temples of pleasure'. Nevertheless notice that Isidore's statement about the lamprey, that it is only of the female sex, is not true in Ireland, where lampreys occur in both sexes. Those who accept Isidore's opinion say that for one month of the year one cannot find a lamprey in Ireland, because it is necessary for them to approach vipers across the sea in order to conceive. Although this opinion is false, it might be understood in a spiritual sense, because adultery is very prevalent in Ireland and because it is contrary to the lamprey's nature,

id est uidue, cursitare per terras ad prouocandum uiros ad
peccandum. Et ualde mirabile est quod in dicta insula, cum
sit frigida et humida et dieta eius ut in pluries sit frigida, unde
1430   homines eius sunt for[n]icarii et adulteri – ita quod nec sententia
excommunicationis nec uerba predicationis possunt ligar[i] eos
uinculis matrimonii.

Dicatur ergo quod tales sunt satyri, qui secundum Isidorum,
libro 11, 'sunt homines syluestres qui nec arte nec natura sunt
1435   dociles. In uoce tamen homines imitantur. Et dicuntur satyri
quia libidine non possunt satiari. Unde mulieres in[ter]ficiunt
coitu quas inueniunt in syluis'. Hec ille. Similiter tales sunt et
rationabiles in uerbis quando reprehenduntur, sed in ex[erc]atione
libidinis excedunt usum rationis. Unde potius dicuntur canes
1440   quam homines, qui secundum philosophum, libro 7 *De animalibus*,
coitu utuntur dum uiuunt canes, sed non discernunt aliquem
gradum nature. Et ideo secundum legem, Deuteronomi 32, equali
immuniditie subiacent meretrices et canes, quia 'de precio canis
et mer[cede] prosti[buli]', que omni libidini seruit, 'non licebat
1445   [of]ferre in domo Dei'.

Quarto, conformantur propter consimilem corruptionem.
Nullum enim uenenum est tante corruptionis sicut uipere. Dicit
enim philosophus, libro 8 *De animalibus*, quod *tyris*, que est
quadam uipera, cum aliquod membrum mordet, statim omnia
1450   putrescunt in circuitu eius. Sic peccatum luxurie magis inficit et
corrumpit et fetere facit quam aliquod aliud. Et hoc intensiue
sicut dictum est supra, et extensiue, quia luxuria est eneruatio

---

1427 id est uidue] *om.* A • uidue] *add* et meretrices CDL **1428** insula] *add* et in
aliis insulis (*with subsequent plurals*) CDGL **1429** sit] *add* naturaliter CDGL
1429 eius] insularum occeani CDGL • in pluries] plurimum S **1430** eius] in
eis degentes CDGL • fornicarii] formicarii p • adulteri] *add* frequenter plus
quam alibi CDGL **1431** ligari] ligare Sp
1435 dociles] docibiles G • imitantur] seruantur (?) A **1436** satiari] saturari S
• interficiunt] inficiunt Sp **1437** quas ... Similiter] *om.* G **1438** rationabiles
in uerbis] multi r. in u. tantum G • quando reprehenduntur] *om.* S • sed]
scilicet L • exercatione] exercendo A, execucione CDL, excusatione Sp
1441 coitu utuntur] coiunctur (?) A, coitu uerentur (?) G **1442** legem] *add*
Moysi AL **1444** mercede prostibuli] meretricule prostitute AGp, meretricis
prostitute CDLS **1445** offere] inferre GSp
1446 conformantur] *add* uipera et luxuria CDL **1447** sicut] *add* uenenum CDGL
1449 quadam] *om.* S • statim] *om.* LS **1450** in circuitu] membra in (*a corr.* C)
circuitu C, membra L **1451** fetere] putrescere et fetere S • aliud] *add* peccatum
CDLS, peccatum G **1452** sicut ... et] *om.* G

that is a widow's nature, to run about through the land inciting men to sin. Because in this island, since it is cold and moist and the food there – as in many islands – is cold, it is particularly wondrous that its men are fornicators and adulterers. This occurs to such an extent that these men may not be restricted within the bonds of matrimony either by a sentence of excommunication or by the words of preachers.

[1433] Therefore one might say that the Irish are like satyrs. According to Isidore, book 11, 'Satyrs are wild men who can not be taught either by nature or by art. Nevertheless they imitate men in being able to speak. And they are called satyrs because their sexual desire cannot be satisfied (*satiari*). For this reason, they kill women whom they find in the woods by raping them'. So he says. Likewise, Irish adulterers are like them in using words rationally when they are chastised, but they exceed any reasonable limit in actuating their sexual desires. For this reason, they might be called dogs rather than men, since dogs, according to Aristotle, *On animals* 7, engage in sex as long as they live, but they do not recognise any distinction in nature. Therefore according to the law in Dt 23:18, both whores and dogs fall in the same category of uncleanness, because 'thou shalt not offer the price of a dog or the hire of a strumpet', who serves anybody's sexual desire, 'in the house of the Lord'.

[1446] Fourth, lechery and the viper agree on account of their similar corruption. For there is no poison that is so destructive as that of the viper. Aristotle says, *On animals* 8, that the kind of viper called *tyrus*, if it bites any limb, all the others around it immediately rot. Likewise the sin of lechery infects and corrupts and makes one stink more than any other sin. And it does this both within, as is said above, and externally, because

+ corporis sensuum. Philosophus in *Ethicis*, 'Concupiscentie uene[ree] corpus transmutant et quasdam insanias faciunt'.

1455   Unde secundum Gregorium, libro 22 *Moralium*, 'Qui uolu[p]tati succumbunt non homines sed iumenta nuncupantur'. Et hoc est quod dicit Aristoteles in epistola ad Alexandrum, 'Coitus est proprietas porcorum, a quo si caueris, grandis erit tibi gloria; si exerceas, bestiarum imitator eris'. Sequitur, 'Crede', inquit, 'mihi

1460   indubitanter quod coitus est destructio corporis, abbreuiatio uite, corruptio uirtutum, legis transgressio, et mores generat femineos'. Hec ibi.

Est etiam fedatio fame et nominis. Unde Ualerius, libro 9, capitulo 1, de gula et luxuria: 'Quid his uiciis fedius? Quid

1465   damnosius? Quibus uirtus atteritur, uictorie languescunt, sopita gloria in infamiam conuertitur, animeque et corporis uires expugnantur. Adeo ut nescias an ab hostibus uel ab illis capi perniciosius'. Hec ibi. Unde Bernardus, epistola 34, 'Amor mulieris eneruauit potentiam Sampsonis, infatuauit sapientiam Solomonis,

1470   fedauit sanctimoniam Dauid regis'. Et quia in hoc uitio fama Christiani nominis exterminatur, solus notorius fornicator uel adulter inter criminosos par est excommunicatis. Ideo prime ad Corinthos 5, 'Cum huiusmodi nec cibum sumere licet'. Quod secundum Augustinum, libro *De penitentia* exponitur sic, 'Quod

1475   quando constat de notorio eius peccato uel confitetur ore proprio, + conuincitur in iudicio, communicare tunc non licet Christiano cum ipso'. Unde male fame sunt religiosi qui communicant cum talibus.

1453 corporis] seminalium corporis siue Sp • sensuum] *om.* G,
sensibilium S 1454 ueneree] *om.* S, ueneno p 1455 uoluptati] uoluntati p
1457 in epistola] *om.* S 1458 porcorum] *om.* S • grandis] magna S
1459 Sequitur] *om.* ACDGL 1460 indubitanter] *om.* CD • corporis]
om. G

1463 nominis] boni nominis CDL • Ualerius] Uasilius G 1465 damnosius]
damnabilius GS 1465–66 atteritur ... conuertitur] *om.* ACDL
1467 expugnantur] expun|gantur D • illis] aliis ACDL 1469 infatuauit]
infatuauit uel infamauit CD 1471 exterminatur] extenuatur G 1473 nec,
licet] nec CD, non LS 1475 eius peccato] *om.* G 1476 conuincitur] *om.* S,
conuenitur ac conuincitur p • Christiano] *om.* G 1477 ipso] *add* Et ideo
(idem dicit CD) glossa super illud Nec cibum sumere (Nec ... sumere] apostoli
Cum huius etc. CD) CDL 1477–78 Unde ... talibus] *om.* CD religiosi] *adds*
et prelati L 1477 qui] *adds* scienter, *and after* talibus, nisi propter eorum
correccionem G

lechery weakens the bodily senses. Aristotle says in his *Ethics*, 'Sexual desires transform the body and create mad behaviours'. For this reason, according to Gregory, *Morals* 22, 'Those who fall victim to their desire are not men, but should be called beasts'. And this is what Aristotle says in his letter to Alexander, 'The sex-act is appropriate for pigs, and if you have been wary about it, your glory will be great; if you practise it, you will just be imitating beasts'. He next says, 'Believe me that, without doubt, sex destroys the body, shortens one's life, corrupts the virtues, breaks the law, and produces feminised behaviour'. So he says.

[1463] Lechery also sullies one's fame and reputation. For this reason, Valerius Maximus 9.1, in the chapter about gluttony and lechery, says, 'What is more filthy than these vices? What condemns a man more completely? By these, virtue is trodden under foot, victories decline, glory is put to sleep and changed into ill-fame, and the powers of the mind and body defeated. Truly, you may not know whether it is more destructive to be conquered by your enemies or by these vices'. So he says. For this reason, Bernard says, letter 34, 'Love of a woman vitiated Samson's power, rendered Solomon's wisdom folly, and sullied the holiness of king David'. Because this vice kills off the fame associated with a Christian's name, a known fornicator or adulterer alone among sinners is considered a match for those who have been excommunicated. Therefore it says in 1 Cor 5:11, 'With such a one not so much as to eat'. And Augustine, in *On penance*, explains the verse, 'Because when his sin is well-known or confessed out of his own mouth, and a judgement has condemned it, it is not permissible for a Christian to communicate with him'. For this reason, those religious who communicate with such people are of ill fame also.

1480 Exterminatio est etiam temporalis substantie, quia secundum philosophum, simul prudentem et [in]continentem non conuenit esse eundem. Regna et imperia exterminata sunt et ad alienos translata per istud uicium. Sicut narrat Orosius de Sardanapallo, ultimo rege Babylonie, qui ita libidinosus et effeminatus fuit quod inter scortorum greges uiuebat et collo purpuram tractabat.

1485 De quo dicit Augustinus, libro 2 *De ciuitate Dei*, quod scribi fecit in sepulchro suo quod soli libidini se mortuum reputabat. Inde tantum ergo demeruit coram Deo ut imperium Babylonie, quod secundum Orosium durauit 164. annis, exterminatum fuisset et translatum ad Medos. Nam Arabatus prefectus + suus,

1490 princeps Medorum, ex casu uidens regem effeminate uiuere inter mulieres, ipsum occidit et urbem spoliauit et deinde imperium fuit translatum ad Medos. Unde libido ista grauiter punita fuit.

Similiter regnum Hibernie finem habu[i]t in Rod[r]ico rege libidinoso, qui dixit quod sex uxores non dimitteret propter

1495 reg[n]i coronam, et ideo regnum translatum est. Uere enim 'regnum de gente in gentem propter peccatum transfertur', Ecclesiastici 10. Et nota quod ecclesia hodie potest comparari domui Sardanapalli, quia greges scortorum commisti sunt gregibus sacerdotum, quorum luxuria multo excedit

1500 incontinentiam laicorum – immo exemplo uite polluunt quicquid sanctitatis est in aliis. Sophonie 4, 'Sacerdotes eius polluerunt sanctum'. Unde Hieronimus, *Epistole*, capitulo 30, 'In te oculi omnium diriguntur; domus tue conuersacio quasi specula sunt constituta. Magist[ra] es publice discipline, et

1505 quicquid feceris hoc sibi omnes faciendum putant'. Hec ille.

1479 Exterminatio] inanicio A, extenuacio G • etiam] *add* coitus ACDL • substantie] *add* uel sciencie CDL   **1480** simul] *om.* G • incontinentem] continentem Sp   **1481** eundem] eorundum AL, iterum G • imperia] *add* secundum Orosium ACDL • exterminata] *om.* G • alienos] alios G   **1482** Orosius] Dionysius (?) G   **1483** libidinosus] luxuriosus CD   **1484** collo] dolo A, colo G   **1487** coram Deo] contra Deum L, Deo G   **1488** quod … annis] *om.* S   **1489** prefectus suus] summus A, *om.* CDGL, suus S, prefectus seuus p   **1490–91** inter mulieres] *om.* A   **1491** Unde] adds patet quod G • Unde … fuit] *om.* CDL

1493 habuit] habut p • Rodrico] Rodico Sp   **1494** sex] Rex C   **1495** regni] regis Sp   **1498** domui] domini (?) L • commisti] coniuncti S   **1500** incontinentiam] luxuriam GS • uite] male uite CDL, *om.* S   **1503** In te] ad sacerdotem scribens ait in te CD • te oculi] oculis S   **1504** sunt] est ACDGL • constituta] conscienda A • magistra] magistratus G, magister Sp • es] est ACDGL

[1479] There is also the destruction of a lecher's worldly possessions, because, according to Aristotle, it is not appropriate that the same person be both prudent and incontinent. Through this vice, kingdoms and empires have been destroyed and passed on to foreigners. This is just what Orosius tells about Sardanapallus, the last king of Babylon, who was so lust-filled and feminised that he lived among flocks of whores and drew purple thread on a distaff. About him Augustine, *On the city of God* 2, says that he ordered to have inscribed on his tomb that he accounted himself dead only to his sex-drive. In this respect, he was so worthless in God's sight that the Babylonian empire, which according to Orosius lasted 164 years, was destroyed and passed to the Medes. For Sardanapallus's own prefect Arabatus, prince of the Medes, by chance seeing the king living effeminately among women, killed him and spoiled the city, and then the empire was passed on to the Medes. For this reason, his desire was heavily punished.

[1493] Similarly, the kingdom of Ireland came to an end in the sex-driven king Rory, who said that he would not put aside his six wives for the kingdom's crown, and so the kingdom passed on to others. For truly, as Sir 10:8 says, 'A kingdom is translated from one people to another [because of sin]'. And notice that the church today may be compared to Sardanapallus's palace, for flocks of whores are mixed with the flocks of priests, and the priests' lechery exceeds by far the incontinence of lay people – indeed, by the example of their life, priests pollute whatever holiness is in other people. So 3:4 says, 'Her priests have polluted the sanctuary'. For this reason, Jerome says in epistle 30, 'The eyes of all are directed toward you, bishop; the behaviour of your household has been established as a mirror. You are the school-mistress of public discipline, and whatever you have done, all people think they are to do'. So he says.

De remediis luxurie.
Capitulum XVI.

Remedium et tyriaca luxurie est continentia, cuius causa est
multiplex. Causa eius effectiua est sola Dei gratia; Sapiencie 8,
'Scio quod non possum esse continens, nisi Deus dederit'. Unde
+ Paulo 'stimulum carnis' patienti, responsum est 'Sufficit tibi
gracia mea', 2 Corinthiorum 12. More ergo piscis homo debet
aperire os cordis ad rorem gratie celestis qui uult continere. Unde
Sorath in libro 8 *De animalibus* dicit quod pisces *elith* per noctem
egrediuntur aquam et in terra ex solo rore matutino concipiunt
et pariunt. Nota quod hec aqua concupiscentia est, eneruans
animam. Iob 23, 'Lapidem excauant aque'. Unde has aquas oportet
egredi qui uult esse lapis solidus et durus per continentiam. Unde
narrat Plynius, libro 29, quod uipera lapidem quendam deglutit,
qui si de uentre eius extrahatur, est optimum remedium contra
uenenum. Sic aliquando est optimus lapis, et solidus per gratiam
effectus, qui aliquando submersus fuit in aquis [Babilonis, scilicet
in fetore et in fluxu libidinis]. Exemplum de Magdalena et + aliis.
Remedium ergo effectiuum continentie est sola gratia.
Remedia continentie conseruatiua sunt multa; primum est
conuersatio bonorum. Narrat enim Hieronymus, *Super Isaiam*,
libro ultimo, quod aquila inter pullos contra uenenum serpentis
ponit lapidem, qui est ametistus, cuius uirtus est temperare
calores uenenosos et resistere ebrietati. Sic societas sancta et uita

1510
1515
1520
1525

heading] Remedium contra luxuriam est continencia CD, De remedio contra
luxuriam L, *om.* AGS
1506 et tyriaca] contra (*with accusative*) CD, *om.* GL   **1507** multiplex] triplex S
• Causa eius] scilicet que CDL   **1508** dederit] det graciam G, det S
1509 Paulo] sancto Paulo p   • carnis] temptacionis S   • responsum] accepit
responsum A, accepit responsum a Deo (Domino CD) CDL   • tibi] *add* inquid
Paule CD, *adds* Paule L   **1510** homo] huiusmodi (?) CD   **1511** aperire] habere S
• qui uult continere] *om.* A   • uult] *add* ueraciter CDL   **1512** Sorath] Socath L,
Sorath p   • pisces] *om.* CDL   **1513** matutino] *om.* CDL   **1514** et pariunt] *om.* S
1520 effectus] *om.* S   **1520–21** Babilonis … libidinis] libidinis AGSp; *add* uel
eciam in aliis peccatis CDL   **1521** Magdalena et] Dauid Magdalena Matheo
Petro et CDL, *add* multis Gp, Magdalena et Augustino et S
1523 Remedia … multa] Remedium uero conseruatiuum est multiplex quorum
(*a corr.* C, *om.* D) CDL   **1524** conuersatio] conseruacio uel (uel eciam CD)
conuersacio CDL, consorcium G, conseruacio S   • enim] *add* Plinius (*add*
quod CD) eciam recitat CDL   • Isaiam, libro] illud Isaie L   **1525** libro
ultimo] *om.* S   **1526** lapidem qui est ametistus] ametistum CDL

On the remedies for lechery.
Chapter 16.

[1506] The remedy and antidote for lechery is continence, which has multiple causes. Its effective cause is God's grace alone; Sap 8:21 says, 'I knew I could not otherwise be continent, except God gave it'. For this reason, God answered St Paul, who was suffering 'a sting of my flesh', 'My grace is sufficient for thee', 2 Cor 12:7–9. Therefore a person who wishes to be continent ought, like a fish, to open the mouth of his heart to receive the dew of heavenly grace. For this reason, Iorath, in *On animals* 8, says that the fish called *elith* leave the water by night and conceive and give birth on land only in the morning dew. Notice that this water is desire that weakens the soul. Iob 14:19 says, 'Waters wear away the stone'. For this reason, the person who wishes to be a firm and hard stone through continence must leave these waters. For this reason, Pliny tells in book 29 that the viper sometimes swallows a rock that, if it is taken out of its stomach, is the best remedy against poison. Likewise the best stone, made firm through the action of grace, is the one that sometime has been submerged in Babylonian water (cf. Ps 136:1), that is in the stench and flow of desire. There's the example of the Magdalen and others. Therefore what makes continence an effective remedy is grace alone.

[1523] There are many remedies that preserve continence; the first is the companionship of good people. For Jerome tells, in the last book *On Isaiah*, that the eagle puts a stone among its chicks to protect them from a snake's poison. This is the amethyst, whose strength is to moderate poisonous heats and to resist drunkenness. Thus, holy companionship

religiosorum temperat arsuram libidinis in alio. Ideo dicitur
Ecclesiastici 37, 'Cum uiro sancto assiduus esto'.

1530   Secundum remedium est meditatio bona. Unde in libro
De simplici medicina dicitur quod caro *tyri* mortui, posita super
locum intoxicatum a uipera, subtilitate sue substantie et proprietate
occulta extrahit ad seips[a]m uenenum. Sic libido luxurie, intellecte
per uiperam, sicut dictum est, curatur et extinguitur, si carnis

1535   uilitas meditetur quoad triplicem differentiam sue mortis. Unde
si consideretur caro in se mortalis et uilis et de mortali genita et
pabulum mortis, mox futura extinguitur libido in meditante.
Unde narratur de sanct[o] Columba, [quando] filia regis Scotie,
puella nimis pulchra, ut magis in [eo] incitaretur libido, fuit

1540   coram ipso [ex] tot[o] denudata, [statim] ad hanc triplicem
meditationem recurrit, dicens, 'Pulchra es sed mortalis, et de
mortali genita, et ad mortem parata. Ideo Deum qui est uita mea
propter [te] non dimittam'.

Tertium remedium est fuga triplicis consortii mulieris, scilicet

1545   in cohabitatione. Prime Corinthiorum 6, 'Fugite fornicationem'.
Glossa Ambrosii, 'Cum aliis uitiis potest expectari conflictus,
sed hanc [fugite]; ne approximetis, quia non aliter melius potest
uinci quam fugiendo'. Unde narrat Hieronymus quod stimulus
quem patiebatur + Paulus fuit propter societatem Tecle, que

1550   sequebatur eum predicando. Si ergo Paulum, fortissimam ecclesie
columnam, ex consortio mulie[bri] permisit Deus tentari,

1528 arsuram] ardorem CD, ardorem siue arsuram S • libidinis] libidinosam
(-um CD) ACDL • alio] aliquo bono (*a corr.* C, *om.* D) uiro CDL, *om.* S
1528–29 Ideo … esto] Psalmus cum sancto sanctus eris etc. S
1531 tyri] uiri CD **1533** extrahit] contrahit CD • seipsam] se S, se ipsum p
1534 sicut dictum est] *om.* LS **1534–35** carnis uilitas] mulier recte ACDGL,
uilitas eius S **1535** meditetur] cogitetur et consideretur CD • triplicem]
duplicem uel triplicem G • mortis] mortalitatis S **1536** caro] mulier ut AG,
ut CDL, uilitas S **1537** pabulum] patibulum G • mox] iam L • libido]
luxuria A • in] in taliter CDL **1538** sancto Columba quando] sancta
Columba (!) Sp • quando] quod CD • Scotie] *om.* CDL **1539** nimis pulchra]
pulcra ualde CDL • eo] ea D, rege p • libido] *int. corr.* C, *om.* D
1540 ex toto] tota p • statim] qui stanti p **1541** meditationem]
medicaminem A • recurrit] cucurrit CDL, occurrit G **1542** Deum … mea]
propter Deum qui est in ea uita et S **1543** te] eam p • dimittam] amittam CDL
1544 triplicis] tripliciter A • mulieris] muliebris S **1547** fugite] *om.* Sp • aliter]
om. G **1549** Paulus] beatus Paulus Sp • societatem Tecle] Teclam ACDL
1550 Paulum] Paulus D, *om.* L • ecclesie] ecclesie \Dei/ G • columnam]
om. A **1551** muliebri] mulieris GS, sancte mulieris p

and life with religious people moderate the burning of desire in another person. Therefore Sir 37:15 says, 'Be continually with a holy man'.

[1530] The second preserving remedy is proper meditation. For this reason, the book *Concerning simple medicines* says that the flesh of the dead snake *tyrus*, if it is put on a place poisoned by that viper, draws that poison to itself through the fineness of its substance and its hidden characteristics. Likewise, lecherous desire, understood here as the viper, as is described above, is cured and extinguished if one meditates on the vileness of the flesh according to a triple distinction about its death. Thus, if the flesh is considered in one's meditation to be mortal and vile in itself, produced from a mortal being, and a food for death, future desire is soon extinguished. For this reason, it is told of St Columba that the daughter of the Scottish king, a very beautiful maiden, was stripped completely nude near him so that she might fire him to greater desire. But Columba immediately remembered this triple meditation and said, 'You are beautiful but mortal, and you were born of a mortal, and you have been prepared for death. Therefore since God is my life, I shall not abandon Him for you'.

[1544] The third preserving remedy is flight from the threefold company of women, that is from sharing a dwelling with one. 1 Cor 6:18, 'Fly fornication'. Ambrose says in the gloss, 'With other vices, you can anticipate the battle, but flee this one; you should not even approach it, because there is no better way to conquer it than flight'. For this reason, Jerome tells that the 'sting' that Paul suffered occurred because of Tecla's company – she followed him while he was preaching. Therefore if God permitted Paul, the strongest pillar of the church, to be tempted by being accompanied by a woman,

quomodo homo peccator et carnalis illi cohabit[e]t? Ideo uere
dicitur Prouerbiorum 25, 'Commorari leoni et draconi magis
expedit quam mulieri nequam'.

1555   Item debet uitari in aspectu. Species enim [o]blata tentat,
et [reten]ta in memoria intoxicat; propter quod uisus custodiendus
est, ne uenenum uel mors intret per fenestras. Nota quod regina
Indorum misit puellam regi Alexandro nutritam penitus ueneno
ita quod aspectu suo, si diu aspiceret, intuentem interimeret

1560   contactu uero libidinoso statim. Unde monitu Aristotelis, magistri
sui, cauebat sibi rex +. In hunc modum debet [ymaginari aspectus]
omnis mulieris que animam oblectant. Ecclesiastici 9, 'Propter
speciem autem mulieris multi perierunt'. Et nota quod caladrius
est quedam auis, cuius natura talis est quod si aliquis detinetur

1565   graui infirmitate, si egritudo fuerit ad mortem, auis auertit faciem
ab illo +. Si uero debet conualescere, auis figit uisum in eum
quasi sibi [ap]plaudens. Et quia certum est quod omnis qui uiderit
mulierem ad concupiscendam eam, iam mechatu[s est eam]
in corde suo, merito custodiendus est uisus a mulieribus. Item

1570   debet caueri a colloquio, quia Ecclesiastici 9 dicitur, 'Colloquium
eius quasi ignis exardescet'.

        Quartum remedium est aduersitas duplex, una assumpta ut
abstinentia et afflictio corporalis. Unde de uipera fit optima tyriaca

---

1552 quomodo] quanto magis S • homo] audet G • et] fragilis et CD
• cohabitet] cohabitetur AL, commoratur (*a corr.*) D, habitare G, cohabitat p
1554 quam] quam habitare cum S
1555 Item] *add* mulier CDL • oblata] ablata uel oblata p **1556** et … intoxicat]
om. S • retenta] oblata Sp **1557** intret] subintret S • fenestras] *add* nostras
ACDL **1558** Indorum] Medorum G • puellam] *add* regi Sp • penitus] *int.*
corr. C, *om.* DS **1559** intuentem] *om.* C, *a corr.* D • interimeret] perimeret L
(*app. corr.* C) **1560** statim] *adds* interficeret S **1560–61** magistri sui] *om.* L
1561 rex] *adds* Alexander eam tangere p • ymaginari aspectus] homo se
custodire ab imaginacionibus et aspectibus p **1564** cuius … quod] est que CDL
1563–69 Et nota … mulieribus] *om.* G **1564–65** detinetur graui infirmitate]
grauiter infirmetur ACDGL **1565** ad mortem] incurabilis L • auis]
expunged C **1566** illo] *add* et tunc sine dubio moritur (morietur S) Sp
1567 applaudens] explaudens p **1568** mechatus est eam] *adds* et moritur S,
mechatur et moritur p **1569** in corde suo] *om.* A • corde suo] cor CD,
corde L, *and add* scilicet secundum sentenciam saluatoris Matheo CD, *and*
adds Matheo L • custodiendus] *corr. from* dicendus CD **1570** debet caueri]
om. A, cauendum est CD • colloquio] *add* mulierum CD, *adds* mulieris L
1570–71 quia … eius] *om.* L eius] mulieris ACD
1573 tyriacha] *add* contra uenenum CDL

how may a sinful and carnal man live with one? Therefore Sir 25:23 truly says, 'It will be more agreeable to abide with a lion and a dragon than to dwell with a wicked woman'.

[1555] Also one ought even to avoid looking at a woman. For her proffered beauty tempts one, and if it is recalled, poisons one; for this reason, sight should be guarded carefully, lest poison or death enter by the windows of the eyes. Notice that the queen of India sent a maiden to king Alexander. She had been fed completely on poison so that she could kill someone looking on her by sight alone, if he looked for a long time, as it were instantly through lecherous contact. For this reason, king Alexander, following the warning of his master Aristotle, was wary of her. One should think about the sight of any woman that might delight one's soul in this way. Sir 9:9 says, 'For many have perished by the beauty of a woman'. And notice that there is a certain bird *caladrius* whose nature is such that, if someone is gripped by a serious illness, and if it is a mortal one, the bird turns its face away from him. But if he is destined to recover, the bird fixes its gaze on him as if congratulating him. Because it is certain that every man who looks at a woman desiring her is then committing adultery in his heart, one should properly preserve one's sight from looking at women. Also one should beware of speaking to a woman, because Sir 9:11 says, 'Her conversation burneth as fire'.

[1572] The fourth preserving remedy is a double hardship, first hardship one takes on oneself, like abstinence and afflicting one's body. For this reason, the best antidote against a viper is produced

quando scilicet caro eius penitus mor[tifica]tur et uenenum ab
1575 ea separatur. Sic caro, flagellis a libidine extracta, fit continens et
munda. Unde fabula est quod Antheus et Hercules pugnabant.
Antheus uero quotiens terram tangebat, totiens ui[gorosius] et
fortior [re]surgebat. Hercules igitur hoc percipiens, tactum terre
sibi negauit et tunc ipsum eleuando a terra, penitus superauit.
1580 Hanc fabulam Fulgentius *Libro mythologiarum* exponit. Per
Antheum intelligitur libido, quia *antheon* Grece idem quod
'contrarium' Latine; libido enim semper est uirtuti contraria. Quia
ergo libido de sola carne concipitur, quotiens carni consenserit,
totiens [ini]quior surgit. Hercules igitur, qui 'uirtutis gloria'
1585 uel 'fortium uirorum fama' interpretatur, sign[ific]at uirtutem
continentie, que libidinem a carne suspendens, a carne triumphat.
Unde Fulgentius, 'Omnem mentem, dum uirtus in altum sustulerit
et carnalibus eam aspectibus denegauerit, uictrix statim exurgit.
Ideo dicitur Hercules multum in illa [pugna] desudasse, quia
1590 rara est pugna que cum concupiscentia uiciisque congreditur.
Unde cum Diogenes dolore animi torqueretur et uidisset homines
ad amphitheatrum concurrentes, dicebat, "O qualis hominum
stultitia, cum concurrunt spectare feris homines repugnantes, et
me pretereunt cum tali dolore pugnantem!"' Hec Fulgentius.
1595   Item aduersitas immissa ualet ad continentiam. Nam
secundum Plynium, libro 8, uipera inter serpentes per hyemem
manet in cauern[is et rim]is terre, quia omnes alii hyemant in
[cauernis] saxorum uel arborum. Et tunc uipera reicit uenenum
per totam hyemem et contrahit caliginem oculorum, quousque
1600 uerno tempore terra perfundatur calore solis. Et tunc uenenum
resumit et uirtute radicis feniculi caliginem deponit oculorum.

1574 caro eius] *om.* A • penitus] punitus AG, *om.* S • mortificatur] moritur p
1575 flagellis] flagellata G, *add* et abstinencia CDL • extracta] exatata (*canc.*)
\<ex>tracta uel exsiccata/ C, exsiccata D, *om.* G   1576 pugnabant] *add* inter
se CDL   1577 uigorosius] uirtuosior AGSp   1578 resurgebat] surgebat GSp
1583 consenserit] appropinquauerit CDL   1584 iniquior] nequior p • surgit]
consurgit AGL, resurgit CD   1585 significat] signat p   1587 in altum] *om.* G
1588 uictrix] nutrix A   1589 pugna] *om.* p   1590 rara] dura S • pugna]
uictoria G   1592 concurrentes] currentes ADL, currentes (? *cut away*), *corr.*
from conquerentes C   1593 feris homines] feminam homini A, feras hominibus
CDL, feris hominibus G
1595 aduersitas] aduersa GL • ad] *add* habendam CDL   1596 uipera] *add*
sola CD   1597 cauernis] cauernis ... rimis A, riuis CL, rymis D, ramis G
• rimis] cauernis ACDGLSp • alii] *add* serpentes CDL • terra] certa G
1601 feniculi] *add* uel alterius herbe CDL

when its flesh has completely deteriorated, and the poison has left it. Likewise one's flesh, when it's removed from sexual desire by scourging, is made continent and pure. For this reason, there is a fable that Antaeus and Hercules fought. And the more often Antaeus touched the earth, the more vigorous and the stronger he raised himself. Therefore when Hercules perceived this, he denied him any contact with the earth and then, raising him above the earth, he conquered him completely. Fulgentius explains this fable in his book *Mythographies*. Antaeus represents the sex-drive because *antheon* in Greek means 'contrary' in Latin, and the sex-drive is always opposed to virtue. Therefore since the sex-drive is born of the flesh alone, the more often one consents to the flesh, the more evilly one raises oneself. Therefore Hercules, whose name means either 'the glory associated with virtue' or 'the renown brave men gain', indicates the virtue of continence; it holds the sex-drive hanging away from the flesh and thus triumphs over the flesh. For this reason, Fulgentius says, 'Every mind rises up immediately as a conqueror, so long as its virtue has endured hardships to the highest degree and has denied itself all carnal sights. Therefore Hercules is said to have sweated a great deal in the battle, because it is an uncommon fight when desire and the vices attack together. For this reason, when Diogenes was tormented by sorrow and had seen men rushing toward the amphitheatre, he said, "O how stupid men are, when they rush to look at men battling wild beasts, and they abandon me while I am sorrowfully struggling against vices!"' So Fulgentius says.

[1595] Also hardship imposed on one strengthens continence. For in book 8, Pliny says that the viper alone among snakes remains in caves and clefts in the earth through the winter; all the others spend their winter in the hollow places of stones or trees. And then the viper casts off its poison for the whole winter, and it contracts a kind of darkening of its eyes, until in the springtime, the earth is suffused with the sun's heat. And then it takes up its poison again and puts off the darkness of its eyes by the strength of fennel-root.

Hec ille. Sic aduersitas seculi et tribulatio que significatur per
frigus hyemale. Matthei 13, 'Orate ut' fuga uestra 'non fiat in
hyeme'. Est magnum remedium contra carnis incendium.

1605   Ecclesiastici 12, 'Malitia unius hore obliuionem facit luxurie
maxime'. Ideo Augustinus, *De ciuitate Dei*, dicit, 'Moribus
infirmis prosperitas nocet; terror anime est eis tutor ad
custodiendum, ne peccent'. Exemplum de Carthagine stante,
quod Romani uirtutibus pollebant; illa autem destructa,

1610   [potentia Romana eos pariter eneruauit, et eorum lima uirtutis
periit. Unde prouerbialiter dicitur de Cartagine, 'Prosperitas
rubigine uoluptatis eos destruxit'. Nota quod Cartago fuit caput
Africe et continue impugnabatur Romam, et tunc Romani,
bellis excitati, pollebant uirtutibus. Sed destructa illa ciuitate,

1615   prosperitas pacis omnimode eneruauit uirtutes eorum, quia
conuersi sunt ad uoluptatem]. In hunc modum multis hodie
confert tribulatio et persecutio [et aduersitas] +.

Remedium incitatiuum con[tin]encie est multiplex
creaturarum exemplum. Primum in modera[m]ine coitus. Unde

1620   narrat *Physiologus* de elephante quod nunquam coit, nisi causa
prolis. Et dicit Plynius, libro 8, quod semper in abscondito coit, et
hoc duobus annis tantum, et illis duobus annis singulis 5. diebus
tantum, et raro die sexto superaddito. Hec ille. Et Aristoteles,
libro 5, dicit quod masculus non tangit feminam postquam

1602 seculi] *om.* G   **1603–4** Mathei ... hyeme] *om.* CD   **1604** hyeme] *adds*
uel sabbato A, *adds* Persecucio uel tribulacio L   •   Est ... incendium] Sunt
in remedium contra luxuriam CD (*both these last two CD variants corr. at
page foot*, contra carnis incendium *still om.* C)   **1606** maxime] magne S
•   Moribus] Mentibus D   **1608** stante] *om.* A   **1609** Romani] Roma (*and
sg. verb*) AG   **1610–16** potentia ... uoluptatem] GSp *have rather*:
non. Nota quod Carthago caput Africe continue impugnabat Romam, et
tunc Romani bellis concitati uirtutibus pollebant. Sed destructa illa ciuitate,
prosperitas pacis omnimode eneruauit eorum uirtutes, quia conuersi ad
uoluptatem fuerunt, et lima uirtutis eorum periit. Unde prosperitas rubigine
uoluptatis eos destruxit, et
1610 potentia ... eneruauit] *om.* A   **1611** prouerbialiter ... Cartagine] *om.* A
1614 excitati] exercitati CD   **1617** et persecutio] *om.* S   •   et aduersitas] *om.* Gp,
p *adds* resistenciam contra libidinem
1618 incitatiuum] incitamentum CD   •   continentie] conscientie p
1619 moderamine] *a corr.* D, moderacione LSp   **1620** narrat] dicit CD, *om.*
at page bound L   **1621** Et ... et] et CDL   **1622** annis[1]] uicibus G   •   et illis ...
singulis] *om.* S   •   annis[2]] *om.* G   **1623** superaddito] *om.* GS   •   Hec ille. Et]
Hoc idem GL   **1624** quod] quod elephas CDL

So he says. Hardship and tribulation in this world work similarly, and winter's cold symbolises this. Mc 13:18 says, 'Pray ye that [your flight] happen not in winter', and this is a great remedy against the burning of the flesh. Sir 11:29 says, 'The affliction of an hour maketh one forget great delights'. Therefore Augustine says in *On the city of God*, 'Prosperity harms those weak in their behaviour; spiritual fear is their instructor, to preserve them, lest they sin'. Consider the example of Carthage: so long as it was standing, the Romans were powerful in virtues; but once it was destroyed, Roman power became equally weak, since the file that had polished their virtue was defunct. For this reason, there's a proverb about Carthage, 'Prosperity has destroyed them with the rust of desire'. Notice that Carthage was the leading place in Africa, and it continually attacked Rome, and then the Romans, stimulated by the wars, became strong in virtues. But once that city was destroyed, peace and good times completely weakened their virtues, because they became converted to voluptuous behaviour. In this way, tribulation, persecution, and adversity still today grant power to many.

[1618] The manifold example given by creatures offers a remedy inciting one to continence. First by moderation in the sexual act. For this reason, *Physiologus* tells of the elephant that it never has sex except to produce offspring. And Pliny, book 8, says that it always has sex in a hidden place, and that only once in two years, and these occasions only on five separate days, and rarely with a sixth day added. So he says. And Aristotle, book 5, says that the male elephant does not touch the female after

1625 concepit, que tamen trahit fetum in utero per biennium. Miser
autem homo [libidinosus; immo] libidinosior est isto bruto +, qui
nec tempus nec modum nec finem illi actui nec debitum a[d]uertit.
Item ad aliud exemplum ad rigorem discipline. Narrat enim
Alexander Nequam, libro *De naturis rerum*, de adulterio ciconie.
1630 Que cubans in nido, masculo per patriam cibum querente,
adulterabatur multis diebus antequam tamen ueniebat masculus.
Ad fontem qui erat ante domum militis se balneauit et sic ad
nidum redibat, et tunc masculus superueniens nihil percipiebat.
Miles ergo cum super hoc admiraretur, fontem penitus fecit
1635 obturari, et ciconia post adulterium una dierum cum balneari non
posset, dolens ad nidum rediit. Tunc masculus fetorem adulterii
sentiens, exiuit et magnam multitudinem ciconiarum secum
adduxit, et post longam disceptationem adulteram discerpserunt.
+ Simile narrat Plynius, libro 8, de le[ena], quod pardus
1640 cum leena adulteratur; unde generatur leopardus. Tunc leo,
fetorem adulterii sentiens, in uindictam surgit, et si femina,
[post adulterium prius quam maritus ueniat], in flumine
balneatur, culpa tegitur. Unde hec duo possunt notari, scilicet
uirtus penitentie et instinctus nature que detestatur adulterium.
1645 Quanta ergo damnatione dignus est qui uiolat matrimonium,
significans Christi et ecclesie coniunctionem, quod peius hodie
seruatur inter Christianos quam inter bruta et quam inter

1625 que tamen trahit] *om.* G • trahit] contrahit ACDL • fetum in utero]
secum CDL   1626 libidinosus immo] *om.* GSp • est] esse comprobatur
(-tus D) CDL • bruto] *add* animali Sp   1628 aduertit] auertit CSp
1628 ad aliud] aliud CD, ad AGLSp • ad²] in ACDGL, et S • discipline] *int.*
corr. C, *om.* D   1629–38 de adulterio … discerpserunt] CDL *have rather*:
de ciconia cubante et adulterante, masculo querente cibum per patriam, que
antequam ueniebat masculus (*a corr.* C, *om.* D) ad nidum, femina adultera ad
fontem qui erat ante domum (portam CD) cuiusdam militis se balneabat. Et
sic ad nidum rediens, masculus (*a corr.* D) nichil percipiebat. Miles ergo hoc
percipiens (aduertens CD), fontem obturauit (*a corr.* D). Cum ergo ciconia
iterum adulterata esset et post adulterium sicut prius se balneare non posset,
dolens rediit ad nidum. Masculus autem ueniens et fetorem senciens, exiuit,
et maximam multitudinem aliarum ciconiarum secum duxit et post longam
disceptacionem adulteram inter se horribiliter disserpserunt.
1632 domum] hostium S   1633 redibat] remeabat S   1635 dierum] die S
1636 fetorem] odorem S   1638 adulteram] ciconiam S
1639 Simile] Similiter p • leena] leone Sp   1639–40 quod … leena] que cum
pardo CDL   1642 post … ueniat] *om.* AGSp   1647 bruta] *add* animalia CDL (*a*
corr. CD)

she has conceived, even though she carries the fetus in her womb for two years. Thus, wretched sex-driven man, who does not pay attention to the time or the manner or the goal appropriate to the act or what is proper, is more lustful than this brute beast.

[1628] Also another example showing firmness in discipline. Alexander Neckam tells in his book *On the natures of things*, about the adultery of the stork. While she was brooding on her nest and the male was seeking food through the countryside, she prostituted herself for many days before the male returned. The guilty female bathed himself in a fountain that was in front of a knight's house and thus returned to the nest, and the arriving male did not notice anything. Therefore the knight, after he wondered about this, had the fountain completely stopped up, and one day after an adulterous encounter when she might not bathe, the female stork returned lamenting to the nest. Then the returning male perceived the stench of adultery and went off and brought back with him a great troop of storks and after a long dispute, they tore the adulterous female to bits.

[1639] Pliny, in book 8, tells a similar story about the lioness, that the panther has adulterous sex with a lioness, from which she produces a leopard. Then the male lion, when he perceives the stench of adultery, rises up to take vengeance, but if the lioness, after the adultery but before her husband comes, bathes in a river, her guilt is hidden. For this reason, one should notice these two things, namely the power of penance and the natural instinct that abhors adultery. For how great a damnation does the person who violates the bond of marriage deserve! This symbolises the union of Christ and the church, and yet today Christians preserve this less strictly than do brute animals or even

paganos, qui sunt diaboli membra! Unde narrat Tullius, libro
De Tusculanis questionibus, quod in India est quedam gens ubi
1650   marito mortuo, uxores eius in [certamen et] iudicium ueniunt, et
illa que + probatur magis eius chara et dilecta ipsi defuncto in uita
ponitur in sepulchro cum ipso uiua, et habet hoc [illa] pro magno,
aliis derelictis. ℂ

1648 membra] *add* quia a fide Christi et ecclesie sunt alieni CDL
1648–49 narrat … *Tusculanis*] narratur libro de tusculariis S   1650 certamen
et iudicium] certamen iudicium AG, certamine coram iudicibus CDL
(in certamine *a corr.* CD), iudicium Sp   1651 probatur] comprobatur S,
comproba|bitur p • probatur … dilecta] probatur magis dilexisse et magis
dilecta CDL (magis … magis] *om. and corr.* CD)   1652 illa] uiua Sp   aliis]
omnibus aliis CDL
1654 *no colophon* AG, Explicit CD, Explicit de ueneno L, Explicit tractatus de
ueneno et eius remediis S; for p's colophon, as well as those of LaV, see pp. 7, 9–10.

pagans, who are the limbs of Satan! For this reason, Cicero tells, in his *Tusculan Questions*, that there is a certain people in India where, when the husband has died, his wives enter into a judged competition, and the one who is proved most dear and beloved to the dead man while he was living is placed alive in the tomb with him, and she has this as a great prize, while the others are simply abandoned. ₵

Appendix:
The extensive interpolations

After 104 musce, pGS[+LaR] *add*:
(*om*. ACDL+BV)

1   Contra ergo uenenum peccati (*om*. S) est remedium curatiuum
     mors Cristi in ligno (signo B). Remedium restauratiuum corpus
     et sanguis pro cibo. Remedium conseruatiuum gracia, scilicet
     cotidiana, cum compunctionis stimulo.

La *adds*:
Insere hic contra nolentes audire uerbum <Dei?> et odientes predicatores
Contra ergo uenenum peccati ... (and then as the others)

R *also adds*, but 1–3 curatiuum ... conseruatiuum] *om*.
4 stimulo] instillacio

After 302 iudicent, pS+R[+GLaV] *add* (in S, the final sentence precedes
the rest):
(*om*. ACDL+B)

5   Item aduocati deteriores sunt quam meretrices, quia meretrices
     uendunt deteriorem et (d.e. *om*. S) uiliorem partem corporis
     sui; aduocati uero meliorem et (m.e. *om*. S) nobiliorem, scilicet
     os et linguam. Item nota quare amittunt aduocati et litigatores
     (*adds* id est *pleidours* S) frequentius sensum in morte quam alii
10   (*adds* Racio est in pronctu S), quia in sanitate (dum uiuerent S)
     uendiderunt eum, et iustum est ut quod uendiderit quis rehabere
     non debet. Item lingue aduocati uel lingua (*only* lingua aduocati
     S) est sicut lingua statere, que ad modicum pondus, scilicet unius
     denarii, statim ad partem alteram inclinatur. Non infletur ergo
15   iudex falsus siue aduocatus malus, si sit ut serpens callidus, quia
     nullam ueram sapientiam habet.

Following its end above at 14 inclinatur, S *continues*:

     Item litigiosi sunt sicut ouis inter spinas, cuius quelibet spina
     retinet, aliquid de lana quod tandem nichil remanet. Sic litigiosi
     multociens deueniunt ad paupertatem; Ecclesiastici 22, 'Obiurgacio
20   et iniurie adnichilabunt substanciam'.

G+VLa *add*: (*the preceding part of G is illegible and was possibly more
extensive*)
only 14–16 Non infletur ergo ... ueram sapientiam habet.

After 104:

[In La only: Here insert this against those who don't wish to hear the word of God and who hate preachers:] Therefore the remedy that cures the poison of sin is Christ's death on the cross. The restorative remedy is his flesh and blood as food. And the preserving remedy is grace, that is daily, together with the goad of compunction.

After 302:

Also lawyers are more wicked than whores, for whores sell the weaker and more vile part of their bodies; but lawyers the better and nobler, namely their mouth and tongue. Also notice why lawyers and the litigious on their deathbeds lose their wit more frequently than other people do; it's because when they were healthy, they sold it, and it is just that someone should not possess again what he has sold. Also the tongues of lawyers are like the beam of a balance which, under a little weight, that of just a penny, is immediately tilted to the other side. Therefore a false judge or an evil lawyer should not puff himself up, for if he is just like a cunning snake, he has no true wisdom.

[S continues:] Also litigious people are like a sheep among thorns, since whatever of theirs catches on a thorn, in the end none of that wool remains for them. Thus litigious people often pass into poverty; Sir 21:5, 'Injuries and wrongs will waste riches'.

After 541 Christi, Sp[+B] *add (with many variants in S, noted below)*:
(*om.* ACDGL+VLaR, *but see collation for ACDGL parallels to the opening sentence*)

Similiter dicit de ueneno illius qui dicitur *seps*. Nota quod inuidia est fel diaboli infusum humano cordi. Actuum 2 (Auicenna 4 S), 'In fel amaritudinis etc.'. Fel est principium putredinis in corpore mortuo, quia quando frangitur cista fellis, noxius humor
25   diffunditur quod est causa putrefactionis (putredinis S). Sic inuidia omnia bona interiora (*om. at line break* S) corrumpit in momento. Prouerbiorum 18, 'Putredo ossium inuidia'. Gregorius (adds *Moralium* 6 S), 'Ossa putrescere est robusta queque inuidia (in mala S) deperire'.
30   Item inuidi sunt 'fluctus feri (tumidi S) maris despumantes suas confusiones', ut dicit Iudas in sua epistola (ut ... epistola] Iudith 2° S). Unde quedam animalia non habent fel in communi loco, id est in splene, sed in (*om.* S) intestinis dicit philosophus. Talis est columba, simplex in uultu (*om.* S) et fel habens in
35   (*om.* S) intestino. Talis est inuidus, humilis in facie et occultam inuidiam portans (habens S) in mente. Prouerbiorum 26, 'Quando submiserit uocem suam ne credideris ei, quia septem nequitie sunt in corde ipsius'. Item inuidia similis est uipere que ut nascitur, prius rodit et penetrat uentrem sue matris; sic inuidia
40   in qua generatur mentem rodit (in ... rodit] est generacionis mente rodit matrem suam S). Item est ursus diaboli. Ursus ad peluim candentem excecatur; sic inuidus ad bonum proximi mente cecatur, ut de eo dicatur illud Ecclesiastici 25, 'Obcecabit (excecauit S) uultum suum sicut ursus'. Item ursus diebus festiuis
45   communiter a mimis (communiter a mimis] *om.* S) magis torquetur, quia trahitur per uicos et uerberatur et a canibus infestatur (dilaceratur S). Sic inuidus in (*adds* diebus S) festis magis affligitur, uidens honorem et decorem (*om.* S) proximi. Unde Seneca, 'Utinam inuidus (oculus inuidi esset S) in omnibus
50   ciuitatibus oculos apertos haberet (in ... haberet] in omni cecitate S) ut de omnium profectibus torqueretur?' Item quanta sunt felicium gaudia, tanti inuidorum sunt gemitus (tormenta S).
Item inuidus est similis talpe, qui lumen solis sine morte diu ferre non potest; habet enim oculos sub pelle ualde debiles.
55   Sic inuidus sine morte anime bonum proximi nequit uidere. Unde Gregorius, 'Qui de bono alterius affligitur quasi de radio solis excecatur'. Item inuidus est ferrum rubiginosum quod assidue consumitur. Ecclesiastici 12, 'Sicut seramentum (fera- S) eruginatum, sic nequicia illius'. Item inuidus est fera pessima,

After 541:

It says the same thing about the poison of the snake that is called *seps*. Notice that envy is the devil's bile poured into a human heart. Act 8:23, 'In the gall of bitterness [and in the bonds of iniquity]'. Bile is the source of rottennness in a dead body, for when the gall-bladder is broken, it pours out a harmful fluid that causes rotting. Likewise envy corrupts all inner goods in an instant. Prv 14:30, 'Envy is the rottenness of the bones'. Gregory, 'For bones to rot is for every powerful thing to perish through envy'.

Also envious people are 'raging waves of the sea, foaming out their own confusion', as Iud 1:13 says. Hence Aristotle says some animals don't have their bile in the usual place, that is in the spleen, but in the intestines. Among these is the dove, simple in countenance and having bile in its intestines. An envious person is like this, meek in countenance and carrying hidden envy in his mind. Prv 26:25, 'When he shall speak low, trust him not, for there are seven mischiefs in his heart'. Also envy is like the viper, which gnaws and pierces its mother's belly so that it can be born; likewise, envy gnaws the mind in which it is produced. Also envy is the devil's bear. A bear becomes blind before a shining basin; likewise the envious person becomes mentally blind before the good of his neighbour, so that Sir 25:24, 'She darkeneth her countenance as a bear' refers to him. Also a bear is commonly tormented by entertainers more on feastdays than on others, because it is drawn through the streets, beaten, and baited with dogs. Likewise an envious person is more afflicted in festivals when he sees the honour and glory accorded his neighbour. Seneca, 'Shouldn't an envious person have his eyes trained upon every city, so that he may be tormented by everyone else's advancement?' Also the more joys befall fortunate people, the more an envious person laments.

Also an envious person is like a mole, which can't endure sunlight very long without dying; for a mole has very weak eyes under a membrane. Likewise an envious person can't look at his neighbour's good without dying a little inside. Hence Gregory says, 'For someone to be afflicted by the good that comes to someone else is like being blinded by the sun's rays'. Also an envious person is like rusty iron that's constantly being eaten away. Sir 12:10, 'As a brass pot his wickedness rusteth'. Also an envious person is the worst wild beast,

60   seuior leone. Qui cum seuissimus sit inter omnia animalia, tamen
predam suam inferioribus relinquit, tanquam a natura edoctus,
quia 'omne bonum in commune deductum pulchrius elucescit',
ut dicit Boetius et Seneca. Nullius rei possessio est iocunda sine
socio, sed inuidus uult potius carere bono quam illud diuidere

65   cum socio (sed … socio] *om*. S). Exemplum de rege quodam,
qui concessit cuidam auaro et cuidam (et cuidam] *om*. S) inuido
munus quod (*adds* etc. *and om. to* Item inuidia est quoddam
speciale S) eligerent, ita tamen quod donum eius qui posterior
peteret duplicaretur. Et cum uterque differret petere, precepit rex

70   inuido ut prius peteret. Quod petiit ut erueretur sibi oculus unus,
uolens quod proximo eruerentur ambo. Noluit enim petere aliquod
bonum, ne proximus illud duplicatum acciperet. Unde poeta,
'Inuidus ut noceat in sua damna meat'. Item inuidia est quoddam
speciale signum discipulorum diaboli, sicut charitas discipulorum

75   Christi. Ioannis 13, 'In hoc cognoscent homines etc. (homines etc.]
omnes quod discipuli mei estis si dileccionem habuitis ad inuicem
S)'. Item inuidi sunt quodammodo peiores demonibus, quia
quidam demones compatiuntur se in uno obsesso corpore, sed duo
(*adds* homines S) inuidi non compatiuntur se sub uno tecto (*adds*

80   manere). Luce 8, 'Quod tibi nomen est? Legio etc.' (Luce 8 [*without
citation*] *follows* 70 corpore S).
    Et nota quod multa mala orta sunt ex pessima matre inuidia,
quia mors anime et corporis ab inicio. Sapiencie 2, 'Inuidia diaboli
intrauit in orbem terrarum'. Postea mors innocentis, scilicet

85   Abel, Genesis 4. Uenditio iusti Ioseph, Genesis 37. Tandem ipse
saluator morti traditus est, Matthei 27: 'Sciebat enim Pylatus
quod per inuidiam tradidisset eum'. Et adhuc inuidia non
cessat communicare malicie molimina, scilicet minas et iurgia,
persecutiones et homicidia. Ideo 'Confundantur zelantes populi

90   etc.', et de ea Esaie 28 uide.
    Sequitur aliqua addicio de speciebus inuidie predictis, quarum
una, scilicet tertia superius posita, fuit dolor de alieno bono.
Cum bonum naturaliter sit materia gaudii, patet quod inuidia
est contraria nature. Ecclesiastici 11, 'Est laborans et festinans et

95   dolens impius, et tanto magis non abundabit'. Item est gaudium de
malo proximi; in quo est specialis imitator diaboli, qui letatur cum
male fecerit. Prouerbiorum 2, 'Letantur cum male fecerint
et exultant in rebus pessimis, quorum uie peruerse et infames
gressus eorum'; et sequitur, 'Inclinata est ad mortem domus eius

fiercer than even a lion. For although the lion is the fiercest of all the animals, it nevertheless leaves its prey, just as it has been taught by nature, for its inferiors to finish eating, because every good that is extended to common use shines forth more beautifully, as Boethius and Seneca say. Without a companion, no ownership is ever joyous, but an envious person would rather lack something good than share it with a comrade. There's an example of this concerning a certain king who granted to a covetous man and an envious one whatever gift they would choose, but with the condition that the gift of the one who asked second would be doubled. And when each of them tried to put off asking, the king commanded the envious man to ask first. And he asked that one of his eyes should be gouged out, wishing that his neighbour should have both his gouged. For he didn't know how to ask for anything good, lest his neighbour should receive it twice over. Hence the poet says, 'The envious person passes on in his losses so that he may do harm'. Also envy is a special sign of the devil's disciples, just as charity is of Christ's disciples. Io 13:35, 'By this shall all men know [that you are my disciples, if you love one another]'. Also envious people are in certain way worse than the devils, for the devils sympathise with one another within a single body they have possessed, but two envious people can't live together under a single roof. Lc 8:30, '"What is thy name?" "Legion", [because many devils were entered into him]'.

And note that many evils take their origin from envy, the worst mother of all, because from the very beginning, she has been the death of both soul and body. Sap 2:24, 'By the envy of the devil, death came into the world'. And afterwards came the death of the innocent, that is Abel in Gn 4. And the sale of the righteous Joseph, Gn 37. And finally the saviour himself was handed over to death; Mt 27:18, 'For Pilate knew that for envy they had delivered him'. And to this day, envy may not stop expressing its vehement malice, in threats, abuse, persecutions, and murders. Therefore, 'Let the envious people be confounded', Is 26:11, and see the rest of that chapter on this subject.

Here's some additional material on the species of envy mentioned above. One of them, namely the third mentioned, was sorrow about the good that befalls another person. Since a good thing is a matter of joy by its nature, it's evident that envy is unnatural. Sir 11:11, 'There is an ungodly man that laboureth and maketh haste and is in sorrow and is so much the more in want'. Also envy is joy about the evil that befalls one's neighbour; in this the envious person proves the special follower of the devil, for he rejoices when he has done evil. Prv 2:14–15, 'They are glad when they have done evil and rejoice in the most wicked things, whose ways are perverse and their steps infamous'. And there immediately follows (2:18), 'For her house inclineth unto death and

100   et ad inferos semite eius'. Unde quia omnia ista sunt uenenosa et
humane nature contraria, transeamus ad fructuosa et odorifera,
scilicet ad caritatem predictam et ad bonam uoluntatem. Unde
Gregorius, omelia 5 *Super euangelium*, 'Uoluntas bona est sic:
aduersa alterius sicut nostra pertimescere, et sic de prosperitate
105   proximi sicut de nostro profectu gratulari. Aliena damna nostra
credere; aliena lucra nostra deputare. Amicum non propter
mundum, sed propter Deum diligere, et inimicum etiam amando
tolerare. Nulli quod pati nos uis facere; nulli quod iuste tibi
impendi desideras. Denegare necessitati proximi, non solum iuxta
110   uires succerrere, sed prodesse ultra uires uelle. Et hoc sacrificium
bone uoluntatis nunquam bene persoluitur, nisi huius mundi
cupiditas perfecte deseratur'.

SB (*the latter without S's variants*) **add**: 21–80 Similiter dicit … 'Legio
etc.'.

After 556 gaudet, **p** *adds*:
(*om.* ACDGLS+BVLaR; B adds a 19-line figure concerning Nero, probably
derived from Boethius, *Philosophiae consolatio* 2 m6)

Unde uitandam est propter septem, uidelicet quia suum
possessorem insanum demonstrat. Ecclesiastes 6, 'Ne sis uelox
115   ad irascendum, quia ira in sinu stulti requiescit'. Item quia ipsam
animam, spiritualiter necat, Iob 5, 'Uirum stultum etc.'. Item quia
diuinum hospitium, scilicet mentem, perturbat. Gregorius, 'Dum
ira animum pulsat, Spiritui Sancto suam habitationem turbat'.
Item quia pulchritudinem imaginis diuine dissipat. Gregorius,
120   'Ira in nobis imaginem Dei dissipat'. Item quia animam multis
uirtutibus priuat. Item quia hominem a generalis iusticie statu
alienat. Iacobi primo, 'Sit autem omnis homo uelox ad audiendum
etc.'; sequitur 'et tardus ad iram'. Ira enim uiri iusticiam Dei non
operatur. Item quia proximum non solum in persona sed etiam
125   quandoque in rebus damnificat. Iob 36, 'Non te superet ira ut
aliquem ui opprimas'. Item quia quod Dei est, scilicet ultionem,
frequenter usurpat. Et ideo dicitur Leuitici 19, 'Non queres
ultionem, nec memor eris iniurie ciuium tuorum'. Et quare? Quia
dicitur in persona Domini, Deuteronomii 32, 'Mea est ultio etc.'.

her paths to hell'. Because all these things are poisonous and contrary to human nature, let us pass on to fruitful and sweet-smelling things, namely charity and a good will. Gregory, in the fifth of his *Homilies on the gospels*, 'A good will acts in this way: it fears the ill-fortune befalling someone else as if it were befalling himself and likewise it rejoices in his neighbour's good fortune just as if it were happening for his own benefit. It believes the losses suffered by others to be his own losses and accounts other people's gains as if they were his. It loves a friend, not on account of the world but on account of God, and it endures even an enemy by loving him. You should not wish to make anyone suffer on our account; you should desire for no one what you might not wish justly to be imposed on yourself. You should refuse [nothing?] to your neighbour in need – not just to wish to aid him according to your power, but do him good beyond your power. And no one ever fulfills this sacrifice of good will unless he has perfectly abandoned worldly desire'.

After 556:

Therefore, wrath is to be avoided for seven reasons. It shows that the person who is possessed by it is mad. Ecl 7:10, 'Be not quickly angered, for anger resteth in the heart of a fool'. Also because it harms the wrathful person's mind spiritually, Iob 5:2, 'Anger indeed killeth the foolish'. Also because it disturbs the soul, God's lodging place. Gregory, 'When wrath strikes the spirit, it disturbs the very lodging place of the Holy Ghost'. Also because it scatters the beauty of the divine image. Gregory, 'Wrath scatters the divine image in us'. Also because it deprives the soul of many virtues. Also because it estranges a man from the state of common justice. Iac 1:19, 'Let every man be swift to hear [and slow to speak], and slow to anger'. Hence a person's anger does not allow him to perform God's justice. Also because it injures one's neighbour, not just in his person but also sometimes in his possessions. Iob 36:18, 'Let not anger overcome thee to oppress any man'. Also because it frequently usurps what is God's alone, namely vengeance. Lv 19:18, 'Seek not revenge, nor be mindful of the injury of thy citizens'. And why? Because scripture says in God's voice, Dt 32:35, 'Revenge is mine[, and I will repay them in due time]'.

After 630 Dei, p[+GSBR] *adds*:
(*om.* ACDL+VLa)

130   Unde Gregorius, super illud euangelium, 'Uenient ad uos in
uestimentis ouium etc.', dicit sic, 'Multi eum regiminis curam
suscipiunt et lacerandos subditos inardescunt, terrorem potestatis
exhibent, et quibus prodesse debeant, nocent. Et quia charitatis
uiscera non habent, domini uideri appetunt, patres se esse minime
135   recognoscunt; humilitatis locum in elationem dominationis mutant,
et si quando extrinsecus blandiunt, intrinsecus seuiunt'. Hec ille.
Est etiam *prester* quidam serpens uomens ignem, ore patenti
currens. Unde poeta, 'Oraque descendens currit fumantia prester'.
Hic est iracundus uomens uerba ignea, quia 'Apertio oris illius
140   inflammatio est', Ecclesiastici 20. Item iracundus a[c]cendit
templum Dei, et est de illis de quibus dicitur, 'Succenderunt igni
sanctuarium tuum', uel Dei. Et si ille qui succendit ecclesiam
Dei incidit in canonem, ut absoluendus mittatur ad sedem
apostolicam, patet quod iracundus qui spirituale templum
145   Dei accendit in se et in proximo grauem meretur penam. 1
Corinthiorum 3, 'Templum Dei estis uos'. Item ira est furia uel
phrenesis mentis que arrepticium facit hominem: aufert enim
homini seipsum. Ut dicit Hugo de Sancto Uictore, 'Superbia aufert
Deum, inuidia proximum, ira seipsum'.
150   Item iracundus hericio comparatur, quia cum tangi debeat,
in spheram se colligit et aculeos erigit. Sic iracundus si corripitur,
rixas agit et contumelias ita quod spine eius non possunt tangi,
nisi cum ferro uel ligno lanceato. Item hericius intrans pomerium
colligit cumulum pomorum et super ea uoluitur donec oneretur.
155   Et postea cum aliquod eorum ceciderit, dum se ad illud uertit et
colligit, alia perdit; tandem ira motus omnia excutit. Hoc modo
factus, impaciens omnia spiritualia bona perdit anime ut posset
tali dici, 'Omnia poma desiderabilia anime tue transierunt a te'.
Item iracundus est similis stulto qui frangit pontem, ne
160   aduersarius suus transeat, cum ipsemet sine ipso nequit saluare
uitam suam. Pons iste est misericordia post peccatum uolenti
transire ad uitam pu[ram]. Hunc pontem frangit iracundus
qui misericordiam perimit. Prouerbiorum 27, 'Ira non habet
misericordiam nec erumpens furor', et qui misericordiam negat,

After 630:

Hence Gregory, in discussing the gospel (Mt 7:15), 'They will come to you in the clothing of sheep[, but inwardly they are ravening wolves]', says, 'Many, however, take up the responsibility of rule and are enflamed with tormenting their underlings; they make evident the fear associated with their power, and harm those whom they ought to help. And because they have no love in their bowels, they desire to appear as lords and scarcely recognise that they are to be fathers; they convert a position of meekness into the pride of domination, and at the same time as they seem to flatter outwardly, they are seething with fierceness within'. So he says.

An angry man is also the *prester*, a snake that passes along with its mouth open, spewing out fire. Hence the poet, 'The prester runs along with its smoking open mouth'. This is the wrathful person, spewing out fiery words, because the opening of its mouth sets things ablaze. This is the angry person, spewing forth fiery words, because 'The opening of his mouth is the kindling of a fire', Sir 20:15. Also an angry person sets God's temple alight, and he is one of those of whom it is said, 'They have set fire to thy sanctuary' (Ps 73:7), that is God's sanctuary. And if someone who sets fire to the church incurs the legal penalty, so that he should be sent to the pope to be absolved, it is evident that an angry person who sets fire to the spiritual temple of God in himself and in his neighbour merits a heavy punishment. 1 Cor 3:16, 'You are the temple of God'. Also wrath is a fury or madness in the mind which makes a person insane, and thus estranges him from himself. As Hugh of St Victor says, 'Pride takes a man away from God, envy from his neighbour, but wrath from his own self'.

Also a wrathful man is compared to a hedgehog, because when he should be touched, he gathers himself into a ball and raises his spines. Thus, if an angry man is corrected, he quarrels and utters scornful words, so that one can't touch his spines except with iron or with the shaft of a spear. Also when a hedgehog enters an orchard, it gathers together a pile of fruit and rolls on top of it until he is completely weighted down [with fruit impaled on its spines]. And afterward, if any of the fruits should fall off, when he turns himself around to pick it up, he only loses some more; and finally, moved by wrath, he just shakes them all off. Having behaved in this way, an impatient person loses all his soul's spiritual goods so that one might say of him, 'The fruits of the desire of thy soul are departed from thee' (Apc 18:4).

Also a wrathful man is like the fool who destroys a bridge lest his enemy cross it, when he himself does not know how to save his own life without the bridge. This is mercy after sin extended to someone wishing to pass to a clean life. The angry person destroys the bridge because he destroys mercy. Prv 27:4, 'Anger has no mercy, nor fury when it breaketh forth', and whoever denies another mercy

165   frustra misericordiam postulat. Matthei 18, 'Nonne oportuit te
       miseri conserui tui sicut et ego etc.'? Et Ecclesiastici 28, 'Dimitte
       proximo tuo nocenti te'. Interlinearis glossa ibidem, 'Indignum est
       Dominum Deum esse propicium ei qui crudelis est in proximum'.
       Et in eodem capitulo, 'Quis orabit pro delictis etc.'. Interlinearis,
170   'Frustra pro peccatis quis orat qui fratri debitam caritatem negat'.
            Secundum Gregorium, 'Per iram multa mala eueniunt'. Primo
       sapiencia perditur, Ecclesiastes 7, 'Ira in sinu stulti requiescit'. Uita
       abbreuiatur; Ecclesiastici 30, 'Zelus et iracundia minuunt dies'.
       Mansuetudo amittitur, que custos est anime; Ecclesiastici 3, 'Filii,
175   in mansuetudine serua animam tuam'. Iusticiam perimitur, Iacobi
       i., 'Ira uiri iusticiam Dei non operatur'. Gracia uite socialis leditur,
       Ecclesiastici 8, 'Cum iracundo non facias rixam, quoniam quasi
       nichil est ante eum sanguis'. Concordia rumpitur, Prouerbiorum 15
       capitulo, 'Uir iracundus parat rixas'.
180   Species ire sunt odium, quo quis inueterato animi rancore
       aliquem habet exosum. Bernardus, 'Odium est ira inueterata'.
       Secunda, discordia qua quis deseritur qui prius amoris uinculo
       colligebatur. Tercia, rixa qua quis in facti iniuriam uerbo procedit.
       Quarta, contumelia qua quis comminatur alicui. Quinta, iniuria
185   cum facto uel uerbo contrarius facit. Sexta, impatiencia qua
       quis impetuosum animi motum non refrenat. Prouerbiorum 26,
       'Sicut qui apprehendit auribus canem, sic qui transit, et impatiens
       commiscebitur rixe alterius'. Septima, proteruitas qua quis subitaneo
       motu in uerba turpia prorumpit. Gregorius, 'Mos est procacium
190   ut recte dicendis semper e diuerso respondeat'. Octaua, furor qui
       aufert iudicium rationis. Nona, clamor qui est confuse mentis
       immoderantia. Decima, blasphemia que est uerborum contra Deum
       inordinata prolacio, que fit tripliciter, scilicet male de Deo sentire,
       uel mala proferre, uel irreuerenter sacra tractare, et pena talium
195   secundum legem est lapidatio. Undecima, obprobrium in quo turpia
       alicui obiiciuntur. Duodecima, comminatio que est post omnia ista
       mortem desiderare propriissime. Ecclesiastici 22, 'Ante sanguinem',
       id est illatam mortem, 'maledicta et contumelie et mine'.

G *adds*: 141–46 et est de illis … Dei estis uos, 150–57 Item iracundus
hericio … factus impaciens, with variants.

S *adds*: 137–46 Est etiam *prester* … Dei estis uos, 150–58 Item iracundus
hericio … transierunt a te, with a few variants.

B *adds*: following an original insertion of about a dozen lines, 137–70 Est
etiam *prester* … caritatem negat.

R *adds*: 150–58 Item iracundus hericio … transierunt a te, with variants.

asks for mercy in vain. Mt 18:33, 'Shouldst not thou then have had compassion also on thy fellow servant, even as I had compassion on thee'? And Sir 28:2, 'Forgive thy neighbour if he hath hurt thee'. And the interlinear gloss on this passage says, 'The person who is cruel to his neighbour is unworthy of finding the Lord God favourably disposed to him'. And in the same chapter (28:5), 'Who shall obtain pardon for [an angry man's] sins'? And the interlinear gloss again, 'A person who denies his brother the love due him prays for his own sins in vain'.

Gregory says, 'Through wrath, many evils come to pass'. First, it destroys wisdom; Ecl 7:10, 'Anger restesth in the bosom of a fool'. It shortens life; Sir 30:26, 'Envy and anger shorten a man's days'. It abandons mildness, the guardian of the soul; Sir 10:31, 'My son, keep thy soul in meekness'. It destroys justice; Iac 1:20, 'The anger of man worketh not the justice of God'. It injures the courtesy associated with social life; Sir 8:19, 'Quarrel not with a passionate man, for blood is as nothing in his sight'. And it destroys harmony; Prv 15:18, 'A passionate man stirreth up strifes'.

There are twelve kinds of wrath, the first hatred, in which someone, because of long-bred rancour in his mind, hates someone else. Bernard, 'Hatred is long-bred wrath'. The second is discord, in which someone abandons a person with whom he was first joined by a bond of love. Third, quarrelling, in which someone proceeds verbally to injure another in deed. Fourth, scornful words, in which someone threatens another. Fifth, injury that a contrary person inflicts in word or deed. Sixth, impatience, in which someone does not restrain the impetuous motion of his spirit. Prv 26:17, 'As he that taketh a dog by the ears, so is he that passeth by in anger and meddleth with another man's quarrel'. Seventh, impudence, when someone bursts forth suddenly in foul words. Gregory, 'It's the way with impudent people that one of them always responds in the contrary to a person speaking properly'. Eighth, rage which carries off any reasonable judgement. Ninth, outcry, the excessiveness of a confused mind. Tenth, blasphemy, which is the unrestrained utterance of statements against God. And this comes about in three ways: to think evilly of God, to utter evil things, or to treat holy things without reverence – and according to the old law (Lv 24:16), the penalty for all these is stoning. Eleventh, reproaches, where nasty things are tossed out about someone. Twelfth, threatening, which is, following the rest of these, to want in the strictest sense someone's death. Sir 22:30, 'Injurious words and reproaches and threats before blood', that is inflicting death.

After 643 uenenum, **p** *adds*:
(*om*. ACDGLS+BVRLa):

       Et quia ira tot mala procurat, debet homo circa ipsam armare
200   se per pacienciam, et hoc propter septem bona que ex paciencia
proueniunt, uidelicet quia per pacienciam imitamur diuinam
mansuetudinem, 1 Petri 2, 'Christus passus est pro nobis, uobis
relinquens exemplum ut sequamini uestigia eius'. Et 1 Petri 5,
'Christo in carne passo, uos eadem cogitacione armamini'. Item
205   quia per pacienciam sustinemus diuinam probacionem, quia
'Tanquam aurum in fornace probauit electos Dominus'. Thobit 12,
'Quia acceptus eras Deo, necesse fuit ut tentacio probaret te'. Item
quia procurat nobis sapiencie illustrationem quoad informationem
rationalis. Prouerbiorum 14, 'Qui patiens est multa gubernatur
210   prudentia'. Item quia procurat nobis ordinatam delectationem
quoad informationem concupiscibilis. Hebreorum 12, 'Omnis
disciplina in presenti quidem non uidetur esse gaudii sed
meroris, postea fructum pacatissimum exercitatis reddet iusticie'.
Romanorum 8, 'Scimus quoniam diligentibus Deum omnia
215   cooperantur in bonum'. Item quia procurat fortitudinem quoad
informationem irascibilis. Prouerbiorum 16, 'Melior est patiens
uiro forti, et qui dominantur animo suo expugnatore urbium'.
Item quia patientibus promittit Deus leticiam et consolationem.
Matthei 5, 'Beati qui lugent, quoniam ipsi consolabuntur'. Psalmus,
220   'Qui seminant in lachrimis in exultatione metent'. Ioannis 16,
'Tristitia uestra uertetur in gaudium'. Item quia procurat nobis
patiencia coronam, et ideo dicit Gregorius, 'Ego quidem uirtutem
patiencie signis et mirabilibus maiorem puto'. Unde dicit Deus
Matthei 5, 'Beati qui persecutionem patiuntur propter iusticiam,
225   quoniam ipsorum est regnum celorum'.
       Item de remediis contra iram propriam et alienam, et
primo alienam. Primum est responsio mollis. Prouerbiorum 15,
'Responsio mollis frangit iram; sermo durus suscitat furorem'.
Unde legitur de quodam monacho qui obuiauit cuidam sacerdoti
230   idolatre, quod cum diceret, 'Quo uadis, de[mon]?', sacerdos
iratus percussit eum et semiuiuo relicto pertransiit. Cui post
obuians, abbas sanctus monachus Macharius ait, 'Salueris,
laborator, salueris', qui compunctus ueniam petiit et conuersus
ab idolatria, monachus est effectus. Item remedium et tiriaca est
235   silentium, Romanorum 12. Prouerbiorum 26, 'Cum defecerint
ligna, extinguetur ignis'. Et nota exemplum, Ecclesiastici 8, 'Ne
litiges cum homine li[n]guato, neque struas in ignem ipsius
ligna', sicut 'Qui non uult comburi, recedit ab igne etc.'.

After 643:

And because wrath brings with it so many evils, a man ought to arm himself against it with patience, and especially because of seven good things that issue from patience. The first is that through patience we may imitate God's mildness; 1 Pt 2:21, 'Christ suffered for us, leaving you an example that you should follow his steps'. And 1 Pt 4:1, 'Christ having suffered in the flesh, be you also armed with the same thought'. Also because through patience we bear divine testing, because 'As gold in the furnace he hath proved his chosen ones' (Sap 3:6). Tb 12:13, 'Because thou wast acceptable to God, it was necessary that temptation should prove thee'. Also because patience gains us the light of wisdom, so far as it forms our reasonable souls. Prv 14:29, 'He that is patient is governed with much wisdom'. Also it gains us an ordered delight, so far as it forms our desiring souls. Hbr 12:11, 'All chastisement for the present indeed seemeth not to bring with it joy, but sorrow; but afterwards it will yield to them that are exercised by it the most peaceable fruit of justice'. Rm 8:28, 'We know that to them that love God all things work together unto good'. Also it gains us fortitude so far as it forms our irascible souls. Prv 16:32, 'The pacient man is better than the valiant, and he that ruleth his spirit than he that taketh cities'. Also because God promises the patient joy and consolation. Mt 5:5, 'Blessed are they that mourn, for they shall be comforted'. Ps 125:5, 'They that sow in tears shall reap in joy'. Io 16:20, 'Your sorrow shall be turned into joy'. Also because patience gains us a [heavenly] crown, and therefore Gregory says, 'Indeed I think patience a very great virtue in its signs and wonders'. And hence God says in Mt 5:10, 'Blessed are they that suffer persecution for justice's sake, for theirs is the kingdom of heaven'.

Also we should discuss remedies against one's own wrath, as well as someone else's, and first of the latter. The first remedy is a mild response. Prv 15:1, 'A mild answer breaketh wrath, but a harsh word stirreth up fury'. Hence we read about a certain monk who met an idolatrous priest while walking. And when he said to him, 'Where are you going, devil?' the priest, angered, struck him and passed on, leaving him half-alive in the road. And a little later, he met the holy abbot Makarios, who said to him, 'May you be saved, labourer, may you be saved'. And, in response, the remorseful priest begged pardon and, converted from his idol-worship, became a monk. Also silence is a remedy and antidote [against wrath], Rm 12[:18–21]. Prv 26:20, 'When the wood faileth, the fire shall go out[, and when the talebearer is taken away, contentions shall cease]'. And notice the example, Sir 8:4, 'Strive not with a man that is full of tongue, and heap not wood upon his fire', which is to say, 'If you don't want to be burned, move away from the fire, etc.'.

240 Romanorum 12, 'Non uos defendentes charissimi, set date locum
ire'. Item remedium est beneficium. Prouerbiorum 25, 'Si esurierit
inimicus tuus, ciba illum'; beneficia que inimico exhibentur sunt
uelut carbones accendentes ad amorem.

Etiam ut dicit Gregorius, ubi supra, scilicet in principio ...

After 680 dignitas, **p** *adds*:
(*om.* ACDGLS)

245 Nota de patiencia Gregorius, *Super Ezechielem*, omelia 1,
'Patiencia uera est que et ipsum amat quem portat'. Item secundum
Augustinum in tractatu *De patiencia*, 'Patiencia est qua equo
animo mala toleramus, ne amino iniquo bona desideremus'.
Sequitur 'Patientia est comes sapientie, non famula concupiscentie;
amica bone conscientie, non inimica innocentie'. Unde ipsa est
250 medicina contra iram, eo quod ira alienet hominem a seipso,
ut non sit compos sui; patiencia uero facit sui esse compotem
et dominari suis appetitibus. Luce 21, 'In paciencia uestra etc.'.
Gregorius super illud, 'Idcirco possessio anime in uirtute patiencie
ponitur, quia radix omnium et custos uirtutum est patiencia'.
255 Hec quidem sufficiant de ueneno ire et de eius malis effectibus ac
contrariis remediis.

B *adds*: 244–52 Nota de patientia ... paciencia uestra

After 713 incineratur, **p[+GSBR]** *adds*:
(*om.* ACDL+LaV)

Accidia saluti anime aduersatur secundum omnem statum
hominis, cum sit eius status triplex, innocenti anime, culpe, et
gratie. In statu innocentie tenebatur ad opus, quia ad Dei laudem
260 et cultum, Genesis 2: 'Posuit eum Deus in paradiso ut operaretur
ibi'. In statu culpe labori addictus est et pene, Genesis 3: 'In sudore
uultus tui uesceris pane, etc.'. In statu gratie ad opera misericordie
siue penitentie, et maxime post lapsum, Apocalipsis 2, 'Memento
unde excideris et age penitentiam et prima opera fac'. Hiis tribus
265 aduersatur acidia.

Beatus Hieronimus comparat acidiosum arbori sterili, dicens,
'Arbor arida et in sterilitatem uersa, nonne mortua est?' Sic qui
inutiliter uiuit mortuus est. Item pene reproborum apud inferos

Rm 12:19, 'Revenge not yourselves, my dearly beloved, but give place unto wrath'. Another remedy against wrath is kindness. Prv 25:21–22, 'If thy enemy be hungry, give him to eat'; the kindnesses you show to an enemy are like hot coals that rise into love. Also as Gregory says, in the citation at the beginning of the chapter ...,

After 680:

And notice what Gregory says about patience, *On Ezechiel*, homily 1, 'True patience is to love those things that one must endure'. Also according to Augustine, in his tract *On patience*, 'Patience is the virtue that allows us to endure evil things with equanimity so that we not desire good things in an evil spirit'. And he goes on, 'Patience is the lord of wisdom, not the serving-maid of desire; the girl-friend of a pure conscience, not the enemy of innocence'. Hence it is the antidote to wrath, because wrath estranges a man from himself so that he is not in control of himself; but patience puts him in control of himself and capable of conquering his desires. Lc 21:19, 'In your patience [you shall possess your souls]'. Gregory says on this passage, 'Thus Christ places the possession of the soul as part of the virtue patience, because patience is the source and guardian of all other virtues'. And these things may suffice about the poison of wrath and about its ill effects and the remedies that are opposed to it.

After 713:

Sloth resists the soul's salvation in every human state – and that is triple, the state of the soul's innocence, of its guilt, and of its grace. In the state of innocence, human beings were committed to work, that is for God's praise and worship, Gn 2:15, 'God put him into paradise to dress it and keep it'. In the state of guilt and of punishment, humans have been appointed to labour, Gn 3:19, 'In the sweat of thy face thou shalt eat bread, etc.'. In the state of grace, humans are appointed to the works of mercy or of penance, and most especially so after his fall, Apc 2:5, 'Be mindful from whence thou art fallen, and do penance and do the first works'. Sloth resists these three.

   Jerome compares the slothful person to a sterile tree, saying, 'Isn't a dry tree, one turned to sterility, dead?' Thus a person who lives uselessly is dead. Also a slothful person resembles the punishment of sinners in hell, for

acidiosus similis est, que pigros facit ponderosos. Matthei 12,
270   'Ligatis manibus et pedibus, etc.'; glossa, 'Ut non bene possent
uelle uel operari'. Ecce, quasi similes damnatis sunt acididiosi
(from Item] *om.* S). Item acidia est sp[iritu]alis paralysis que
totum hominem dissoluit et (*adds* tollit S) usum membrorum,
impedit meritum, et tollit premium, 1 Machabeorum 9, 'Alchimus
275   percussus est paralysi, et impedita sunt omnia opera eius'.

Item acidiosus comparatur turdo et turturi, et dicitur turdus
a tarditate uolatus. Auis est pigra et ponderosa, et eius stercus est
uiscus. Unde in proprio fimo inuiscatur, secundum Papiam. Sic
desidiosus cum sua desidia et tristitia ab omni bono retardatur,
280   et sic 'Requiescit Moab in fecibus suis', Ieremie 44. Unde fit
ei comminatio Sophonie, id est, 'Uisitabo super uiros defixos
in fecibus suis'. Item acidiosus est seruus iniquus, qui negligit
multiplicare talenta domini sui et ideo auferetur ab eo non solum
quod habet sed quod habere uidetur, Matthei 5. Id est qui non
285   habet uoluntatem operandi, auferetur ab eo gratia intelligendi;
Iob 12, 'commutans labium ueracium'; glossa, 'Argenti seruitio
subtrahitur, ut loqui non audeat quod non operatur, et iusto Dei
iudicio perdit linguam qui bonam recusat habere uitam'. Item
acidiosus est asinus diaboli qui graui onere premitur, pungitur,
290   uerberatur, in fine diei asperis cardonibus pascitur. Hec patitur
acidiosus; ad omnia enim mala fit insensibilis, et si nihil operis
extra faciat, tamen sub cordis sui pondere desudat.

Nota ergo tria mala que sequuntur acidiam. Paupertas,
Prouerbiorum 28, comminatur piger quod 'Ueniat ei quasi
295   cursor egestas et mendicitas, quasi uir armatus', quasi dicat
'Modo est paupertas lenta et inermis, sed in morte erit uelox
et inexpugnabilis'. Uilitas, Ecclesiastici 22, 'De stercore boum
lapidatus est piger', uiliter tractandus et obiurgandus. Penalitas,
acidiosus enim cum intra sit uacuus a bono, extra querit unde
300   consoletur, et non inueniens affligitur. Et hoc est quod 'Desideria
occidunt pigrum', Prouerbiorum 21. 'Ipse est puer paralyticus qui
male torquetur', Matthei 4.

Item acidia est tepiditas in operando bonum siue ociositas.
Apocalipsis 3, 'Utinam frigidus esses aut calidus, sed quia tepidus
305   es, incipiam te euomere ex ore meo'.

Et est uitandum propter septem mala que procurat homini que
homo summopere debet curare. Uidelicet insaniam quantum ad
cerebri malam dispositionem. Prouerbiorum 12, 'Qui sectatur

this makes sluggards heavy. Mt 22:13 'Bind his hands and feet[, and cast him into the exterior darkness], where the gloss says, 'so that they might neither wish or work well'. Look: sluggards are, as it were, likenesses of the damned. Also sloth is a spiritual paralysis that destroys the whole man and takes away the use of his limbs; it impedes gaining merit and takes away any reward, 1 Mcc 9:55, 'Alcimus was struck with palsy, and all his works were hindered'.

Also a slothful person is compared to the thrush and the turtledove, and the former is called *turdus* because of the slowness (*tarditas*) of its flight. It is a fat and heavy bird, and its shit is sticky. Hence it gets stuck in its own shit, as Papias says. Likewise, an idle person is held back from any good work by his own idleness and sorrow. Ier 48:11, 'Moab hath rested upon his dung'; hence he is threatened, So 1:12, 'I will visit upon the men that are settled on their dung'. Also sloth is the evil servant, who neglected to increase his lord's talent, and therefore, not just what he has, but what he seemed to have was removed from him, Mt 25[:26–30]. That is, the grace of understanding will be removed from the person who doesn't have the desire to work, Iob 12:20, 'He changeth the speech of the true speakers'; the gloss says, 'Because he does not work, he is drawn down into the service of silver so that he might not dare to speak, and by the just judgement of God, the person who refused to have a good life loses the power of his tongue'. Also the slothful person is the devil's ass, who is pressed down with a heavy load, is goaded, beaten, and fed sharp thistles at the end of the day. The slothful person endures such things, because he is made insensitive to all evils. If he did no external work, he should nevertheless sweat under the weight of his own heart.

Notice that three evils follow sloth. First, poverty; Prv 24:34, where the sluggard is threatened that 'Poverty shall come upon thee as a runner, and beggary as an armed man', as if he had said, 'Now your poverty is slow and peaceful, but in death it will be speedy and irresistible'. Second, vileness; Sir 22:2, 'The sluggard is pelted with the dung of oxen', to be treated vilely and rebuked. Punishment: for a slothful person, since he is devoid of all good within, seeks outside himself something that might console him, and finding nothing such, he is further pained. And this is because 'Desires kill the slothful', Prv 21:25. 'My servant is sick of the palsy and is grievously tormented', Mt 8:6.

Also sloth is lukewarmness in performing good deeds or laziness. Apc 3:16, 'Because thou art lukewarm and neither cold nor hot, I will begin to vomit thee out of my mouth'.

And it is to be avoided because of seven evils that come to a person that one ought to take care about to the height of one's power. First, madness so far as the evil disposition of his brain. Prv 12:11, 'He that

ocium stultissimus est', et tamen dicitur Prouerbiorum 15,
310   'Sapientior sibi uidetur piger septem uiris loquentibus sentencias'.
        Item inopiam quantum ad rerum temporalium egestatem.
Prouerbiorum 18, 'Qui sectatur ocium replebitur egestate'.
        Item lasciuiam quantum ad luxurie iniquitatem, Ezekielis 16,
'Hec fuit iniquitas Sodome sororis tue, saturitas panis et abundancia
315   aque, et ocium eius'. Et Ecclesiastici 32, 'Seruo maliuolo tortura et
compedes; multam enim maliciam docuit ociositas'.
        Item inconstantiam quantum ad mentis leuitatem.
Prouerbiorum 13, Uult et non uult piger; anima autem operantium
impinguabitur', scilicet pinguedine gratie.
320   Item infamiam quantum ad bone opinionis uacuitatem,
Ecclesiastici 22, 'In lapide luteo lapidabitur piger, et omnis loquetur
super aspernationem eius'.
        Item indignationem diuinam quantum ad extremi iudicii
terribilitatem. Et de hoc potest exponi illud quod dicitur in
325   Matthei 25, 'Serue male et piger, sciebas quod meto ubi non
seminaui, etc.'.
        Item maledictionem eternam ad penarum inferni acerbitatem,
Hieremie 48, 'Maledictus qui opus Dei facit fraudulenter', uel
secundum aliam literam 'negligenter'. Et propter omnia ista
330   maledicitur acidioso.
        Ecclesiastes 9, 'Quodcunque potest manus tua instanter
operare', et hoc propter septem bona, uidelicet quia dum
hic sumus, adest nobis ad bene operandum loci et temporis
oportunitas. Galatarum ultimo, 'Dum tempus habemus, operemur
335   bonum ad omnes'.
        Item quia ad hoc nos inuitat laboris quem Christus sustinuit
continuitas, 2 Timothe 2, 'Labora sicut bonus miles Christi'.
Unde in persona Christi dicitur in psalmo, 'Pauper sum ego et in
laboribus, etc.'.
340   Item quia ad hoc nos inducit futura necessitas. 2 Corinthiorum 4,
'Unusquisque secundum suum laborem mercedem accipiet'.
Matthei 22, 'Uoca operarios et redde illis mercedem etc.'.
        Item quia ad hoc nos eleuat premii immensitas, Romanorum
4, 'Non sunt condigne passiones huius temporis ad futuram
345   gloriam que reuelabitur in nobis'. Et quare dicitur Sapientie 3,
'Bonorum laborum gloriosus est fructus'.
        Item quia ad hoc nos confortat premii securitas. Gregorius,
'Sancti uiri quot labores nunc uirtuti commodantes exhibent, tot
remunerationis sue pignora intra spei cubiculum clausa tenent'.

pursueth idleness is very foolish'. And nevertheless Prv 26:16 says, 'The sluggard is wiser in his own conceit than seven men that speak sentences'.

Second, lack of wealth extending to his poverty in worldly things. Prv 28:19, 'He that followeth idleness shall be filled with poverty'.

Third, wantonness extending to the iniquity of lechery. Ez 16:49, 'This was the iniquity of Sodom thy sister, fullness of bread and abundance [of water] and her idleness'. And Sir 33:28–29, 'Torture and fetters are for a malicious slave, for idleness hath taught much evil'.

Fourth, inconstancy extending to a frivolous mind. Prv 13:4, 'The sluggard willeth and willeth not, but the soul of them that work shall be made fat', that is with the fat of grace.

Fifth, infamy, extending to the lack of a good name. Sir 22:1, 'The sluggard is pelted with a dirty stone, and all men will speak of his disgrace'.

Sixth, God's wrath, extending to the horror of the last judgement. And what it says in Mt 25:26, 'Wicked and slothful servant, thou knewest that I reap where I sow not' should be interpreted in this way.

Seventh, an eternal curse, extending to the sharpness of the punishments of hell. Ier 48:10, 'Cursed be he that doth the work of the Lord deceitfully', or according to a variant reading 'negligently'. And on account of all these the slothful person is cursed.

Ecl 9:10, 'What so thy hand is able to do, do it earnestly', and this is because of seven good things. First, so long as we are here, we have a present opportunity, in both space and time, to work well. Gal 6:10, 'Whilst we have time, let us work good to all men'.

Second, because the continuous labour that Christ endured invites us to do so, 2 Tim 2:3, 'Labour as a good servant of Christ'. Hence it says in Ps 87:16, speaking in Christ's voice, 'I am poor and in labours [from my youth]'.

Third, because our future necessity impels us to do so. 1 Cor 3:8, 'Every man shall receive his own reward, according to his own labour'. Mt 20:8, 'Call the labourers and pay them their hire'.

Fourth, because the immensity of the reward raises us to do so. Rm 8:18, 'The sufferings of this time are not worthy to be compared with the glory to come that shall be revealed in us'. And for this reason, it says in Sap 3:15, 'The fruit of good labours is glorious'.

Fifth, for our confidence in the reward comforts us to do so. Gregory: 'However many labours holy men now exhibit as conducive to their virtue, they hold just so many pledges of repayment closed within the chamber of their hope'.

350   Item quia ad hoc nos efficit premii delectabilitas. Psalmus,
       'Quorum magna multitudo dulcedinis tue, Domine, quam
       abscondisti, etc.'.

G *adds*: 257–80 Accidia saluti … suis Ieremie 44, 293–302 Nota ergo tria
mala … male torquetur

S *adds*: 257–80 Accidia saluti … suis Ieremie 44, 288–90 Item acidiosus
est asinus … pascitur, 293–302 Nota ergo tria mala … torquetur Matthei 4

BR *add*: 257–302 Accidia saluti … torquetur Matthei 4

After 823 meliora, p *adds*:
(*om.* ACDGLS+BVRLa)

       Similiter ouis in pascuis quasi nunquam satiatur – immo quod est
       mirabile, cum tota die fuerit in pascuis, auidius comedit in sero et
355   uespere quam in mane seu meridie. Sic in mundo cupidi nunquam
       satiantur, immo auidius congregant et retinent in sero senectutis
       quam in mane iuuentutis. Unde Seneca, 'Cum cetera uitia in
       homine senescant, sola auaricia in senibus iuuenescit'. Hec ille.
       Unde est de auaris sicut de puero paruulo tenente panem in manu,
360   cuius manum canis capit propter panem. Sic diabolus auarum
       capit propter pecuniam male acquisitam.

After 872 Hibernia, CDL *add*:
(*om.* AGS+BRVLap)

       … illa scilicet pars que dicitur Ultonia, ubi antiquitus de Egipto
       exiens filia Pharaonis cum marito suo, nomine Gaiel et maxima
       comitiua. Audierant enim mala que superuentura erant Egipto,
365   et hoc per responsa deorum fugientes, eciam plagam uenturam
       (superuenturam L) miserunt se in mare, comittentes se deorum
       suorum gubernaculo. Qui taliter diebus plurimis fluctuantes,
       tandem cuidam litori propter maris intemperiem (temperiem L)
       leti applicuerunt. Et quia ipsa ducissa eorum nobilissima inter
370   eos (*adds* omnes qui fuerant L) Scota uocabatur, ipsam partem
       terre ubi applicuerunt a sue ducisse nomine Scociam uocauerunt
       (a … uocauerunt] \ducisse nomine Scociam uacuerant/ D).
       Et ideo falsum dicunt aliqui, \scilicet/ quod Ybernia Scocia

Sixth, for the delightfulness of the reward causes us to do so. Ps 30:20, 'How great is the multitude of thy sweetness, O Lord, which thou hast hidden [for them that fear thee]!'

After 823:

Likewise, with a sheep it's as if it were never fulfilled in its grazing. Indeed, it is wondrous that, although it has been grazing for the whole day, it gobbles more hungrily in the evening and at sundown than in the morning or at midday. Likewise, avaricious people are never fulfilled in this world; indeed, they gather and hoard goods with greater hunger in the evening of old age than they do in the morning of youth. For this reason, Seneca says, 'Although other vices may grow old and wane in a person, avarice alone becomes vigorously youthful in old people'. So he says. For this reason, avaricious people are like a little boy holding a piece of bread in his hand; a dog will grab his hand while trying to seize the bread. Similarly, the devil seizes an avaricious person because of the money he has acquired through evil practices.

After 872:

[Greater Scotland, that is Ireland, is similar to this Greek island], and particularly that part called Ulster, settled very long ago by Egyptian exiles, Pharoah's daughter and her husband Gael, with a large retinue. For they had heard of the evils that were to come upon Egypt, and fleeing them as a result of a message from the gods, they embarked on a further plague, a sea voyage, entrusting themselves to guidance from their gods. After being driven about in this way by the violent sea for a great many days, at last they joyfully arrived on a shore. Because this very noble woman leader was named Scota, they called that part of the world where they landed Scotia 'Scotland'. Therefore, those who say that Ireland is

uocatur (uocita\n/tur L). Scoti enim quasi a principio regnum
375   ab aliis distinctum et semper regem proprium habuerunt. Scoti
autem qui de parte Ybernie sunt, uolentes Normannis Angliam
prius inuadentibus subici (*a corr.* CD, *om.* L), et post Yberniam
sunt subiecti.

And following 876 animali, **they add further (on this occasion +V):**

Et hoc est uerum de Scocia que nunc (*a corr.* C, quomodo L)
380   dicitur Ybernia, et hoc non propter ipsam terram uel propter
colonos (colones DV, *corr.* C) eius qui modo sunt in ea, set
oracionibus sanctorum (illorum L) qui quondam degentes in
ea per spiritum cognouerunt uenturos illic esse homines eciam
uenenata (ue|neta D) corda habentes, repletos omni dolo et
385   nequicia, \omni feditate/ et spurcicia (sui (*expunged*) spurcia|
D), iniustos nequiter seruientes (s'uientes C, se\./uientes (*corr. by
erasure*) D, seui|entes L) et innoxios condempnantes. Sunt amota
uenenosa animalia ab illa insula, ne multiplicatis uenenosis
hominibus, iustus iudex uenenum cordium malorum hominum
390   (*om.* L) se daret intoxi\cans/ (*a corr.* C, intoxicatos L) per uenenum
talium animalium.

For **384–88** repletos ... insula] iniustos spurcicia repletos et feditate. Unde
forsitan dicunt ab illa insula uenenata extirpata V (as well as a few other
uariants)

After 1060 uirtutis] pGS[+B] *add* (in G *after* **1127** Plinio 19):
(*om.* ACDL+RVLa)

Item auarus est similis equo gestatorio qui portat thesaurum
alicuius diuitis, et in fine diei et itineris sui pecunia sublata ab eo
portatur in thalamo. Equus uero in stabulum ducitur cum fracto
395   dorso (*om.* S) et pede claudo et costis excoriatis. Sic auarus post
multa pondera metalli et graues curas seculi et multa pericula
corporis sui, spoliatis bonis omnibus et graui tormento afflictus,
damnum portabit (pertulit S) perpetue paupertatis. Isaie 13, 'Onus
iumentorum austri'. Iumenta austri sunt auari qui portant pondera
400   seculi a peccatis onusti, et portant 'gibbis camelorum', id est in
cruciatibus (-iantibus S) temporalium. Item auarus similis est cani
ueteri, qui decubans super fimarium, et non patitur sine latratu
asportari unum pugillum, et tamen non sinitur uti nec potest.

called Scotland are mistaken. For the Scots from the very beginning have had a kingdom separate from all others and have always had their own king. However, those Scots who are from a part of Ireland and who wished to be subjects of the Normans, who had previously invaded England, have later become subjects of Ireland.

After 876:

And this freedom from poison is true of that Scottish territory that is now called Ireland. But it is not because of the land itself, nor because of those now settled there. Rather, it is the result of the prayers offered by holy men who once lived there. For they learned through divine inspiration that the coming invaders would be people with poisoned hearts, people filled with every kind of trickery and vice, with every sort of foulness and turpitude. They would evilly serve unjust people and would condemn harmless ones. For this reason, the just judge (in response to the holy men's prayers) removed poisonous animals from the island, lest their poison spread to men. In place of the poison of such animals, he gave poison to those already infected with the hearts of evil men.

After 1060:

Also an avaricious person is like a baggage-pony that carries some rich man's treasure. At the end of his day and journey, the money he's borne up under is carried away from him into a private chamber. And the horse is led to the stable with a broken back, a lame hoof, and lacerated sides. Likewise the avaricious person, after many metal weights and the grievous cares of this world and many dangers to his body, stripped of all his goods and afflicted with grievous torment, will endure the loss of endless poverty. Is 30:6, 'The burden of the beasts of the south'. The beasts of the south are avaricious people who weighted down with their sins, carry the weights of this world and carry them with 'the bunches of camels' (ibid.), that is in the torments of temporal things. Also an avaricious person is similar to an old dog lying on a dungheap that won't allow anyone to carry away even a fistful of shit without barking, and nevertheless has no power to use it.

Tales sunt qui pecuniis incumbunt loculis, et baculis defendunt,
405   nec ad alicuius utilitatem cedere permittunt. Abacuch 3,
'Turbabuntur pelles terre Madian'.

Item auarus similis est stulto qui habens nouos sotulares,
abscondit eos in sinu suo et incedens per aspera loca, cum
grauiter pedem lesisset, gaudebat quod sotulares essent illesi.
410   Sic auarus omni lesioni se exponit anime et corporis ut res suas
conseruet illesas. Non formidat terre longa itinera, nec maris
pericula, nec corporis supplicia; et inter hec nihil aliud efficitur
auarus nisi bursa principum, cellarium latronum, rixa potentium.
Hec Gregorius. Item apis non sibi mellificat sed aliis; sic omnes
415   auari non sibi sed aliis. Unde Ambrosius, 'Res nostre non sunt
quas nobiscum ferre non possumus. Sola misericordia comes est
defuncti'.

Nota quod ualde stultus esse qui naufragium patiens, deberet
mergi, sed adhereret sacculo auri uel argenti qui ut traheret
420   eum ad profundum, et non magis arriperet tabulam uel remum
quibus supernataret. Sed auarus potest dicere illud T[re]norum 4,
'Inundauerunt aque super caput meum, etc.'. Item auarus similis
est molendinario qui obstruit currentes aquas, donec superfluant
ripas aluei, et tamen (tandem S) apertis alueis suis, fluunt aque
425   cum impetu, cum eas ultra (amplius S) prohibere non potest.
Aque sunt temporalia que diu retineri non possunt, quia aut
distribuuntur, aut auferuntur, aut in seipsis putrescunt et (*om.*
clause S) deficiunt, aut ipse possessor morte preoccupatur (occu-
S). Et tunc ostium ianue aperitur et ab inimicis omnia diripiuntur
430   et fluunt ab ipso 'sicut torrens raptim transit in conuallibus', Iob 2.

Item auarus similis est perdici, qui furatur oua alterius
perdicis et cum produxerit ex eis pullos, illi audientes propriam
matrem, currunt ad illam et dimittunt nutricem suam. Propria
mater diuitiarum est mundus; nutrix uero earum est auarus qui
435   furtiue et (*om. phrase* S) curios[e] incumbit super illas. Sed in fine
clamabit earum mater, id est mundus (*om. phrase* S), et aduocabit
ad se omnia usque ad nouissimum quadrantem. Hieremie 17,
'Perdix fouit que non peperit; fecit diuitias et non in iudicio', id est
non discernit quomodo acquirat (quando adquireret S), dummodo
440   habeat. Item auarus stultus est nuncius qui propter trium dierum
uel duorum expensas secum defert decem annorum, cum possit
corpore grauari et a latronibus spoliari. Talis est auarus quod uix

These are the people who lean on their moneybags, and defend them with cudgels, rather than allow them to pass to anyone's use. Hab 3:7, 'The curtains of the land of Madian shall be troubled'.

Also an avaricious person is like a fool who, having new shoes, hid them in his bosom. When he passed on through rough places so that he hurt his feet grievously, he rejoiced that his shoes were unharmed. Likewise the avaricious person exposes himself, body and soul, to any sort of injury so that he may he preserve his things unharmed. He's not afraid of long journeys across the earth, nor of the danger of the sea, nor of injuries to his body, and among all these, an avaricious person makes himself nothing except a purse for princes, a storehouse for thieves, a quarrel for the powerful. Gregory says all this. Also the bee does not make honey for itself, but for others. Likewise, all avaricious people make riches for others, not themselves. Hence Ambrose, 'Those things that we cannot take with us are not ours. Mercy alone is the guardian of the dead'.

And notice how stupid it is for a person suffering shipwreck and threatened with drowning to hold on to a sack filled with gold or silver that would only drag him down to the depths. He should rather have grabbed hold of a plank or an oar, with which he could have floated. But an avaricious person may cite Lam 3:54, 'Waters have flowed over my head'. Also an avaricious person is like a water-mill, which stops the running water until it flows over the edges of the weir, and then, once the weir is opened, the water flows on with such a force that the mill can no longer stop it. The water represents temporal goods that cannot be held onto for long, because they are either given away, or taken away, or they rot within and fail, or death forestalls their owner himself. And then the passage in the millgates is opened and everything is seized by enemies, and the things flow away from their owner 'as the torrent that passeth swiftly in the valleys', Iob 6:15.

Also an avaricious person is like a partridge; it steals another partridge's eggs and, when it has hatched the chicks and they hear their own mother, they run to her and abandon their nurse. The world is the proper mother of riches, and the avaricious person is only their nurse, who furtively and delicately broods on them. But at last their mother, the world, will cry out and will call to herself all of them, down to the very last farthing. Ier 17:11, 'The partridge hath hatched eggs which she did not lay; so is he that hath gathered riches, and not by right', that is, he does not understand that he may have them in just the same way he first gathered them. Also an avaricious person is a foolish messenger, who carries with him ten years worth of expense-money just to cover two or three days so that he may suffer bodily injury and be robbed by thieves. An avaricious person is just like this, because he has scarcely

habet duos uel tres dies ad uitam, et tamen non cessat cumulare
pecuniam. Ideo Seneca, 'Auarus similis est monstro; quanto minus
445   restat uie, tanto magis uiaticum querit'.

Rex quidam gentilis et potens ac diues ualde (*om.* S), cum
sentiret mortem, fecit deferri in lancea per ciuitatem pannum
uilem in quo erat sepeliendis et uoce preconis fecit clamare, 'Hoc
cilicium est de omnibus bonis meis, et de omni gloria sua defert
450   secum'. Rex moriturus quantum ad hoc fuit sapiens in nouissimo
suo (*adds* Prouerbiorum 29 S). Item Socrates, ueniens ad Athenas
secum detulit pondus auri, quod submersit dicens, 'Submergam te,
ne submergar a te'. Item data erat cuidam heremite pecunia quam
abscondebat apud caput lecti. De nocte uero uenerunt predones,
455   ut sibi pecuniam auferrent; hoc uidens, heremita proiecit eis
pecuniam dicens, 'Accipite tremorem capitis mei'.

Canis sequitur duos homines (*adds* in uia S), sed cuius sit
canis donec separentur ignoratur. Sed cum uterque uadit uiam
suam, tunc patet cuius sit canis, quia ipsum sequitur cuius est
460   (quia ... est] *om.* S). A simili de diuitiis. Diuitie enim non sunt
hominis, sed mundi, sed non apparet in presenti donec homo uiam
uniuerse carnis ingrediatur. Sed tunc bene patet quod mundi sunt,
quia tunc mundo remanent et hominem non sequuntur (donec ...
sequuntur] donec separentur et homo moriatur S). Unde Beda,
465   *Super Lucam*, 'Non sunt bona hominis que secum fer[r]i non
possunt'. 'Sola misericordia etc.', ut supra (*concludes citation* sola
misericordia comes est defunctorum S). Unde quidam uersificator,
'Ludus fortune uariatur imagine lune. / Crescit, decrescit, in
eodem sistere nescit'. Item uersus, 'Cui satis est, quod habet satis
470   illum constat habere. / Cui nihil est, quod habet satis illum constat
egere. / Ergo facit uirtus non copia sufficientem, / et non paupertas
sed mentis hiatus egentem'. Et sic patet de ueneno auaricie.

GR *add*: 407–13 Item auarus similis est stulto ... potentium,
422–30 Item auarus similis est molendinario ... Iob 2,
446–51 Rex quidam ... nouissimo suo (+ the S addition),
457–60 Canis sequitur ... de diuitiis

S *adds*: 392–414 Item auarus est similis equo ... Hec Gregorius,
422–41 Item auarus similis est moldendinario ... dummodo habeat,
444–51 Ideo Seneca auarus ... in nouissimo suo, 457–69 Canis sequitur ...
sistere nescit, 472 Et sic ... auaricie

B *adds*: not entirely in the order elsewhere, the full passage except for
450–56 quantum ad hoc ... capitis mei, 466–72 Sola ... ueneno auaricie

two or three days to live, and nevertheless he doesn't stop heaping up money. Therefore Seneca says, 'A miser is like a monster; the less life remains for him, the more he looks for resources for this journey'.

A noble and powerful and very rich king, when he knew he was about to die, had carried on a spear through his city the wretched cloth in which he was to be buried, and he had a herald cry out, 'This hairshirt is the sum of my goods, and it bears with it all my glory'. In this regard, this dying king was wise about his end. Also Socrates, travelling to Athens, carried with him a golden weight which he sunk in a stream, saying, 'I will submerge you, lest I be submerged by you'. Also a hermit, when he had been given money, hid it at the head of his bed. And thieves came there in the night to carry away his money; seeing this, the hermit threw them the money saying, 'Take this fear from my head'.

A dog follows two men, but one can't tell which of them the dog belongs to until they separate. But when each of them goes his own way, it's evident which one owns the dog, because it then follows its master. And it's just the same with riches, for riches are not man's, but the world's, but this isn't evident until a person at last enters the way of all flesh. But then it is quite evident that riches are the world's, because now they remain with the world, and they don't follow the person. Hence Bede says, *On Luke*, 'Those goods which he can't carry with him are not man's'. 'Only mercy', as above. Hence some versifier says, 'Fortune's game is varied, like the shape of the moon. It waxes, it wanes, and it never knows how to stay in the same state'. And there's another verse, 'For the person who feels satisfied, the enough he has is enough. For the one who feels he has nothing, the enough he has makes him feel needy. Therefore it is virtue, not plenty, that creates a sufficient amount, and it's not poverty but a gaping spirit that creates need'. And this is evident with the poison of avarice.

After 1653 derelictis, **p** *adds* (p+illeg. V only):

Utinam sic esset inter Christianos suas uxores dimittentes, et qui
alias suis habent uxoribus magis charas! Hec igitur dicta sufficient,
475   secundum mei tenuitatem ingenii, de predictis ad aliqualem
instructionem simplicium qui habent populum informare. Pro
quibus sit mihi Christus premium et merces, qui cum Patre et
Spiritu Sancto uiuit et regnat in secula seculorum. Amen.

After 1653:

If only the same were true among Christians, who go about divorcing their wives and who hold other women more dear than them! Therefore, the things I have said here, so far as the slenderness of my wit allows, should be enough for some instruction of simple men who are appointed to teach the people. For which, I hope for reward and payment from Christ, who lives and rules with the Father and the Holy Ghost forever.

Editorial notes

On textual divisions, extensively marked in p, but generally foreign to both αβ, see the introduction, p. 26, n. 44.

8 *quam carnalium*: p *corporalium siue carnalium* represents what I consider 'a doublet of doubt' (here in part inspired by deviant reading of p's source S, and the majority confirmed by Augustine's repeated use of *carnis*). Such readings, rife in the tradition, are provided as a service to readers. Scribes routinely have difficulty distinguishing similar tachygraphic forms; while many such are utterly conventional, a great many can be construed as ambiguous, as reflected in competing fuller renditions. The doublets signal that the scribe has found an abbreviated reading in his exemplar ambiguous, and that the reader should choose the variant s/he finds most appropriate in context. Examples of the technique, usually joined by *uel* (and in other textual traditions by *aliter*), are particularly frequent in C. On occasion the effort remains unsignalled; G, for example, at line 105, reads *primum omnium principium*, reflecting a doubt as to whether the source reads p^m ('primum') or pn^m ('principium'). Another early example appears at line 78 (in p). More usually, however, such difficulties of interpretation become evident in varying scribal responses to what, by implication, were similar archetypal readings, e.g. at 81 *illuminationis* or 93 *stimulantem*. On such occasions, either the readings of Malachy's sources (as here) or the general argumentative context, frequently repetitive (as at 105), directs one to the anterior reading.

22 *in testimonium*: See the introduction, p. 31. Throughout the Middle Ages, particularly in writing English, the conventions for word-spacing differ from those customary in modern type-face. Prepositions are routinely joined with their objects, and prefixes written separately from the root-word. These conventions are distinctly recessive in Latin copying, where scribes have been trained 'grammatically' in that language and thus have a fixed sense of word-boundaries. Nevertheless, the convention routine for English appears widely in D's text, and it here has tripped up S (and necessarily, his inheritor p). S has read an unspaced (and customarily abbreviated) Latin form *ints-* as if *intl-*; this would imply that his exemplar was written in textura, where 'long s' sits on the writing line, rather than exhibiting the descender usual in anglicana. The same kind of error occurs again at 1273, here in p only, where the unspaced 'inore' has been construed as 'more' and has stimulated a disastrous reduction of the sentence; and cf. S, in Appendix 29, where 'inuidia' is reported as 'in mala' (similarly 399 inuidia] in malicia S). For a few further plausible examples, see 409 uise] in se ADGL (se p), 501 compari] cum pare L; 619 in mitra] mitra CDL; 633 impatiencia] paciencia CDLS; 1216 magne] in agro parue S.

57 *secundum philosophum*: In BA, the opinion is ascribed to Pythagoras; *philosophum* may represent an abbreviated form, misread in the archetype underlying all copies.

63 *significat*: In the MSS, the verb is rarely written in full, but as the ambiguous – it might equally represent *signat* – abbreviated *sig(n)ᵃt*.

92 *faciem*: Confirmed by BA 1127/19: 'he lepeþ vpon his face … and craccheþ', as well as by the description of Virgil's flea *in fronte* 101.

95 *ad animam … dormientem*: Just as most such omissions, this is an entirely mechanical error – and one with a remarkably minor stimulus. The archetypal scribe behind AGS has taken up one run of copying ending *clamantem* and returned to his copy in search of a word ending *-ntem*, but at the second instance, rather than the first. Repeated mistakes like this imply that copyists did not 'mark' their exemplars (as we would, with a piece of paper under the line copied) with any care. Fifteenth-century illustrations of scribes at work often show the exemplar being copied placed on a nearly vertical stand and at eye-level for a sitting copyist (analogous to our computer screens); the copying proceeds on a below-eye-level desk-top or slanted writing board. In such a context, without careful marking, the succession of eye-movements between text and copy predictably produces only approximate returns to the exemplar. Here, however, one might be surprised that a scribe apparently took as his key for returning to the exemplar a case-ending, rather than the verbal root. But his second omission, the loss of 99–100 *gratuita … uulnerantem* (central to the argument, where grace is at issue), another example of finding the wrong accusative of the present participle on resuming copying (here with the additional stimulus of 'notional homeoteleuthon', **uenenosum …** **uulnerantem**), confirms that this was his normal practice. In general, as here, γ's frequent small textual intrusions can be identified as potentially authorial only by noticing possible underlying eye-skips that have removed them from other copies.

104 *musce*: For discussion of the following interpolation (Appendix 1–4), a rather vapid effort to bring a greater degree of conclusiveness than Malachy had provided, see the Introduction, pp. 36–37.

105–9 Augustine's text, which lacks it, indicates that αβ *omnium* is a scribal intensifier. But Augustine offers no help in dealing with the remaining variation, as *omnia mala famulantur* in the final clause paraphrases 'primumque vitium ejus naturae'. For 108 *ducisse sue* Gregory has 'suis ducibus … tradit'; CD's feminine form has probably doubled *sue*, i.e. *ducesse sue*', while in αβ the possessive has become absorbed in the preceding *(duc)es*.

114 *statum*: *gradum* has been attracted to the following verb.

119 *potestatibus*: Intruded in βγ as if a doublet of *principibus*, but simply an echo of earlier *potestas*. The paragraph offers several further examples of γ fastidiousness and qualification. In particular, their archetypal scribe seeks to soften Malachy's universal condemnation. But authorial 'usus scribendi' elsewhere is frequently totalising.

134, 143 I take the γ readings here as interpolation. The first certainly misses the drift of the argument, which is that even the *perfecti* have become powerless to effect change, not because they are oppressed but because lords are too poisoned to heed them. Thus, the gloss on clerical power follows directly from what precedes. I take the second expanded γ reading, with an additional example of *-ficere*, as similarly intrusive.

148 *154*: Comparable variation recurs, at 1488. Orosius gives the figure as a mere 'sexaginta et quatuor'.

157 *rubeta*: BA's form at 1154/25 (both ME and Latin), as all MSS here. *rudeca* is the form in Pliny, probably an example of p consulting the source. I have not been able, in the case of isolated superior readings in p, to eliminate the possibility that they result from such fastidiousness.

162 *inspicit*: I retain the copy-text, although isolated among the variants. Both the competing readings potentially reflect attraction to surrounding material, the majority *respicit* to earlier *recipit*, *inspicit* to subsequent *interimit*.

168 *a dieta*: The reading is confirmed by reference to Isaac's title and the source in BA. The γ intrusion earlier in the line is vacuous, a doubling of preceding materials.

174 *qui et basilicus*: α MSS follow the reading of the gloss.

193 *sanctitatis*: Gregory reads 'humilitatis'.

199 *derelictis*: BA 1128/33, 36–37 'schoueþ [shows] his hornes aboue ... setteþ hem [the horns] bare aboue þe sond', both imply the presence of a verbal form, pointing to α.

203 *interimit*: BA 1179/10 cites the gloss in the form of α, without the final clause, but β's apparent addition 'et sic ... cadit' concludes the biblical verse.

204 *cordis*: γ offers an honest 'doublet of doubt', the abbreviated form misinterpreted elsewhere. A similar error occurs at 224, on this occasion in γ.

205 *auctoritatis*: The genitive echoes the core of the gloss: the interlinearis, 'cerastes, cornibus potestatis armatus'; the marginal, 'Cerastes enim Grece cornua dicuntur ... [Anticristus] ... morsu pestifere predicationis et cornu potestatis armabitur' (*cerastes* armed with the horns of power ... *Cerastes* is the Greek word for 'horns' ... Antichrist will be armed with the bite of pestilent preaching and the horn of power). Lδ here, in addition to differing in case, intrude a typically fussy gloss. As the citation indicates, Malachy offers an original moralisation, as the gloss sees the serpent's danger as 'veneno consumens eos ad vite latitudinem prouocat' (Antichrist, while his poison consumes them, incites them to an undisciplined life), not extorting bribes.

221 *scitalis*: BA 1126/19 confirms that this is the snake under discussion; CD, responding to the medieval loss of distinction between classical *sc* and *s*, have confused it with the snake that kills through desiccation (see 408).

245 *Hypocrita*: Various copies assimilate to the usual reading of Vulgate Is 9:17.

252 *sublimitate*: αβ have misinterpreted an abbreviated form, but *sublimi* 253, everywhere but in G, indicates that γ preserves the correct reading.

254 *uota et uita repugnant*: 'their vows and their behaviour are opposed'. γ *tota* is vacuous and clearly *facilior*. The *uota* 'vows' must refer to the religious men's *magisterium*, their alleged devotion to instruction. Like the γ reading here, the insertion 174 *quoad corpus* appears to me obtuse: grace, after all, isn't physical?

257 *adurit*: In spite of majority *admittat*, L is probably correct: cf. BA 1127/37–38 'and brenneþ nought in fuyre but abateþ ... the brennynge'. Again, an abbreviated form has stimulated variation; all the scribes seem to have seen a reading of the type 'ad + minims + suspension + t', but only L recognised the superscript i (= ri), while the rest read it as superscript t (= it).

264 *lacteam*: That the word should appear in the natural description is confirmed by its use in the moralisation at 267, as well as by BA 1128/5–6 'and casteþ out of his mouþ white quyttere'.

267 *per prauum exemplum*: Apparently construed by γ as anticipating the similar statement in the following lines.

274 *prauus*: In spite of the attractive *facundus*, γ probably inserts here. This may have been stimulated by the subsequent quotation, which opens with an account of a good preacher.

284 *uelare*: Gregory's text confirms this reading, as well as 286 *subiecti et timidi* and *quod ipsi nesciunt*. Similarly, 291 *uentositatis* is Augustine's reading.

292 *falsi iudices*: Answers forms of *iudico* twice in the proof-texts cited in 298–302.

299–301 *illos, nullis*: Both readings are confirmed by the source texts, here the Vulgate and Gregory's comment.

318–20 *quod … uincitur*: The α readings are probably confirmed by BA 1153/18–19 'sleeþ also alle þing þat haþ lyf' and 21 'he is ouercome'. The intruded γ *et occiditur* is probably what remains from these MSS's earlier omission.

339 *muro oppositum*: Although the γ addition may have fallen victim to a skip *-situm … -situm* in other copies, the source, *De preliis*, offers no comparable description.

348 *adustus*, **350** *contuitus*: The print has accommodated its forms to earlier uses.

354 *mortem*: Has probably suggested the *montem* of the subsequent γ interpolation. Another apparent γ intrusion, at 1112–13, introduces a *collem* 'hill', again alien to the discussion.

361 *salamandre*: Cf. BA 1243/28–29 'a certeyn kynde of *salamandra* haþ row3 skynne and hery'.

366 *Dei*: In γ, succeeded by another vapid bit of clarification (here with a mirroring effort at overspecification earlier in the sentence in α).

370 *perniciossimus*: At 706, A again confuses the loop that indicates either terminal *-us* or initial *con-* with an abbreviation involving words in *qu-*. The same confusion appears in CD at 871 and apparent confusion of *con-* and *d-* in S at 388 *coguntur*.

386 *somno*: Confirmed by BA 1135/8–9 'as it were by slepe'.

397-98 *Fascinatio uulgo*: Following the gloss; the βγ intrusion *proprie* seems particularly silly.

400 *hominis*: The γ addition *mali* is an echo of earlier *malitia*. Similarly, 432 *malum aduersum* anticipates *aduersitatem*.

421-22 *sugit ... sugit*: BA 1135/10 'soukeþ blood of him þat he smyteþ' shows Sp to have skipped between adjacent uses of the verb, also misrepresented in other copies.

448 *in gemmam preciosam*: Cf. BA 1222/3 'But þere it is þe sonner harde and turneþ into stoon'.

458 *corpus*: Cf. BA 1135/20-21 'And þis serpent destroyeþ and rendeþ nought oonliche þe body but also he destroyeþ ... boþe bones and senewes' (with a comparable verse from Lucan on 'body and bones', 1125/23).

463-65 *Detractor ... dicit*: αβ have skipped between a pair of biblical quotations, since the gloss refers to the widely cited verse about the deaf serpent. The passage provides a further example of Malachy's innovative moralisations, as the gloss makes the obvious point of the *coluber* as one resistant to a corrective preacher, not Malachy's specification of the specific precept.

470 *furiositatem*: Cf. BA 209/2 'for þe wood humour and venemous', translating Latin 'humorem furiosum et venenosum'.

482 *philosophum*: The entire discussion in BA is ascribed to Avicenna, suggesting that this may be an archetypal error: there the more familiar 'Aristotelem' was read for 'Auicennam', perhaps in an abbreviated form, and the usual synonym 'philosophum' represents a substitution later in the tradition.

485-86 *Unde ... malorum*: The βγ formulation of this material seems to miss the point, which is not that the episode in Daniel shows envy but that 'inveterate' old men are more prone to its venom than are the young.

488 *quam in pratis*: Rather than BA 428/24 'nyʒe cleues and bankes of watris' (Latin 'iuxta litora et iuxta aquas'), but 428/23-24 'ham þat hooueþ in hilles ... is worse þan of hem þat woneþ' might suggest following CDL in a second use of 'habitancium'.

499 *circa*: Scribal misinterpretation of the similar abbreviations for *contra* and *circa* is endemic throughout the text; here cf. BA 1136/25 'aboute þe ryuer Eufrates'.

500-1 BA 1136/28 confirms GSp, 'of oþere naciouns, what nacioun it euere be'.

502–4 *ut perimat … noscens*: This corresponds to BA 1136/5–9 'And knoweþ þe sleer and reseþ on him, be he in neuer so gret companye … and fondeþ for to slen him and passe all difficultees and space … oþer by watres oþer by ryueres'. This is a complicated case of what I have described above as 'mixed blessings' (pp. 33–34): split transmission in which fragments of an original reading appear isolated in various copies (most evident in the varying reductions of *perimat*; *permeat*).

513 *perdit*, **515** *regios*: Both corresponding to the Latin readings underlying BA 209/6 'lesiþ' and 209/10 'kynges'. The first reading is confirmed by difficulties with the later, apparently repetitive, *prodit*; the synonymous substitution *amittat* is an effort at addressing this issue.

529 *recte*: *directe* might seem preferable as reiterating the language of the previous sentence. But, as usual in this editorial situation, the reading could well represent assimilation to what has already been stated, and Malachy's point seems to be wilful *mis*judgement of the envious, not their misinterpretation of evidence.

538 BA 429/24 'violent' confirms the majority reading, but in **539** *interficit* is right, cf. BA 'sleeþ'. The erroneous second reading has been attracted to the earlier use of *inficit*.

541 *Christi*: All six primary MSS here include at least the opening of an additional sentence, also at the head of the large addition, only in Sp+B. This appears to be a bit of marginalia, in some copies, where it has been cancelled, rejected from the text. BA 1135/17–23, the source of 456–59, while it emphasises the virulence of this snake's poison, includes no comparable information.

546 *amantius*: Confirmed by Seneca's text.

547 *Differentie*: Gregory only introduces the parts as 'haec singula exercitum suum'. Certainly, A *differen*tie probably underlies CD *diuerse*, and *species* is a clarification of that reading. While GSp accord with the later discussion, where these are *effectus*, they have probably incorporated their reading from there.

554–55 Seneca confirms the order of AGSp; CDL have removed the contrastive structure (*ira* opposed to other vices) and grouped the effects. But the problem appears to have been stimulated by an archetypal scribalism; Seneca reads 'impendit(, paucis gratuita est)' (only pays out), not 'incendit' (burns [its goods] up).

559 *se prepedit*: The isolated p reading is confirmed by Gregory's text; this might be an example of the printer confirming readings against Malachy's sources.

562 *igneos*, **575** *claros oculos*: Confirmed by BA 1155/2 'yhen as þough it were fyre' and BA 1155/4 'clere yhen'.

581 *dorso* (CDL): A doublet inspired by the correct *dextro*; cf. BA 1155/30 'in þe right syde'. In the following line, BA 1155/31 'seþynge' represents his Latin 'feruentem' (and cf. 583 *feruere*).

584 *excitat ... extinguit*: The MSS fairly frequently agree in offering singular verb forms with compound subjects.

587–99 The source here, *De ira* 1.18.3–6, although partly paraphrased, confirms αβ throughout.

612 *quasi*: While the various γ qualifications are interpolations, this reading is correct; cf. BA 1154/32–33 'stonyeþ þerfore eche membre þat he toucheþ and makeþ it lese feelynge as þough it were frore'. Another good example of a 'mixed blessing', part of it compelling, part silly; γ copies have construed 'quasi' as introducing a simile.

623 *aliquando*: Confirmed by BA 430/21 'somtyme', amid a passage marked by extensive γ intrusions.

641 *et ... doctores*: The clause is probably authorial; cf. BA 1155/28: 'And schal be take and kepte to þe vse of medicyne'. Although omitted in most of the MSS collated, it also appears in BRLaV (in V largely illeg.).

649–54 The paraphrase in p has at least been stimulated by skipping between two uses of the phrase 'contra iram'. A similar omission produced the paraphrase at 1610–16.

688 *totaliter* (ACDL): Unparalleled in BA and echoing *hyeme tota* (just as most MSS include an echoic *omni* in the preceding line).

702–4 A paragraph littered with 'mixed blessings'. βγ share a common eyeskip, *nituntur ... uruntur* 707–8, but elsewhere offer readings superior to GSp, including the lengthier conclusion at 712–13.

732 *iuuenes*: However plausible, *innubes* p is wrong, a dissimilation from the use earlier in the line; cf. BA 1148/6 'ʒonge and virgine'.

739 *ratio*: Confirmed by BA 1204/25–26 'Þey taken gret charge of here comune profyte and hauen þerof resoun and mynde'.

742–44 The CDL addition only extends the biblical citation, but it explains the transition to *hyem-* in the following sentence.

748–50 *Est ... instinctu*: This omission appears to be an eye-skip between uses of *torper-* or some confusion based on repeated *-iam*.

768 *grossitiem*: cf. BA 1140/27–28n 'propter grosciciem'.

781 *auarus*: The long addition, in most copies, is an echo of 775.

821 *u.*: BA 1184/31–32 reads 'foure oþer fyue of hem'.

825 *mercator*: Cf. 'Omnis ergo negotiator dici potest Mercurius' (Fulgentius 1.18, Helm 29/9). The source also confirms 'pennas ad talos' (i.e. only wings on his heels, not fully winged, like an angel, as the variant 'usque ad' implies). For 829 *mercium curius*, although Helm offered 'merciumcurum' and cited the variants 'cyrum' and 'curam' (29/8), Herebert knew better. At this point, A reads *cirrus*, with Herebert's marginal note *kirios*; he recognised the word as the transliterated Greek that it is, 'lord, master', probably from something like *Remigii* 66/21 'mercatorum kyrios, id est dominus' (similarly 194/22–23).

898 *innocentibus ... sibi*: The γ omission is an eye-skip between the two uses of *uite*.

907 *cibum*: I am completely baffled by the γ addition about 'red earth'.

918 *prophetans*: The collated copies are unanimous in reading *procrastinans*, but I think Neckam's suggestion more compelling: 'Certissimum item nuntius est corvus mutationis aeris et alia crocitationis modulatione *prophetat* auram salubrem fore, alia tempestatem futuram praedicit' (It is also most certain that the crow is a messenger about changes in the atmosphere, and at some times prophesies, through the inflections of its cawing, that the weather will be pleasant, and at others, predicts a coming storm; 1.61, p. 110). Neckam offers this information in the service of an entirely different moralisation, the raven as preacher, gathering authorities to sway his audience to seek the joys of heaven and avoid the pains of hell.

929 *uentres pigri* (CDL): The phrase simply concludes a full citation of the verse, but one germane to Malachy's moral, that flatterers are seeking a free meal.

951 *Arionem*: I assume the myth well enough known that Malachy will have communicated the name accurately, although he might well not have known that of Arion's city, Methymna. In the following lines, AG reproduce Cicero's text.

964–68 In general, I have accommodated the variation here to BA. 965 *maiores* may be a back-formation from the following *minores* and a substitution for an adjective parallel to *certas* (cf. BA 1204/9 'makeþ hem priuey weyes euen and strei3t', the Latin ' redeunt per semitas certas et expeditas'). Here I am guided by the moralisation of the following paragraph, with its description of prelates sweeping in to gather up tithes collected by others; reading thus requires construing *transeunt* as the verb of the two resulting clauses. 968 *condant* ('before they store it away') is confirmed by BA 1204/27 'þat þey doon togideres'; the abbreviation con̄dat has been construed as indicating not the plural but a more extensive abbreviated form. The additional sentence in p is answered by a parallel addition at 981. These appear to have been generated in response to 969 *quattuor* and a difficulty in identifying the four intended separate moralisations (cf. the variation at 975 *Tercio*).

999 *in*: The ADL intrusion, potentially omitted through a small eyeskip elsewhere, probably only accidentally answers BA 1125/35–36 'tweye hedes, oon in þe oon ende and anoþer in þe oþer ende'.

1014 *cito*: The lengthy following reading, in γ only, may represent an eyeskip; the other scribes might have jumped from *disparent* to *disperguntur*. But, as in some other γ readings (see 354n), the intrusion of a metaphor alien and extraneous leads me to think this an interpolation. These MSS again intrude a *uentus* at 1038–39 (there stimulated by *inflati*).

1028 *inimicus*: Certainly the additional citation may have been skipped in many copies (*Unde dicitur … inimicus Ideo dicitur … inimicus*). Given his recourse to the orator and philosopher, Malachy is a good deal more likely than the scribes to have known an outstanding example of twelfth-century Ciceronianism. But I am more inclined to see this widely cited proverbialism as an interpolation, stimulated by the echo *inimicus … amici*.

1035 *cum*: The ACDL addition is attractive, and other scribes may have assimilated to the reading of the Vulgate.

1047 *deuastata*: S has inserted the Vulgate reading of the clause, but *deuastata* also appears proximately in Ex.

1055–57 The reading printed follows G, which most closely approximates Ambrose. The MSS vary in the repetitive context of the comparatives. Cf. BA 625/7–8, paraphrasing Ambrose, 'þe more clere eyre sche draweþ, þe more clerelich sche syngeþ' (the Latin 'quo puriorem aerem id temporis attrahunt spiritu, eo cantus resonant clariores').

1101–3 I have generally followed those variants that most closely accord with Ambrose's text (where 200 *lingua*, in A only, is notable as directing one toward to authorial reading).

1103–5 For this concluding citation, see p. 21. In ASp, it has probably fallen victim to eyeskip on the final syllables in -*r(i)a*.

1114–15 The grammar follows BA, that 'anoþer spiþere of þe same kynde' should be shown to the victim.

1129 *ipsum*: Cf. BA 1186/16–17 'Also libro xxviii° Plinius seiþ'. Sp have a doublet of doubt, hesitating between reading *Pli* and *phi*. In 1132, the additional citation has been suggested by earlier *mundat* (and cf. the earlier γ elaboration). 1135 *eam* p probably duplicates *eam* in the following citation, and *eos* refers to the tongue and gall, not, as in γ, to dragons in general.

1153 *et putrescit*: Perhaps an archetypal error; cf. BA 434/18 'idreynte oþir isode' (the Latin 'submergitur uel decoquitur').

1163 *piscatus*: A sees what is at issue; cf. BA 434/20 'ibrused' (the Latin 'contritus siue pistatus').

1172 *quandoque*: Cf. BA 1205/6 'somtyme'. As the context demonstrates, the γ elaboration here is categorically wrong-headed.

1208 *ascendit*: The reading of the received Vulgate, Ps 77:30–31; the variant is a 'common-sense' substitution to accord with following *super*.

1209 *accuratius*: Cf. Gregory, 'quae sumenda sint praeparari accuratius expetit'.

1238–42 The varying reproductions of the text are predicated upon slightly different eye-skips, both depending upon the similar sentence openings, 'Hec ergo fabula ostendit … Hec igitur fabula et consimiles'. Because the first has a moral local to the preceding fable, the Sp placement is probably correct; the other MSS have recognised their omission relatively immediately and inserted the omitted material out of order. However, Sp have completely skipped the second sentence, 'Hec igitur fabula et consimiles … quedam uera', probably in the belief that it was the material just copied. In addition, they have dropped a clause from the subsequent Augustine material, probably because of a notional skip between two uses of 'ueritatem'. A similar mess, again predicated on skipping between similar copy, occurs at 1608ff.

1243 *et uilia* (CDL): Intruded to assimilate the text to the conclusion at 1259.

1273 *more* (p): The mistake, for *in ore* (written as one word) has produced massive and senseless abbreviation. Cf. BA 1244/10 'in his mouþe is a pype wiþ þe whiche he sowkeþ blood'.

1276 *nimium excessum* (CDL): 'The excessive excess', probably the most vacuous of all those intrusions that typify γ.

1285 *fumositatibus*: Cf. BA 432/16–17 'signes … imade and ibred of fumosite of herte'.

1294 *lacerta*: An archetypal error; cf. BA 207/27 'þe strenges of þe tonge may not strecche and sprede'.

1296–98 I have generally accommodated the variants to Seneca's text, which confirms both *incendit et detegit* and *remouet*. 1297 *detentus* may be an archetypal scribalism for Seneca's *devinctus*.

1303 *uicium* (p): Probably anticipating *u^m*, i.e. the later *uenenum*. One of a number of examples of 'mixed blessings' here. For p's 1309 *nouatur*, cf. BA 1130/16 'and bycomeþ ȝonge aȝein' (the Latin 'ut in iuuentutem *redire*') and unanimous 1326 *renouare*. But p's isolated 1310 *primo* is confirmed by BA 1131/4–5 'first anon to þe yhen', and it arguably refers to the correct biblical book in 1307, where the citation amalgamates features of Mt 17:20 and Mc 9:28.

1316 *Physiologo*: BA has 'philosophus', and this is an archetypal error. G, having misunderstood the form, accidentally returns to the source reading.

grauatam: The unanimous MS reading accords with BA 1130/23–24 'þe addre feleþ him ygreued wiþ yuel oþer wiþ eelde'; and p's addition appears simply generated by *morbo* (just as the γ insertion later in the line by *senio*). In 1324 *tunicam*, AG is confirmed by BA's Latin; cf. BA 1130/34 'a nou skynne' (the Latin 'nouum cutem'). However, BA discusses the snake-skin as a 'tunica(m)' in the surrounding discussion, and, in that context, I have let the copy-text stand.

1330–35 See the discussion above, pp. 33–34.

1345 *annuerunt*: The competing reading, *consenserunt*, has been assimilated to *senserunt* in the following line.

1371 *ore inserto cum*: Cf. BA 1266/27–28 'doþ his mouþe into þe mouþe' (the Latin 'ore inserto in os'). Although 1380 *extenuatiua* may simply represent p's lucky guess, the reading is at least apt for the following citation, as *excecatiua* is not.

1397–1402 That the viper and lamprey must represent the same species does not seem to lead to the moral that supposes this a figure for adultery. That conclusion, in its turn, must be recalling the earlier discussion of the viper shedding its venom before intercourse (as does the head of the following paragraph); were the snake to retain its venom, the two would be similar and thus, as it were, wedded.

1413–14 *inferiori ... superiori*: Following BA 1248/20–21 'schapen as a mayde fro þe nauel vppeward and as a fisshe fro þe nauel dounward'. For 1415 *siccum* (BA 1248/25 'a drye place', the Latin 'ad locum siccum'), see pp. 27–28. In 1419, p has skipped between two citations marked 'Is''.

1436 *interficiunt*: Cf. BA 1199/11 'þey sleeþ wommen'.

1443–45 Dt 23:18, to which I have assimilated the text, reads, 'Non offeres mercedem prostibuli nec pretium canis in domo Domini'. Cf. BA's discussion, 1170/32–36, with a double reference to 'offrynge of þe prise'.

1465 *atteritur* ...: βγ have omitted a good deal of the passage through an eye-skip *-itur* ... *-itur.* Valerius's text also confirms that the same copies err in offering 1467 *aliis.*

1484 *collo*: While I follow the MSS in printing *-ll-*, the word is, of course, *colo* 'a distaff'. The subsequent Augustine quotation is probably scribally truncated across all the copies; cf. 'ea sola se habere mortuum, quae libido ejus etiam, cum viveret hauriendo, consumpserat' (now dead, he had only those things that his lust had consumed, drinking them in, while he lived).

1489 *suus*: p proves over-ingenious in offering a contextually plausible reading; Orosius confirms the printed text.

1504 *Magistra*: Jerome's reading.

1513 *matutino*: Confirmed by BA 679/29 'of þe morowe dewe'.

1538ff. Not recognising an Irish saint, p has taken him to be a woman on the basis of his name's terminal *-a* and has, consequently, misreported the anecdote.

1544 *triplicis*: Although rather submerged, the threefold division encourages avoiding *cohabitatio, aspectus* (1555) and *colloquium* (1570–71).

1564–65 *graue detinetur infirmitate*: Following BA's Latin, which p has perhaps consulted.

1597–98 Cf. BA 1266/35–37: 'he huydeth himself oonliche in þe chynes and dennes of þe eorþe, and oþere addres and serpentes huydeþ hemself in holowe stones and trees' (the Latin 'in terre cauernis ... alii omnes cauernis saxorum aut arborum'). Trevisa's copy must have read something like 'in rimis et terre cauernis', and Malachy's copy appears to have had the same additional phrase, although the MSS report it in the following clause.

1609–17 I print the passage in the form provided by βγ. The disorder in the other copies is predicated upon having skipped between 'destructa (non)' and 'destruxit', the omission partially restored at a later point. This partial report may reflect a further bit of oversight, a skip between 'prouerbialiter' and 'prosperitas'.

1630–38 Both sets of MSS paraphrase Neckam's account – and both omit Neckam's detail that the knight's wife tries to unstop the well.

1642 *post ... ueniat*: The additional clause in γ is confirmed by BA 1218/5 'but if þe leonesse be ywaisshe ... ar sche come to þe leoun' (similarly BA 1218/8–9).

1650 *certamen et iudicium*: Following Cicero's 'in certamen iudiciumque veniunt'.

Appendix: The extensive interpolations

21 Among the earliest MSS, S provides the most proximate source of p. However, a passage such as this one indicates both this copy's deviance and that p followed a fuller and more cultivated version now extant in the later B.

362 On the γ intrusion here see the Introduction, pp. 30–31.

Malachy's sources

6–8 *De civitate Dei* 14.3 (*PL* 41:406).

11–15 BA 1131/19–22, 1245/22–25. For the 'naturalis astutia' of the next line, cf. BA 1129/28–31.

19–20 BA 1125/1–3, 1245/15–18. With the following line, indeed with 6–38 generally, cf. Neckam 2.105 (p. 188), 'Reducere autem debet homo ad memoriam maledictionem divinam serpentem datam, quociens ad memoriam revocat partum viperae. Fuit enim serpens materialis, organum antiqui serpentis, a quo venenum infusum in radicem ramos in posteritate infecit' (Everyone ought to remember the divine curse laid on the serpent, just as frequently as they recall the viper's birthing. The viper, a material snake, is just a limb of the old serpent, whose poison, spread about in the root, infects its offspring, the branches, as well).

23–26 BA 1129/11–14, 21–27.

27–28 Cf. BA 93/29–31. So far as I can see, neither Isidore nor Papias says anything of the sort, and the ascriptions may derive from misreadings of abbreviated forms in BA.

38–40 Unfound.

54–56, 62–65 The gloss here, *Biblia Latina* 1:324a, paraphrases Isidore, *Quaestiones in vetus testamentum* 36.2 and 3 (*PL* 83:355), subject to further paraphrase here. The second selection on Christ as brazen serpent appears in Neckam 2.109 (p. 192), cited at pp. 19–20 above.

56–61 BA 1131/8–18.

69–73 From a MS gloss (there is no continuous example contemporary with Malachy); the gloss usually printed, ascribed to Aquinas, while provocative, does not offer comparable information: 'Notandum Socrates magnus, qui primus vniuersam philosophiam ad corrigendos componendosque mores fecisse memoratur tempore [in fact, a citation from John of Salisbury, *Polycraticus* 7.5] … Eo autem tempore cum sapientes plurimi a vulgaribus persequerentur, quoniam vnum deum predicabant, Socrates ipse deprehensus est atque ab Aueto Athenienium duce eiusque discipulo, sibi dato mortis poculo, ipso non aliter quam quodam immortalitatis, assumpto medicamento, interijt' (One should notice that the great Socrates is still recalled as the person who first made all philosophy the study of constructing and correcting human behaviour ... But at the time when many wise men were persecuted by the mob because they preached that there was but a single god, Socrates was taken by Avetus, the ruler of Athens and his student. Having been given a deadly drink, nothing other than a kind of immortality, he took the poison and died', sig. C iiiᵛ).

74 *Epistulae morales* 67.7.

80–82 *Etymologiae* 4.9.8 (*PL* 182:193), but probably from an unidentified locus in BA; cf. Neckam 2.108 (p. 189).

83–84 *De Genesi ad litteram* 9.15 (*PL* 34:404); cf. Sermo dubius 374.3 (*PL* 39:1668).

88–93 BA 1127/12–22. However, Neckam's moralisation of the following Virgilian anecdote, while provocative, offers a contrasting moral: '[Virgil's] serpens antiqui serpentis typum gerit, qui somnolentos et desides et otio effoeminatos persequi dedignatur, sed vigilantes infestat. Si torporem ignavia excutis, qui prius somno desidiae torpuisti, aderit serpens antiquus, paratus venenum suggestionis infundere' (p. 191) (This snake is a type for the old serpent, who disdains persecuting sleepy people and lazy ones and those made weak through leisure, but assaults those who are awake. If you cut away the sleepiness with its accompanying neglect, in which you have previously lazed about sleepily, the old serpent will come, prepared to pour in his poison that incites one to sin).

100–4 This refers to the central narrative of the ps.-Virgilian 'Culex', probably from Neckam 2.109 (pp. 190–91).

105–6 *De civitate Dei* 12.6 (*PL* 41:353).

108–9 *Moralia* 31.45.87 (*PL* 76:620).

111–14 *De casu diaboli*, cf. chapter 3 (*PL* 158:329–30).

114–16 *De similitudinibus* 7 (*PL* 159:607, actually Alexander of Canterbury).

121–23 BA 1153/15–21. Cf. Neckam 2.120 (p. 198).

124–26 Cf. *Biblia Latina* 3:27b, a reduced version of Jerome, *Commentarii in Isaiam* 5 (*PL* 24:166), on Is 14:29 'de radice enim colubri egredietur regulus, et semen ejus absorbens volucrum' (Out of the root of the serpent shall come forth a basilisk, and his seed shall swallow the bird).

126–28 Although there is no overt reference to Pliny, all the detail, including 'semipedem longitudinis', appears in Neckam 2.120 (p. 198).

135–36 *Biblia Latina* 2:573a offers nothing relevant, but cf. *PL* 113:1000: '*Super aspidem*. Post humanam infirmitatem, divina virtus ostenditur, quae tantis imperat. Et agit de Christo secundum membra. *Et conculcabis*. (AUG.) Serpentem calcat Ecclesia, quae cavet astutiam ejus' (*Upon the asp.* After human weakness, divine virtue shows itself and controls such things. This verse shows Christ being referred to through the acts of his limbs. *And thou shalt trample*. The church tramples the snake, because it is wary of his subtlety).

140–41 As *Biblia Latina* 3:115a, from Jerome, *Commentarii in Jeremiam* 2 (*PL* 24:740).

144–47 *Commentarii in Isaiam* 5 (*PL* 24:163).

147–49 Orosius, *Historiae* 2.2 (*PL* 31:745–46). On the duration, see the text note.

154–56 *Regula pastoralis* 2.6 (*PL* 77:34).

157–63 Although BA 1154/25 provides the form *rubeta* and ascribes all his material to Pliny, he includes nothing like what is alleged here, nor does Neckam.

166–68 ? Epistola 130.6 (ad Demetriadem, *PL* 22:1111): 'Solent miseri parentes, et non plenae fidei Christiano, deformes et aliquo membro debiles filias, quia dignos generos non inveniunt, virginitati tradere' (But wretched parents, not ones filled with Christian faith, are accustomed to grant their deformed daughters, ones weak in some limb, as virgins, because they do not find their wellborn sons worthy of this status).

168–69 BA 322/26, but not the extension that describes poor children improved.

173–74 As *Biblia Latina* 3:23a.

177–89 Cf. 'Romulus vulgaris' 1.7 (1:197–98); an allusion to the fable appears at Neckam 2.58 (p. 165).

192–93 Based on *Regula pastoralis* 3.17 (*PL* 77:78).

196–201 BA 1128/32–1129/2, 1178/37–1179/4.

201–3 As *Biblia Latina* 1:108b; cf. BA 429/9–13, 1179/7–13.

212–13 *Epistulae morales* 17.11.

215–18 BA 203/32–204/5, 1180/9–15.

221–26 BA 1126/19–25.

229–31, 237–38 BA 1159/28–29.

231–36 *De trinitate* 11.2.5 (*PL* 42:988): 'Et si tam violenta [voluntas] est, ut possit vocari amor, aut cupiditas, aut libido, etiam caeterum corpus animantis vehementer afficit. Et ubi non resistit pigrior duriorque materies, in similem speciem coloremque commutat. Licet videre corpusculum chamaeleontis ad colores quos videt facillima conversione variari' (And if the will is so powerful that it may be called love or desire or lust, it strongly effects even the rest of the lover's body [reading *amantis*]. And where more resistant and harder material does not resist it, the will turns the appearance and the colour into something like itself. You can see the chameleon's body changed by very easy stages into the colours that it sees.)

237–41 BA 1160/16–17 (the references to Isidore and Avicenna at 1159/31).

242–43 BA 1160/37–1161/1, with reference to both exegete and glossa.

245–47 BA 1160/30–33.

250–51 *Moralia* 18.7.13 (*PL* 76:44).

255–58, 262–65, 270–74 BA 1127/28–1128/8.

274–76 Alexander, *De similitudinibus* 38 (*PL* 159:619).

278–79 BA 1129/29–31.

282–86 *Moralia* 10.29.48 (*PL* 75:947).

288–91 *De civitate Dei* 9.20 (*PL* 41:244).

294–96 Cf. the rather more general formulations at *Moralia* 2.46 and 5.34 (*PL* 75:589, 713), but perhaps simply paraphrase or summary of *Moralia* 32.23 (*PL* 76:665–66).

300–2 *Moralia* 19.25 (*PL* 76:125).

304–6 BA 1129/38–1130/2 (the Isidore reference at 1129/32).

309–11 *De officiis* 2.51.

315–16 ? Cf. *Enarratio in Psalmos* 70.2.6 (*PL* 36:896), in a discussion of the Fall and the divine image.

319–25 BA 1227/34–35, 31–33, 16–17; similarly BA 1153/21–25, 1154/10–19.

327–29 Unfound, although elsewhere proverbially ascribed to Augustine.

331–33 Neither this nor the reading at 413–16 corresponds to the gloss either in *PL* 113 or *Biblia Latina*, but cf. the source, Ambrose, *In Psalmum David*

CXVIII expositio 10.23 (*PL* 15:1338–39): 'Nam si est tanta vis in naturalibus, ut animal visum prosit ictericis; ita ut mortui quoque cornu ejus animantis prodesse dicatur, si fuerit demonstratum iis, qui hujusmodi inciderint passionem: dubitare possumus quod justi sanet aspectus? Ergo vile animal irrationabile tantam virtutem habet, ut sanare possit hominem momento exiguo, quo videtur: homo justus, si tamen cum fide ab eo aspiciatur, qui utilitatem ab eo percipere desiderat, nihil confert? An non vel ipsi oculorum radii virtutem quamdam videntur infundere iis, qui fideliter eum videre desiderant'? (For if there is such strength in natural beings that seeing an animal benefits those with jaundice, that it may be said that those who have been struck by this kind of disease also benefit from an animal's dead horn, if they are shown it – can we doubt that the sight of a righteous man may heal? For a worthless irrational animal has so great power that it may heal a man in the brief moment in which it is seen. Then a righteous man, if he is looked upon with faith by a person who desires to see something useful in him – will he confer no benefit? Won't those rays from the eyes appear to pour some strength into those who wish to see him in faith?).

334–40 *De preliis Alexandri magni.*

344–47 Although unascribed, from BA 1154/20–23.

359–60 Cf. R. Stegmüller, *Repertorium Biblicum Medii Aevi*, 7 vols (Madrid, 19[5]0–61), no. 211.5 'Dionysii Areopagita epistola ad Timotheum de martyrio S. Pauli'.

360–65 Again unascribed, but BA 1243/28–35.

368–69 *De civitate Dei* 14.3 (*PL* 41:406).

370–72 BA 1134/37–1135/3

372–76 BA 1136/10–14. Cf. Neckam 2.111 (p. 193).

379–80 *Moralia* 31.45 (*PL* 76:621).

383–87 BA 1135/3–5, 8–10. Cf. Neckam 2.112 (p. 193).

396–99 The gloss here, *Biblia Latina* 4:359a, also includes the citation from Sap 4, here in 404–5.

402–3 Certainly from BA, but unfound.

406–8 BA 1135/5–6. Cf. Neckam 2.116 (p. 195).

410–13 John of Salisbury, *Polycraticus* 5.15 (1:345/16–19).

413–16 See 331–35 above.

420–21 BA 1135/9–12.

423–32 *De preliis Alexandri magni.* The physician is there named Phillip.

437–39 BA 1135/12–14, with Papias, s.v. prester, largely a restatement of Isidore. Cf. Neckam 2.117 (pp. 195–96).

440–42 Not Seneca (and I have found examples ascribed to 'philosophus' and to Socrates); see, most appositely, (ps.-)Caecilius Balbus, *De nugis philosophorum* 10.2 (p. 22) 'Socrates dixit, "Dignos esse invidos, qui, si fieri posset, in omnibus civitatibus aures vel oculos haberent, ut de omnium profectibus torquerentur"' (Socrates said, 'If it might be so, it would be appropriate for the envious to have ears or eyes in every city, so that they might be tormented by everyone else's successes'). The editor's note there indicates another, more proximate version ascribed to Seneca in Vincent of Beauvais, *Speculum morale.*

442–43 Horace *Epistulae* 1.2.57.

443–50 BA 1221/34–1222/4. Cf. Neckam 2.138 (p. 219).

451–54 *Moralia* 5.46 (*PL* 75:728).

456–59 BA 1135/17–21, which includes the final sentence, not in Isidore. Cf. Neckam 2.119 (pp. 197–98).

460–61 BA 1136/1–3 (preceded by a Pliny reference, 1135/35).

465–66 *Biblia Latina* 2:523b.

468–71 BA 208/36–209/3.

473–75 BA 1129/38–1130/2.

476–78 'Tractatus de interiori domo' 23.49 (*PL* 184:533).

480–92 passim BA 428/18–26, but Trevisa lacks the antifeminist remark at 482–83, here ascribed to Aristotle. However, BA's Latin here continues, 'et ideo putantur deteriores, ut dicit Auicenna' (and therefore women are considered weaker, as Avicenna says). Cf. Neckam 2.110 (p. 192), with a bit of the Avicenna material Malachy ignores.

495–505 BA 1136/16–21, 24–28, and 3–9; the cited Martianus is an otherwise unknown classical naturalist, whose opinion is reported by Pliny (and further transmitted by BA).

510–16 BA 209/4–10.

522–25 *Gregorius*: Seems rather to be based upon Bede, *Super parabolis Salomonis* 2.24 (*PL* 91:1009): 'Quomodo autem justus appellatur, qui cadere, id est, peccare memoratur? nisi quia de levibus quotidianisque loquitur peccatis, sine quibus nec justorum quispiam esse in hac vita potuit?

Quia nimirum per ignorantiam, per oblivionem, per cogitationem, per sermonem, per surreptionem, per necessitatem, per fragilitatem carnis, singulis diebus, vel inviti vel volentes frequenter reatum incurrimus. Et tamen resurgit justus, videlicet quia justus est, nec justitiae ejus praejudicat lapsus fragilitatis humanae' (For how is a person called righteous who is said to have fallen, to have sinned? Isn't it because one speaks here of easy and commonplace sins, without which no righteous person may exist in this life? For it is no wonder that we frequently run into guilty acts, whether it is through ignorance, forgetfulness, thought, word, deceit, necessity, or weakness of the flesh – and it happens daily, whether we want it to or not. Nevertheless, a righteous man rises again, precisely because he is righteous, nor is a slip due to human weakness prejudicial to his being righteous).

525–28 BA 1136/10–13, in BA's simplified formulation.

536–39 BA 429/23–30, reduced. For the following fragmentary reference to *seps* in the collations, see 456 above.

544–46 *De ira* 1.5.2.

546–48 *Moralia* 31.45 (*PL* 76:621).

549–51 BA 1154/33–35.

552–56 *De ira* 3.5.3–5.

557–66 *Moralia* 5.45 (*PL* 75:724).

561–63 BA 1155/2–3.

566–68 Cf. the end of *Philosophiae consolatio* 4 p3: 'Ita fit ut qui probitate deserta, homo esse desierit, cum in diuinam condicionem transire non possit, vertatur in beluam' (Thus it happens that the person who has abandoned uprightness has ceased to be a human, and since he cannot pass into a divine state, he is turned into a beast), or Boethius's restatement of the proposition at head of 4 p4.

570–72 Gregory, continuing from 557–66 above.

573–76 BA 1155/3–8, 12–14.

578–79 Gregory, continuing from 570–72, and providing the biblical citation in 585–86.

580–83 BA 1155/29–34.

587–99 *De ira* 1.18.3–6.

600–1 Again *Moralia* 5.45 (*PL* 75:724).

605–6 I have not found the Bernard citation. The phrase 'odium inueteratum' occurs only three times in *PL*.

606–8 Again *Moralia* 5.45 (*PL* 75:724).

610–12 BA 1154/31–33.

616–18 Unascribed, but cf. BA 861/5–11. BA there describes the stone 'noset', bred in a toad's head; however, he presents this as a proof *against* poison – it grows hot in its presence – and includes no detail about the erect toad.

621–25 BA 430/19–23.

627–29 BA 755/16–18.

632–34, 644–45 *Moralia* 5.45 (*PL* 75:726).

635–41 BA 1155/22–28 (the reference to Pliny at 1155/30).

645–47 As *Biblia Latina* 2:460b.

649–57 Except for the overt citation, also from this locus, largely a reduction of *Moralia* 5.45.81 (*PL* 75:726).

658–70 *De ira* 2.34.1, 3.24.3–4, and 3.6.1.

672–74 *De clementia* 1.19.3.

674–79 BA 1144/5–10, although it is not so specific about disagreement of Pliny and Aristotle.

681–82, 691–94 *Moralia* 31.45 (*PL* 76:621).

685–89 cf. BA 1129/10–17.

695–708 BA 1198/12–16, 4–5, 22–25, 30–33, 1198/36–1199/5, in BA's language and including a comparable moral.

717–19 Unfound in BA, but cf. Albertus 7.2.5 (p. 552).

721–23 *Homiliae in evangelia* 11.2 (*PL* 76:1115).

729–36 BA 611/13–30, much abbreviated, and 1143/12; cf. Pliny's account BA 1142/14–20, 1143/16–18. Followed by BA 1148/6–7, BA 1147/13–15.

736–37 *Franciscus: Scripta Leonis ...*, ch. 62 (198–99); cf. 526–27.

738–40 BA 1204/20–22, 25–26.

744–47 BA 1131/26–30.

751–52 *secundum Augustinum*: Actually Bernard, *Sermones in Cantica* 35 (*PL* 183:962).

754–55 *Homiliae in evangelia* 1.16 (*PL* 76:1136).

760–61 BA 1136/35–1137/1. Neckam also associates the spider with avarice, at 2.113 (pp. 193–94).

761–62 BA 1138/13–14, contextually ascribed to Aristotle.

765–69 BA 1140/25–29; cf. 1138/32, 1139/3–6.

772–73 cf. BA 1137/14.

774, 790–92 As *Biblia Latina* 2:502a.

776 Unfound. Cf. the Francis citation at 736–37. The order's founder persistently refers to worldly riches as 'musce'; cf. *Scripta Leonis*, chs 20 and 59 (122–23, 196–97).

778–81 BA 1140/29–33, although not the final detail.

782–83 Not apparently Seneca, although often so ascribed, but cf. Gregory, *Moralia* 15.23 (*PL* 75:1095): 'Formidat potentiorem alterum, ne hunc sustineat violentum; pauperem vero cum conspicit, suspicatur furem' (He fears another person more powerful than himself, lest he should have to endure his aggression; when he sees a poor person, he imagines him a thief).

784–85 Cf. *Hexameron* 5.5 (*PL* 14:211).

796–97 BA 1137/17–21.

800–3 Unfound, but cf. *Moralia* 8.44–45 (*PL* 75:845–47).

808–9 BA 1185/29–32, 35–36.

811–17 BA 1185/13–19, including the biblical citation.

820–24 BA 1184/31–33. Cf. Neckam 2.147 (pp. 226–27), including a moralised reading of the verse Malachy cites at 1015 and 1135 (and cf. 627–29).

825–37 Fulgentius 1.18 (Helm pp. 29–30).

838–56 BA 1141/5–24.

860–64 The gloss, *Biblia Latina* 2:385b, here cites Gregory, *Moralia* 5.20 (*PL* 75:700).

865–67 BA 748/22–25 (the author references at 749/6–7).

867–71 BA 748/33–34, 749/4–6.

872–73 Unfound in BA.

874–79 BA 768/20–24, without reference to Bede. For his discussion, see *Historia* 1.1 (*PL* 95:27): 'nullum ibi reptile videri soleat, nullus vivere serpens valeat: nam saepe illo de Brittania adlati serpentes, mox ut proximante terris navigio, odore aeris illius adtacti fuerint, intereunt: quin potius omnia pene quae de eadem insula sunt contra venenum valent. Denique vidimus, quibusdam a serpente percussis, rasa folia codicum qui de Hibernia fuerant, et ipsam rasuram aquae immissam ac potui datam, talibus protinus totam vim veneni grassantis, totum inflati corporis absumsisse ac sedasse tumorem' (One never sees a crawling beast there, and no snake is strong enough to live there. Often snakes brought there from Britain, as soon as the boat is nearing the land, die once they have been touched by the scent of the air; indeed, nearly every thing from this island is a powerful antidote to poison. For we have seen that, for people bitten by snakes, just shavings from the leaves of a book that had been in Ireland, put in water and taken as medicine, have destroyed immediately all the strength of the attacking poison and restrained all the bodily swelling).

880 *Sed prothdolor!*: Such lamenting comparisons, juxtaposing animal sagaciousness and human sin, have provocative analogues in Neckham. Cf., for example, his appeal to human shame, 1.121 (p. 199).

884 The association of Celtic peoples and theft is long-lived ('Taffy was a Welshman …') and also prompts discussion in Walter Map, Gerald of Wales, and *Piers Plowman*.

884–89 BA 1138/20–23.

894–97 BA 635/6–9, ascribed there to Aristotle.

904–6 BA 622/14–16.

906–11 BA 1263/11–17, 20; and cf. 1253/19, 1254/9–15.

918–20 BA 621/34–36 (inherited, as other references to Fulgentius are not). See further the textual note to 918.

921–24 BA 621/25–27, 30–31, 32–33, 36–622/4.

933–38 BA 1224/34–1225/2, similarly 606/13–20. For Malachy's Pliny, BA 'Aristotil seiþ', implies that this may be archetypal example of confusing *Pli* and *phi*. For parallel information, but only about the eagle, see Neckam 1.24 (p. 75).

942–46 BA 681/35–682/4 (in 681/32 Trevisa's 'Ysider' is a scribal reading for BA's Iorath). Cf. in part Neckam 2.28 (p. 146).

948–50 BA 680/2–5.

950–54 *De civitate Dei* 1.14 (PL 41:28).

955–58 *De officiis* 3.21.

960–68 BA 1204/2–3, 31–39, 9–11, 26–28.

983–88 BA 1204/12–16.

997–1001 BA 1125/34–36, 1126/3–5. Cf. Neckam 2.118 (p. 197).

1007–9 BA 1126/8–11.

1019–21 BA 1248/35–37.

1021–22 *Homiliae in Ezechielem* 1.9 (*PL* 76:879).

1022–24 BA 1249/18–20.

1027–28 Epistola 22.3 (*PL* 22:395).

1028 col Although frequently assigned to Seneca in various proverb collections, indeed William of Conches, *Moralium dogma philosophorum* 1A.1 (False friends bring forth flattery, rather than counsel, and their single contention is who deceives most ingratiatingly).

1028–33 John of Salisbury, *Polycraticus* 3.4 (1:177/20–26).

1039–41 Neckam 2.180 (p. 316).

1043–45 *Satyra* 4.70–71.

1048–51 Cf. *Moralia* 31.25 (*PL* 76:599–600).

1051–59 *Hexameron* 5.22 (*PL* 14:237), partially as reported BA 625/4–10.

1065–66 This is early, strict Franciscan practice, as mandated by Lc 9:3, 10:4 and 7.

1072–78 BA 602/10–18.

1080–81 The ascription to Seneca in CDGL is certainly wrong, but I have not found the proverb. Perhaps it is a garbled reference to Richard of St Victor, *In Apocalypsis Ioannis* 7.8 (*PL* 196:817–18), a discussion of Apc 14:20 'sexcenta'.

1084–87 BA 1140/35–1141/4.

1092–97 *De diuinatione*: A wrong reference; see *De officiis* 2.55.

1098–1103 *De officiis* 1.30 (*PL* 16:65–66).

1114–16 BA 1141/10–13.

1119–21, 1123–25 BA 1141/26–30.

1128–30 BA 1186/16–18, but not quite what BA reports Pliny as having said.

1132–35 BA 1185/27–35, including the biblical reference.

1141–43 Cf. the full discussions above at 997 and 1007; and cf. for the hydra, BA 1126/3–15.

1144–45 BA 1248/34–35.

1148–49 BA 1250/3–4.

1151–53 BA 434/17–19; cf. 1250/1–3.

1153–55 *Enarrationes in Psalmos* 140.13 (*PL* 37:1824).

1159–60 BA 625/10–13 (following upon the citation at 1057–59).

1162–65 BA 434/19–21.

1170–76 BA 1250/4–10.

1181–86 Although not source-marked (and according to some MSS, 'evidenter'), cf. BA 1130/2–4 (and its continuation) or 1124/35–1125/5.

1188ff. The chapter, to a degree approached elsewhere only with envy and wrath, is carefully patterned after Gregory's discussion, *Moralia* 30.18 (*PL* 76:556–57). The following biblical examples are also derived from Gregory's discussion.

1202–4 BA 1132/5-6, there ascribed Pliny and Avicenna, another likely example of confusing *pli* and *phi*.

1211–13 BA 1133/23-26.

1215–17 BA 1129/3–6.

1221–38 Cf. 'Romulus vulgaris' 2.11 (Hervieux 1.208–9).

1240–42 *Contra mendacium* 13.28 (*PL* 40:538).

1243–59 Again extensively from Gregory, *Moralia* 30.18 (*PL* 76:557). The additional biblical references in 1255–58 are to 3 Rg 17:6, Gn 3:6, and Mt 4:3, respectively, and, like the Ezechiel citation, are again taken from Gregory's discussion.

1245–49 BA 1126/37–1127/1.

1264–66 BA 1131/6–9 (ascribed to both Pliny and Avicenna).

1269–70 *Secreta secretorum* 13 (p. 38).

1270–75 BA 1244/7–11, 5–7.

1278–80 BA 1133/22–23.

1283–88 BA 432/11–22 (and the next but one).

1289–91 Rather loosely summarising *Epistulae morales* 95.16–19.

1291–95 BA 207/25–31.

1295–98 *Epistulae morales* 83.16, 19.

1300–2 Again *Moralia* 30.18 (*PL* 76:556).

1304–5 BA 1131/21–22. The opinion is there ascribed only to Pliny; the addition of Aristotle may thus represent an archetypal 'doublet of doubt'.

1308–12 BA 1130/14–16, 1131/2–6.

1312–14 The gloss here, *Biblia Latina* 4:38a, cites a reduced version of Augustine's discussion. Because this, *De doctrina Christiana* 2.16 (*PL* 34:47), 'bares the device' that underlies Malachy's entire work (not to mention Neckam's and BA's), it deserves full citation: 'Rerum autem ignorantia facit obscuras figuratas locutiones, cum ignoramus vel animantium, vel lapidum, vel herbarum naturas, aliarumve rerum, quae plerumque in Scripturis similitudinis alicujus gratia ponuntur. Nam et de serpente quod notum est, totum corpus eum pro capite objicere ferientibus, quantum illustrat sensum illum, quo Dominus jubet astutos nos esse sicut serpentes; ut scilicet pro capite nostro, quod est Christus, corpus potius persequentibus offeramus, ne fides Christiana tanquam necetur in nobis, si parcentes corpori negemus Deum! vel illud, quod per cavernae angustias coarctatus, deposita veteri tunica vires novas accipere dicitur, quantum concinit ad imitandam ipsam serpentis astutiam, exuendumque ipsum veterem hominem, sicut Apostolus dicit, ut induamur novo; et exuendum per angustias, dicente Domino, *Intrate per angustam portam*! Ut ergo notitia naturae serpentis illustrat multas similitudines quas de hoc animante dare Scriptura consuevit; sic ignorantia nonnullorum animalium quae non minus per similitudines commemorat, impedit plurimum intellectorem' (Ignorance about things renders [the Bible's] figurative locutions obscure, when we do not know the natures of animals or stones or plants or any other thing. For many such things are put forward in biblical similes in place of something else. Because the snake is known to expose its whole body, instead of its head, to those striking it, what more illustrates the sense than that the Lord commands us to be as wise as serpents [Mt 10:16]? That is, for our head, which is Christ, we should rather offer our bodies to those who persecute us, than in a sense the Christian faith be killed in us, and we deny God in the interests of sparing our bodies. Or another example with the snake: it is said to take on new powers, once it has cast off its old skin, having pressed itself through narrow places in its cave. How closely this accords with imitating the snake's cleverness in shedding 'the old man', as Paul says, so that we may be clothed in the new one [e.g., Eph 4:22, 24] – and that is the same casting off through narrow places as when the Lord says, 'Enter ye in at the narrow gate' [Mt 7:13]. Thus, noticing the nature of the snake illuminates many similes that Scripture regularly offers about this beast, and thus, ignorance of many animals, not less frequently invoked in such similes, impedes understanding a great deal).

1315–25 BA 1130/23–1131/2. BA ascribes this passage to Aristotle, whose 'philosophus' has apparently been scribally assimilated to the title of the popular bestiary. Perhaps surprisingly, no such information appears in that text.

1330–31 Unascribed, but BA 432/24–26.

1333–35 *Homiliae in evangelia* 2.40 (*PL* 76:1302); he is discussing Lc 16:20–21.

1343–44 BA 1133/9–12.

1349–55 BA 1132/33–1133/2 (on its venom, BA 1125/30–31, 1267/15–19; cf. 424–25).

1358–60 BA 1135/7; see the discussion at 383.

1363–64 Cf. *Moralia* 15.15 (*PL* 75:1090). Gregory's discussion, which includes the subsequent anecdote of baby vipers killing their mother to be born, together with a proposed etymology for the snake's name, provides another source that may have suggested to Malachy his topic.

1367–68 'Senecan' only; cf. Xystus/Sixtus, 'Enchiridion' 12, 'Non manus aut oculus peccat aut aliquod huiusmodi membrum, sed male uti manu vel oculo' (Neither the hand nor the eye nor any other limb sins, but one uses the hand or eye evilly).

1369–77 BA 1266/22–31.

1381–82 *Chrisostomus*: unfound.

1383–85 Cf. *Contra Iulianum* 4.13 (*PL* 44:768–69).

1385–87 A rather inexact memory of *Biblia Latina* 4:326a: 'Contra honorem sui corporis est. Corpus enim maxime propagationis causa creatum fuit. Contra huius honorem facit qui fornicatur' (It is opposed to honouring his body, for the body was mainly created for propagating the species. The person who fornicates acts against the honour due to the body).

1388–94 (reprised at 1403–4) BA 1267/19–29, whose text appears to fuse Ambrose with original detail; cf. *Hexameron* 4.7 (*PL* 14:213), and see further BA 679/6–14 and Neckam 2.41 (p. 154).

1394–96 Apparently not in BA, but cf. *Etymologiae* 12.6.43 (*PL* 182:455).

1397–98 BA 678/16–19.

1412–16 BA 1248/19–27, including the ascription to *Physiologus*.

1420 As 1394–96 above.

1433–37 BA 1199/6–15.

1439–42 BA 1170/29–36, including an allusion to the subsequent citation from Dt.

1447–50 BA 1267/15–19.

1453–54 Unfound; probably from Grosseteste's translation of the *Nicomachean Ethics*.

1455–56 *Moralia* 24.8 (*PL* 76:294).

1457–61 *Secreta secretorum* ch. 14 (p. 38).

1463–68 *Facta et dicta* 9.1 (ext).1.

1468–70 Cf. Epistola 1.3 (*PL* 182:727), but Malachy may be thinking of the common reduction to a verse couplet, Walther *Sprich.* 519.

1474–77 Augustine: Unfound. Some MSS here have an added reference to the gloss; rather than *Biblia Latina* 4:326a (simply 'vt erubescens corrigatur' [so that, ashamed, he may be corrected]), it probably paraphrases *PL* 114:527, 'Dicendo *nominatur*, ostendit satis non temere, et quolibet modo, sed per judicium auferendos esse malos ab Ecclesiae conjunctione' (In saying, *Any man named a brother*, it shows well enough that evil people are not to be removed from the union of the church precipitately or in any old way, but through judgement).

1479–81 Again unfound, as 1453–54.

1482–84, 1486–92 Orosius, *Historiae* 1.19 and 2.2 (*PL* 31:734–35, 745–46).

1485–86 Augustine, *De civitate Dei* 2.20 (*PL* 41:66).

1493–95 Rory O'Connor [Ruaidhri Ó Conchobhair], king of Connaught 1166–98 and intermittently High King 1166×89. The Irish *Annála Connacht* 1233.3 (46–47), describing the destruction of his successors at the hands of other Irish leaders, offers much the same information.

1502–5 Epistola 60.14 (*PL* 22:598–99).

1512–14 BA 679/27–30.

1517–19 BA 1260/30–33.

1524–27 *Commentarii in Isaiam* 18 (*PL* 24:662), not apparently from BA.

1530–33 Cf. BA 433/15, 19–23 (the same information and reference, but a little distant in detail).

1538-43 *sanctus Columba*: The anecdote does not appear in the materials assembled by the Bollandists, *Acta Sanctorum: June II* (Paris and Rome, 1867), 179–233, and Richard Sharpe tells me that there is no sign of it in Irish materials either.

1546-48 As *Biblia Latina* 4:326a.

1548-50 Cf. Epistola 42.5 (*PL* 30:290).

1557-61 *Secreta secretorum* ch. 25 (p. 52), summarised.

1563-67 BA 632/35–633/5.

1573-75 cf. BA 1267/33–37.

1576-94 Fulgentius 2.2 and 4 (Helm pp. 41 and 43).

1596-1601 BA 1266/34–1237/8.

1606-8 Cf. *De ciuitate Dei* 1.28 (*PL* 41:42).

1608-12 This material probably falls under 'general common knowledge', although there is certainly an analogue at *De civitate Dei* 3.21 (*PL* 41:102–3). Augustine does not cite, nor have I yet to find Malachy's 'proverb', but tribulation as a file that removes the rust of sin is a pulpit commonplace (following from extended readings of Sap 3:6, Sir 2:5, etc.). For one example, cf. Augustine, sermo ad fratres in eremo 10 (*PL* 40:1252).

1620-25 BA 1196/20–21, 1192/34–1193/1, 1194/1–5. Cf. Neckam 2.144 (p. 225).

1625-27 Such speculations on man's brutality, of course, underwrite the use of natural imagery throughout the work. Cf. Neckam 2.121 (p. 199), a discussion of the toad.

1628-38 Neckam 1.64 (pp. 112–13); for a nonequivalent parallel, see BA 619/22–27.

1639-43 BA 1218/2–6, cf. 1214/32–35.

1648-53 *Tusculanae* 5.27.78.

Appendix: The extensive interpolations

9 *pleidours* (S only): One of only two examples of the vernacular in texts surveyed here (the other the gloss of 'cicada' 1060, cited in the collations from CDL only). Here the word may well be English, rather than Anglo-Norman, since it appears as a surname in thirteenth-century records.

23-25 not apparently from BA.

27–29 *Moralia* 5.46 (*PL* 75:728), as well as *Regula pastoralis* 3.10 (*PL* 77:64). Note the S variant 29 *in mala*, another example of error created by confusion over word-boundaries (the noun *inuidia* construed as preposition + noun).

32–33 BA 249/6–8.

38–39 Unascribed, but BA 1266/23–25, cited more fully at 1373. For the gnawing infants as a figure for envy, see Neckam 2.105 (p. 187).

44–47 Unascribed, but BA 1262/7–9.

49–51 *Seneca*: from (ps.-)Caecilius Balbus; see 440–42 above. The citation provides a good indicator of the non-authorial nature of this material, since, like 38–39 above, it appears elsewhere in the authorial text.

53–54 BA 1252/34–1253/5; there ascribed to Isidore (*Etymologies* 12.3.5, *PL* 82:441). A citation like this offers strong evidence for access to the unmentioned BA, rather than to his cited sources, since Isidore lacks BA's added detail of hating the sun and dying in the light.

56–57 Perhaps cf. *Moralia* 25.9 (*PL* 76:334): 'Tunc enim coactus in tenebras exteriores mittitur, quia nunc in interioribus excaecatur voluntarie. Rursum in nocte iniquus conteritur, cum peccatorum praecedentium confusione damnatus, veritatis lumen non invenit, et quid deinceps agere debeat non agnoscit' (Then he is compelled into outward darkness, because he has now wilfully blinded himself internally, he is condemned in the destructiveness of his past sins, he has not found the light of truth, and as a result, has not recognised what he ought to do).

60–61 BA 1216/32–34.

62–63 The proverb appears in Geoffrey of Vinsauf, 'Summa de arte dictandi', cited Hallik 487 (no. 59).

63–64 This leonine hexameter does not appear in Walther *Sprich.*

72–73 Walther, *Sprich.* 12804.

102–12 *Homiliae in evangelia* 1.5.3 (*PL* 76:1094).

117–18 *Moralia* 5.45 (*PL* 75:724), again cited in Malachy's text, at 607 (with 'claudit').

119–20 Unfound.

130–36 *Homiliae in evangelia* 1.17.4 (*PL* 76:1140).

137–38 BA 1135/12–15 (including the verse, Lucan, *De bello civili* 9.722). Again, in Malachy's original, at 437.

148–49 *Summa sententiarum* 3.16 (*PL* 176:114).

150–56 Cf. BA 1211/11–20. However, BA offers no detail on the hedgehog's frustration, once it loses its apples.

167–70 As *Biblia Latina* 2:773b.

171–79 The entire paragraph represents *Moralia* 5.45 (*PL* 75:724), which also provides most of the cited proof-texts – and which, again, has been extensively cited in Malachy's text.

181 *Bernardus*: Unfound, as is Malachy's parallel citation at 605–6.

189–90 *Moralia* 10.2 (*PL* 75:919).

222–23 *Dialogi* 1.2 (*PL* 77:161).

229–34 *Verba seniorum* 127 (*PL* 73:784–85), much reduced.

244–45 *Homiliae in Ezechielem* 1.7 (*PL* 76:864); similarly 2.5, 2.8 (cols 993, 1037).

245–49 *De patientia* 2 and 5 (*PL* 40:611, 613).

253–54 *Homiliae in Evangelium* 2.35 (*PL* 76:1261).

266–67 Cf. *Commentarius in Marcum* 11 (*PL* 30:622–23).

270–71 As *Biblia Latina* 4:69a.

276–78 Papias offers, 'Turdae aues a tarditate dictae; hyemis enim confinio se referunt. *Turdela* quasi maior turdus, cuius stercus generare viscum dicitur'. The information is not apparently from BA. Given its biological difference and general applause for that bird, 276 *turturi* must be an archetypal error for *turdele*.

286–88 As *Biblia Latina* 2:401b.

289–90 Unascribed, but cf. BA 1120/14–18, 1124/20–21.

313–15 Ez 16:49, which Malachy cites at 1262.

347–49 *Moralia* 8.7 (*PL* 75:809). One might note that Étienne's compositor has apparently omitted one of the seven promised commendations.

353–55 Unascribed, but cf. BA 1233/33–34.

357 *Seneca*: In fact, although also frequently ascribed to Jerome, apparently Augustine, sermo ad fratres in eremo 48 (*PL* 40:1330).

392–95 In spite of the resemblance of this discussion to materials like those in BA, this appears pure observation. It does, however, resemble the material on the devil's ass at 289–90 above.

401–3 Again, probably simple observation, but cf. BA 1170/37–1171/13.

411–14 ? A rather general reference to *Regula pastoralis* 3.20 (*PL* 77:86).

415–17 *Expositio Luce* 7 (*PL* 15:1730).

431–33 BA 637/22–27, ascribed there to Isidore and Ambrose. Similar information appears at Neckam 1.44 (p. 96).

444–45 *Seneca*: From one of the several versions of Publilius Syrus, *Sententiae*, 'Monstro similis est avaritia unica'.

446–50 Tubach 4355 (of Saladin).

451 S's variant probably alludes to Prv 23:17–18.

451–53 Tubach 2343 (of Craton the philosopher), repeated several times by John of Wales.

453–56 At least a similar story, Pelagius, *Verba seniorum* 16.13 (*PL* 73:971).

464–66 *Beda*: Actually Ambrose, as in the earlier citation at 415–16.

467–69 Walther, *Sprich.* 14070.

469–72 Walther, *Sprich.* 3913.

Indexes

All entries are non-inclusive and refer only to the only onset of the reference or citation. Starred entries mark materials in the Appendix.

Biblical references

Fontes: Malachy's first-hand sources

'in *Apologijs Aesopi*' = 'Romulus vulgaris', *Fabulae*, perhaps in a derivative
   version, ed. Auguste L. Hervieux, *Les Fabulistes latins depuis le siècle
   d'Auguste jusqu'à la fin du moyen âge*, 2nd edn, 5 vols (Paris, 1893–99)
   cf. 1.7 (1:197–98) 177
   cf. 2.11 (1:208–9) 1221

Alexander the Great = *Historia Alexandri regis macedonie de preliis*
   ([Grenoble?], 1490) [the 'J³ version'; Bod-Inc-A-174] = *The Wars of
   Alexander*, ed. Hoyt N. Duggan and Thorlac Turville-Petre, Early English
   Text Society ss 10 (Oxford, 1989)
   sigs i i^{va}–i ii^{ra} (summarised) 334 = *Wars* 4961–84
   sig. d ii^{rb}–^{vb} (summarised) 423, 1167 = *Wars* 2684–2707
   See also ps.-Aristotle

Alexander Neckam, *De naturis rerum: Alexandri Neckam De naturis rerum
   libro duo*, ed. Thomas Wright, Rolls Series 34 (London, 1863)
   cf. 1.24 (p. 75) 933
   cf. 1.44 (p. 96) *431
   cf. 1.61 (p. 110) 918n
   1.64 (pp. 112–13) 1628
   cf. 2.28 (p. 146) 942
   cf. 2.41 (p. 154) 1388
   cf. 2.58 (p. 165) 177
   cf. 2.105 (p. 187) 19, 54; *38
   cf. 2.108 (p. 189) 80
   2.109 (pp. 190–91) 104, cf. 88
   cf. 2.110 (p. 192) 480
   cf. 2.111 (p. 193) 372
   cf. 2.112 (p. 193) 383
   cf. 2.113 (pp. 193–94) 760
   cf. 2.116 (p. 195) 406
   cf. 2.117 (pp. 195–96) 437
   cf. 2.118 (p. 197) 997
   cf. 2.119 (pp. 197–98) 456
   2.120 (p. 198) 121, 126
   cf. 2.121 (p. 199) 1625
   cf. 2.138 (p. 219) 443
   cf. 2.144 (p. 225) 1620
   cf. 2.147 (pp. 226–27) 820 (and see the note)
   2.180 (p. 316) 1039

Ambrose of Milan
De officiis 1.30 (*PL* 16:65–66) 1098

De doctrina Christiana 2.16 (*PL* 34:47) 1312
De Genesi ad litteram 9.15 (*PL* 34:404) 83
De patientia 2 and 5 (*PL* 40:611, 613) *245
De penitentia see glossa below on 1 Cor 5:11
De trinitate 11.2 (*PL* 42:988) 231
Enarrationes in Psalmos
   ? cf. 70.2.6 (*PL* 36:896) 315
   140.13 (*PL* 37:1824) 1153
sermones ad fratres in eremo
   10 (*PL* 40:1252) 1608
   48 (*PL* 40:1330) ('Seneca') *357
sermo dubius 374.3 (*PL* 39:1668) 83
   see also Bernard *In Cantica*, glossa (751)

Avicenna: all citations second-hand from BA, one unfound; see notes ad loc.

Bede
Historia 1.1 (*PL* 95:27) 874
Super parabolis Salomonis 2.24 (*PL* 91:1009) ('Gregory') 522
See also Ambrose

Bernard of Clairvaux
Epistola 1.3 (*PL* 182:727) 1468
Sermones in Cantica 35 (*PL* 183:962) ('Augustine') 751
'Tractatus de interiori domo' 23.49 (*PL* 184:533) 476
unfound 605; *181

Boethius, *Philosophiae consolatio*: ed. Ludwig Bieler, Corpus Christianorum
   94 (Turnholt, 1984)
   4 p2 and p3 566
   See also Geoffrey

ps.-Boethius, a commentator on *De disciplina scolarium*: the text ed. Olga
   Weijers, Studien und Texten ... 12 (Leiden, 1976)
   A gloss on 2.6 (Weijers 101/4), cf. *De consolatione* (Lyons: Jean de Pré,
   1488), sig. C iii^v 69

(ps.-)Caecilius Balbus, *De nugis philosophorum quae supersunt*, ed.
   E. Woelfflin (Basel, 1855), ('Seneca') Munich version 10.2 (p. 22) 440; *49

Cicero
De diuinatione 1092, see the next
De officiis
   2.51 309

on Nm 21:7 (1:324a) 54
on Iob 4:11 (2:385b) 860
on Iob 12:20 (2:401b) *286
on Ps 4:5 (2:460b) 645
on Ps 38:12 (2:502a) 774, 790
on Ps 57:5 (2:523b) 465
on Ps 90:13 (2:573a), cf. *PL* 113:1000 135
on Ps 118:74, see Ambrose, *In Psalmum* 331
on Sir 28:2, 5 (2:773b) *167
on Is 14:29 (3:27b) 124
on Is 59:5 (3:23a) 173
on Ier 8:17 (3:115a) 140
on Mt 10:16 (4:38a) 1312; see also Augustine, *De doctrina*
on Mt 22:13 (4:69a) *270
on 1 Cor 6:18 (4:326a), cf. *PL* 114:527 1385, 1474, 1546
on Gal 3:1 (4:359a) 396

Gregory the Great
Dialogi 1.2 (*PL* 77:161) *222
Homiliae in evangelia
    1.5.3 (*PL* 76:1094) *102
    1.11.2 (*PL* 76:1115) 721
    1.16 (*PL* 76:1136) 754
    1.17.4 (*PL* 76:1140) *130
    2.35 (*PL* 76:1261) *253
    2.40 (*PL* 76:1302) 1335
Homiliae in Ezechielem
    1.7 (*PL* 76:864); similarly 2.5, 2.8 (cols 993, 1037) *244
    1.9 (*PL* 76:879) 1021
Moralia in Iob
    cf. 2.46, 5.34 (*PL* 75:589 and 713) 294
    5.20 (*PL* 75:700) ('glossa') 860
    5.45 (*PL* 75:724–26) 557ff. (scattered citations to 650); *117, *171
    5.46 (*PL* 75:728) 451; *27
    8.7 (*PL* 75:809) *347
    cf. 8.44–45 (*PL* 75:845–47) 800
    10.2 (*PL* 75:919) *189
    10.29.48 (*PL* 75:947) 282
    15.15 (*PL* 75:1090) 1363
    15.23 (*PL* 75:1095) ('Seneca') 782
    18.7.13 (*PL* 76:44) 250
    19.25 (*PL* 76:125) 300
    24.8 (*PL* 76:294) 1455
    cf. 25.9 (*PL* 76:334) *56
    30.18 (*PL* 76:556–57) 1188ff. (to 1260 and at 1302)

'Iorath', *De animalibus*: both citations (942, 1512) from this otherwise
   unknown Arabic writer second-hand from BA; see notes ad loc.

Juvenal, *Satyra* 4.70–71 1043

Martianus (not Capella, but an otherwise unknown classical natural
   historian cited by Pliny): the unique citation (495) second-hand from BA;
   see note ad loc.

Orosius, *Historiae*
1.19 (*PL* 31:734–35) 1482
2.2 (*PL* 31:745–46) 147, 1482

Papias, *Elementarium* (Milan: Dominicus de Vespolate, 12 December 1476
   [Bod-Inc-P-021]), unfoliated
s.v. prester 437
s.v. turdae and turdela *276
Two citations (28, 705) second-hand from BA; see notes ad loc.

Pelagius, see *Vitae patrum*

Physiologus [the standard bestiary]: the unique certain citation (1412)
   second-hand from BA; 1316 is an archetypal error for 'philosophus', i.e.
   Aristotle, and also from BA

Pliny, *Historia naturalis*: all citations second-hand from BA or Neckam; see
   notes ad loc.

poeta
See also Horace, uersus

Publilius Syrus, *Sententiae*, this citation not in the standard edition of this
   variable text, ed. Wilhelm Meyer (Leipzig, 1880) *444

? Richard of St Victor, *In Apocalypsis Ioannis* 7.8 (*PL* 196:817–18) 1080

Seneca (minor)
De clementia
   1.19.3 672
De ira
   1.5.2 544
   1.18.3–6 587
   2.34.1, 3.24.3–4, and 3.6.1 658
   3.5.3–5 552

Epistulae morales
   17.11 212
   67.7 74
   83.16, 19 1295
   cf. 95.16–19 1289
See also Augustine sermo, Caecilius, Geoffrey, Gregory *Moralia*, Publilius,
   Xystus

Solinus, *De mirabilibus mundi*: all four citations (808, 960, 983, 1132)
   second-hand from BA; see notes ad loc.

Valerius Maximus, *Facta et dicta* 9.1 (ext).1 1463

Verba seniorum, see *Vitae patrum*

uersus
Walther, *Sprich.* 519 1468n
Walther, *Sprich.* 3913 *469
Walther, *Sprich.* 12804 *72
Walther, *Sprich.* 14070 *467
not in Walther, *Sprich.* *63

ps.-Virgil, 'Culex', probably second-hand from Neckham; for the text, see
   Emil Baehrens, ed., *Poetae Latini Minores 1* (Leipzig, 1879), 46–72 100

Vitae patrum
Verba seniorum 127 (*PL* 73:784–85) *229
Pelagius, *Verba seniorum* 16.13 (*PL* 73:971) *453

William of Conches, *Moralium dogma philosophorum*, ed. John Holmberg
   (Uppsala, 1929), 1A.1 1028col

Xystus/Sextus, 'Enchiridion': *The Sentences of Sextus*, ed. Henry Chadwick
   (Cambridge, 1959, 2003), cf. 12 (p. 13) ('Seneca') 1367

Similitudines

agnus (coagulum agni) 1121
ametistus 1526
amphibena 997, 1140
apis 729; *414; rex apis 672
aquila 936, 1072, 1525
aranea 756ff., 880ff., 1084, 1114
asinus (diaboli) *289
aspis 379ff.

basiliscus 120ff., 314ff.
boas 1215
bufo 158, 542ff., 636ff.

caladrius 1563
cameleon 229
canis 621 (rabidus); 1439; *360, *457;
    (uetus) *400
cerastes 196
cicada 1052, 1159
ciconia 1629
columba *34
coruus 905

delfinus 942
dipsas, see situla
draco 807, 1128

elephas 818, 1620
elith 1512
equus gestatorius *392
eruca 695

fel (diaboli) *22
ferrum rubiginosum *57
formica 738, 959ff.
formicoleon, see myrmicoleon

hemorrhois 420
hericius *150
hydra 1007, 1140
hypnalis 383, 1358

lanuginosa 846, 901
leena 1639
leo *60
lingua statere *12
linx 443
locusta, see cicada
lupus 933

margarita 720
miluus 894
molendinarium *421
murena 1390ff.
musca 737, 774, 796, 1124
mustela 318
myrmicoleon vel formicoleon 851,
    930

nuntius stultus *440

ouis 934; *353; inter spinas *17

papilio 702
perdix *431
pons *159
prester 437; *137

regulus 120ff.
rubeta, see bufo

salamandra 254, 357
sanguissuga 1270
satyrus 1433
saura 88
scitalis 221
scorpio 1017, 1141ff.
seps 456; *21
serpens 35, 51ff., 277, 304, 373, etc.
serpens antiquus 5
serpens eneus 52ff., 653
sirena 1412
situla 408

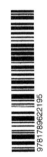